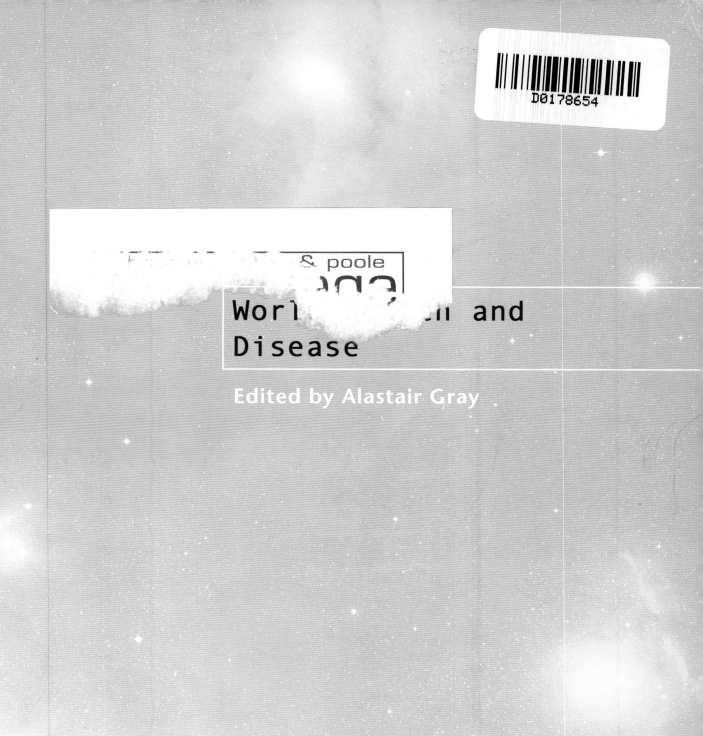

& poole

World   and
Disease

Edited by Alastair Gray

Published by Open University Press

Written and produced by The Open University

Health and Disease Series, Book 3

OPEN UNIVERSITY PRESS

Buckingham   •   Philadelphia

The Open University

The U205 *Health and Disease* Course Team

The following members of the Open University teaching staff have collaborated with the authors in writing this book, or have commented extensively on it during its production. We accept collective responsibility for its overall academic and teaching content.

Basiro Davey (Course Team Chair, Senior Lecturer in Health Studies, Department of Biological Sciences)

Robin Harding (Senior Lecturer and Regional Staff Tutor, Science)

Kevin McConway (Senior Lecturer in Statistics)

The following people have contributed to the development of particular parts or aspects of this book:

Steve Best (graphic artist)

Mark Bridge (BBC producer)

Teresa Dowsing (course manager)

Sheila Dunleavy (editor)

Phil Gauron (BBC producer)

Rebecca Graham (editor)

Celia Hart (picture researcher)

Pam Higgins (designer)

Jim Iley (critical reader) Senior Lecturer in Chemistry

Jean Macqueen (indexer)

Jennifer Nockles (designer)

Harriet Pacaud (BBC producer)

Rissa de la Paz (BBC producer)

John Taylor (graphic artist)

Geoff Wheeler (BBC producer)

Joy Wilson (course manager)

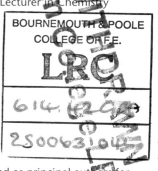

Authors

The following people have acted as principal authors for the chapters listed below, but have also contributed extensively to the structure and philosophy of the book as a whole.

Chapters 1–3 and 5–10

Alastair Gray, Director, Health Economics Research Centre, Institute of Health Sciences, University of Oxford.

Chapters 4 and 11

Philip Payne, Visiting Professor of Nutrition, Department of Nutrition and Food Sciences, School of Biological and Molecular Sciences, Oxford Brookes University.

External assessors

Course assessor for third editions

Professor John Gabbay, Professor of Public Health Medicine, University of Southampton, and Director of the Wessex Institute for Health Research and Development.

Book 3 assessors for third edition

The Course Team and authors gratefully acknowledge the contribution of the following specialist assessors who have commented on particular aspects of this book:

Mr H. Brammer, former FAO Agricultural Development Adviser, Bangladesh.

Dr Philip Clarke, Health Economics Research Centre, Institute of Health Sciences, University of Oxford.

Dr Edward Clay, Senior Research Associate, Overseas Development Institute, London.

Professor Barbara Harriss-White, Wolfson College, Queen Elizabeth House, University of Oxford.

Professor C. Jeya Henry, Department of Nutrition and Food Sciences, School of Biological and Molecular Sciences, Oxford Brookes University.

Dr Michael Murphy, Director of the ICRF General Practice Research Group, Institute of Health Sciences, University of Oxford.

We gratefully acknowledge the contributions made by the external assessors for the previous edition of this book:

The late Professor Brian Abel-Smith, Professor of Social Administration, Department of Social Policy, London School of Economics and Political Science.

Professor James McEwen, Henry Mechan Chair of Public Health and Head of Department of Public Health, University of Glasgow.

Professor James Whitworth, Professor of International Public Health, London School of Hygiene and Tropical Medicine.

Acknowledgements

The Course Team and the authors wish to thank the following people who, as contributors to previous editions of this book, made a lasting impact on the structure and philosophy of the present volume.

Nick Black, David Boswell, Alan Cockburn, Gerald Elliott, John Greenwood, Mary Griffiths, Richard J. Hayes, Richard Holmes, Betty Kirkwood, Andrew Learmonth, Tom F. De C. Marshall, Perry Morley, Jennie Popay, John Rivers, Steven Rose, Peter Smith, Phil Strong, Charlotte Ward-Perkins.

Cover images

Background: Nebulae in the Rho Ophiuchi region (Source: David Malin/Anglo Australian Observatory). *Middleground*: Globe (Source: Mountain High Map™, Digital Wisdom, Inc). *Foreground:* Child smoking a cigarette, Sichuan Province, China, 1998 (Photo: Gang Feng Wang/Panos Pictures)

Open University Press, Celtic Court, 22 Ballmoor,
Buckingham, MK18 1XW

e-mail: enquiries@openup.co.uk

website: www.openup.co.uk

and

325 Chestnut Street, Philadelphia, PA 19106, USA

First published as *The Health of Nations*, 1985.
Completely revised second edition published as
World Health and Disease, 1993. This full-colour
completely revised third edition published 2001.

Copyright © 2001 The Open University

A catalogue record of this book is available from the
British Library.

Library of Congress Cataloging-in-Publication Data

Edited, designed and typeset by the Open University.

Printed and bound in the United Kingdom by the
Alden Group, Oxford.

ISBN 0 335 20838 X

This publication forms part of an Open University level 2
course, U205 *Health and Disease*. The complete list of
texts which make up this course can be found on the
back cover. Details of this and other Open University
courses can be obtained from the Call Centre, PO Box 724,
The Open University, Walton Hall, Milton Keynes,
MK7 6ZS, United Kingdom: tel. +44 (0)1908 653231,
e-mail ces-gen@open.ac.uk

Alternatively, you may visit the Open University website
at http://www.open.ac.uk where you can learn more
about the wide range of courses and packs offered at all
levels by the Open University.

3.1

CONTENTS

A note for the general reader

World Health and Disease examines contemporary and historical patterns of health and disease in the United Kingdom and the rest of the world. The book draws on the disciplines of demography, epidemiology, history, the social sciences and biology to describe and explain its subject matter.

The book contains eleven chapters, grouped around the following broad themes. After an introductory chapter, Chapters 2 to 4 provide an epidemiological and demographic survey of the contemporary world, discussing population trends and structures, birth and mortality rates and causes of death in different parts of the world, and recent trends in life expectancy. Chapter 4 offers a case study of the way in which these patterns manifest themselves in the lives of the rural population of Bangladesh.

Chapters 5 to 8 are concerned with the links between health, population, and social and economic development. Chapters 5 and 6 examine population history and theories about the forces that lead to population growth, before exploring the impact of the Industrial Revolution on the health and the size and structure of England's population. Chapters 7 and 8 then consider the way in which health and population change are related to the process of development in low- and middle-income countries. The main theme of these chapters is that world patterns of health and disease can only be understood properly within a social and economic context.

In Chapters 9 and 10 the focus changes to the United Kingdom, in order to examine in more detail the nature and causes of health and disease patterns within a nation. Chapter 11 concludes the book with a case study of food and health, which brings together the various perspectives adopted elsewhere, and shows as vividly as possible the many factors that influence what we eat, as well as the complex relationship between diet, nutrition and health, and the impact of food production on the environment.

The book is fully indexed and contains an annotated guide to further reading and to selected websites on the Internet. You will also find details of how to access a regularly updated collection of Internet resources relevant to the *Health and Disease* series on a searchable database called ROUTES, which is maintained by The Open University. This resource is open to all readers of this book.

World Health and Disease is the third in a series of eight books on the subject of health and disease specially written for the Open University for the level 2 course U205 *Health and Disease*. The book is designed so that it can be read on its own, like any other textbook, or studied as part of this course. General readers need not make use of the study comments, learning objectives and other material inserted for OU students, although they may find these helpful. The text also contains references to a collection of readings (*Health and Disease: A Reader*, Open University Press, second edition 1995; third edition 2001) prepared for the OU course: it is quite possible to follow the text without reading the articles referred to, although doing so should enhance your understanding of this book's contents.

Abbreviations used in this book

AFP	alpha-fetoprotein
AIDS	acquired immune deficiency syndrome
BSE	bovine spongiform encephalopathy
CHD	coronary heart disease
DALY	disability-adjusted life year
DH	Department of Health
DOTS	directly observed treatment short-course
ESR	European Standardised Rates
FCE	finished consultant episodes
FSA	Food Standards Agency
FSEs	former socialist economies of Europe
GAVI	Global Alliance for Vaccines and Immunizations
GHS	General Household Survey
GNP	Gross National Product
GP	general practitioner
HDI	Human Development Index
HIPC	heavily indebted poor countries
HIV	human immunodeficiency virus
HMSO	Her Majesty's Stationery Office (subsequently The Stationery Office)
ICD	International Statistical Classification of Diseases and Related Health Problems (formerly International Classification of Diseases)
IMR	infant mortality rate
MAFF	Ministry of Agriculture, Fisheries and Food
MSSG	Medical Services Study Group
NGO	non-governmental organisation
NHS	National Health Service
ODA	Official Development Assistance
ONS	Office for National Statistics
OPCS	Office of Population Censuses and Surveys
ORS	oral rehydration solution
ORT	oral rehydration therapy
PMR	proportional mortality ratio
PNMR	perinatal mortality rate
SMR	standardised mortality ratio
TB	tuberculosis
TPFR	total period fertility rate
UN	United Nations
UNICEF	United Nation's Children's Fund (formerly the UN's International Children's Emergency Fund)
vCJD	variant Creuzfeldt-Jakob disease
WHO	World Health Organisation

Study guide for OU students

(total of around 80 hours, including time for the TMA, spread over 5 weeks)

Chapters 9–11 are the longest in the book and since they occur at the end you should make sure to allow enough time to study them before completing the TMA. There is an audiotape and two videos associated with this book; you will be asked to view the video on health in South Africa again later in the year while studying Book 6. Most of the Reader articles (those by Strassburg, Engels, Diamond, McKeown, Szreter, Epstein) are referred to again later in the course, so by studying them here you are also preparing for Books 4–6.

1st week

Chapter 1	**Introduction**
Chapter 2	**World patterns of mortality**
Chapter 3	**Mortality and morbidity: causes and determinants** Reader article by Strassburg (1982); video, 'South Africa: Health at the crossroads'; audiotape, 'Smoking: A global health problem'

2nd week

Chapter 4	**Livelihood and survival: a case study of Bangladesh**
Chapter 5	**The world transformed: population and the rise of industrial society** Reader articles by Engels (1844) and Diamond (1992)
Chapter 6	**The decline of infectious diseases:** **the case of England** Reader articles by McKeown (1976) and Szreter (1988)

3rd week

Chapter 7	**Health in a world of wealth and poverty** Reader article by Drèze and Sen (1989)
Chapter 8	**Population and development prospects**

4th week

Chapter 9	**Contemporary patterns of disease in the United Kingdom** video, 'Status and wealth: the ultimate panacea?'; revise the audiotape, 'Smoking: A global health problem'
Chapter 10	**Explaining inequalities in health in the United Kingdom** Reader article by the Medical Services Study Group of the Royal College of Physicians (1978); video, 'Status and wealth: the ultimate panacea?'

5th week

Chapter 11	**Food, health and disease: a case study** Reader article by Epstein (1999) is optional here, but set reading for Book 4

TMA completion

World Health and Disease emphasises that epidemiology, anthropology, history, the social sciences and biology can each contribute to an integrated descriptive, comparative and explanatory account of health and disease patterns. It therefore draws on a number of different methods of studying health and disease, all of which were discussed in the first two books of the course, and it provides some empirical foundations for later books. The structure of the book is outlined in 'A note for the general reader' (p. 6), and is described further in Chapter 1. Study notes, where appropriate, are given at the start of chapters. These primarily direct you to important links to other components of the course, such as the other books in the course series, the Reader, and audiovisual components.

Many chapters in this book involve the interpretation of data about populations, their lifestyles and their health status. All this material is discussed in some way in the text, although you may wish to refer back to relevant parts of *Studying Health and Disease* if you have difficulty in working through the exercises we have included to strengthen your skills in data interpretation. However, we do not expect you to *memorise* the data: they have been included primarily to illustrate and to help explain the patterns and relationships that the text is exploring.

The index includes key words in orange type (also printed in bold in the text) which can be looked up easily as an aid to revision as the course proceeds. There is also a list of further sources for those who wish to pursue certain aspects of study beyond the scope of this book, either by consulting other books and articles or by logging on to specialist websites on the Internet.

The time allowed for studying *World Health and Disease* is about 80 hours spread over 5 weeks. It is the *longest* book in the course. The schedule (left) gives a more detailed breakdown to help you to pace your study. You need not follow it rigidly, but try not to let yourself fall behind. If you find a section of the work difficult, do what you can at this stage, and then return to reconsider the material when you reach the end of the book.

There is a tutor-marked assignment (TMA) associated with this book; about 5 hours have been allowed for writing it up, *in addition to* the time spent in studying the material it assesses.

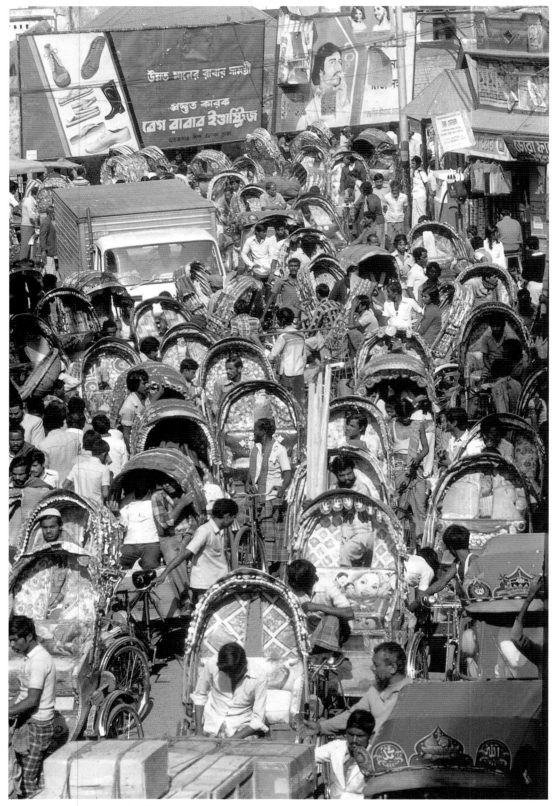

Figure 1.1   *The 'full tide of human existence' on display in this street scene in Dhaka, Bangladesh in 1993. (Photo: Mark Edwards/Still Pictures)*

CHAPTER 1

Introduction

1.1 Description and explanation

This book is about the patterns of health and disease that exist around the world and the factors that influence their magnitude and cause them to change over time. It has two broad aims — to describe and to explain these patterns.

In fulfilling the first aim, we describe the patterns of health and disease in some detail and draw comparisons between the situation that currently prevails in different places around the world: for example, the length of life which people in different countries or social groups can expect, and the commonest causes of death, illness or disability. We also look back to the past, in particular to the period before and after the Industrial Revolution in England, so that we can compare the health profile of the population in the eighteenth and nineteenth centuries with the health experienced in England today. Another aspect of the descriptive task in this book is to look at how birth and death rates influence population size and structures.

The second aim of the book is to consider why these health and disease patterns exist, and to assess which factors can best explain the ways in which they have changed over time. This endeavour also enables us to look into the future and attempt some predictions about the main health issues of global importance in the twenty-first century, and their underlying causes. As you will see again and again, the causes always turn out to be *multiple* and *interconnected* in many complex ways. The evidence does not support linear explanations of 'cause and effect' for the health problems that beset the world. If you look at Figure 1.1 and attempt to count how many possible influences on health and disease this single photograph suggests, you cannot avoid the conclusion that they are many, varied and interacting.

The attempt to explain the patterns of world health and disease raises three overarching questions, which run throughout the book:

1   To what extent have world patterns of health and disease been shaped in the past, and continue to be shaped in the present, by large-scale social, economic and environmental changes, such as the agricultural and industrial revolutions?

2   Do the poorer countries of the world today have health and disease patterns similar to those of developed countries in the past, before they became industrialised? To what extent can today's poorer countries anticipate the same kinds of epidemiological and demographic changes as those that accompanied industrialisation elsewhere?

3   To what extent can the patterns of health and disease we observe in a given country, or region, be related to the social and economic structure of that place and its people (for example, its housing, sanitation, income levels, employment, health care system), and how much to individual biology or personal lifestyle? What part is played by geographical, political or cultural factors in explanations for who gets sick and why?

This is not a book about the development of medical science, or about the people whose discoveries, skills and work helped to elevate medicine to the position of power and influence it holds today.[1] The broad approach of this book emphasises the social, economic and environmental characteristics of societies, and the ways in which these characteristics influence the health and disease of individuals. It covers a huge territory in both time and space, and attempts to draw many comparisons between countries around the world.

1.2   Categorising the world's countries

A comparative approach requires a method of 'grouping' countries that have something in common so that we can more easily refer to them, but this creates a problem. There are many different terms in current usage for categorising the countries of the world.

● Note down some of the ways in which countries can be categorised.

■ You might have thought of some of the following: rich and poor; North and South; East and West; First World and Third World; developed and developing; advanced and backward; industrial and non-industrial; modern and traditional; capitalist and socialist; democratic and authoritarian.

All such groupings tend to suffer from two big problems. First, the *similarities* between countries on which these groupings are supposedly based may be *less* important than the differences between these same countries. For example, Iceland and Russia are both in the 'North', but their cultures, histories, size, politics and roles in today's world are totally different.

Second, the range of health experience between different groups *within* a single country may be so wide that to call the country as a whole 'developed' or 'poor' becomes meaningless. South Africa illustrates this difficulty very clearly. The health profile of the majority black population has many similarities with the poorest African countries, such as Mali, Sierra Leone or Burkhina Faso, whereas the white population has health characteristics that resemble most Western European countries and North America.

Third, the ways in which countries are grouped and the labels attached to them are not 'value neutral'. The choice of terminology indicates a particular view of the world, which may have been overtaken by events or with which many might not agree. For example, the term 'Third World' came into use in about the 1960s to convey the sense of a group of countries who were not members of either the First World (the West) or the Second World (the communist bloc). However, the Second World fragmented during the 1980s and 1990s, when East and West Germany re-unified, the former Soviet Union broke up into its constituent nations, and neighbouring countries like Poland and Yugoslavia underwent huge political changes. Thereafter, the concept of a 'Third World' became less useful. Similarly, to talk of the 'developing' countries is to imply that these countries are undergoing progressive changes that in time will make them like the currently 'developed' countries. A quite different view is implied by the word 'underdeveloped', which somehow implies

---

[1] The medical and historical dimensions are discussed in two other books in this series, *Medical Knowledge: Doubt and Certainty* (Open University Press, 2nd edn 1994; colour-enhanced 2nd edn 2001), and *Caring for Health: History and Diversity* (Open University Press, 2nd edn 1993; 3rd edn 2001).

that these countries are not as developed as they should be, or could have been, or even that their condition has been imposed on them by outside forces.

There is no simple solution to these linguistic difficulties. In general, we have categorised countries simply according to whether their national income per person is 'low', 'middle' or 'high'. This has the advantage of being in line with many official statistics, for example those published by the World Bank. Again, following official statistics, we sometimes refer to the low-income and middle-income countries together as the 'developing countries' or regions, and to the high-income countries as the 'developed countries' or regions, without meaning to imply that the developing countries are following a particular path or that developed economies have reached some final stage of development.

Broadly, the low-income countries are in Sub-Saharan Africa and in Central, East and South Asia; the middle-income countries are in Eastern Europe, Central and South America, the Middle East and North Africa, and the high-income countries include those in Western Europe, North America, Japan, Australia and New Zealand.

We also sometimes use the distinction between 'industrialised' countries, which broadly correspond to the developed countries, and the 'non-industrialised' (low-income) and 'industrialising' countries, which broadly corresponds to the middle-income groups. But it is important to remember that grouping together such a large number of countries is fraught with difficulties: some low-income countries such as India or China have substantial industrial sectors and may export aircraft or other advanced technology around the world. Others are virtually prostrate economies, without natural resources and heavily dependent on foreign assistance and food aid.

We will return to this question of classification at various points, for an important aim of the book is to examine the connection between the economic and social characteristics of countries and their disease burden, mortality rates, and demographic structure. Chapter 2 begins that task by examining world patterns of mortality. By the time you reach the end of Chapter 11, you will have been on a journey which stretches back to archaic hunter-gatherer societies and forward to a projected global population of over 9 billion by 2050 (3 billion more than at the turn of the new millennium). You will have learnt a great deal about the health of many different countries around the world, but the picture we draw of England and of Bangladesh are particularly detailed. And you should be convinced of the complexity of interacting influences on health and disease, at all levels from the individual, local, national, international, and the global.

CHAPTER 2

World patterns of mortality

Study notes for OU students

This chapter builds on some of the basic concepts of epidemiology and demography introduced in another book in this series, *Studying Health and Disease* (Open University Press, second edition 1994; colour-enhanced second edition 2001). When interpreting epidemiological data from populations with different age profiles you will need to recall the rationale for *age-standardisation*. You should also be clear about the distinction between *incidence* (the number of new cases arising in a given period, e.g. a year) and *prevalence* (the total number of cases — new and continuing — in the population at a certain timepoint, e.g. on a specified date).

2.1 Introduction

Neither is the population to be reckoned only by numbers. (Francis Bacon, 1561–1626)

In this chapter we shall be looking at the population of the world and how it is distributed. You will see what proportions of the world's population live in low-income, middle-income and high-income countries, and how these proportions are changing. We will then examine the age- and sex-structure of the populations in different countries, and explore the ways in which birth and death rates influence, and are in turn influenced by, population structure. Finally, you will see whether the mortality differences that separate the low-income and high-income regions of the world are narrowing.

2.2 Measuring health

Before embarking on a comparison of the levels of health of different populations we must be quite clear how we are going to measure **health**. In its constitution, the **World Health Organization (WHO)**, an agency of the United Nations, has defined health as 'a state of complete physical, mental and social wellbeing' (WHO, 1958, Annex 1). You can probably see that the use of this famous and frequently quoted definition leads to considerable problems in actually measuring the health of a nation or even that of an individual. Using this definition, what proportion of your own life is 'healthy'? Most of us would have some difficulty in answering this question, even though the state described seems a desirable one to strive towards.

The WHO definition has been criticised on many grounds: for example, because of the difficulty of defining 'complete wellbeing'. So, for practical purposes, we are forced to use other surrogate or 'proxy' measures that are closely correlated with health or its absence, in particular the level of disease and death. (It should be noted, however, that when the WHO defined health, they pointed out that it was 'not merely the absence of disease and infirmity'.) Therefore, instead of looking at world patterns of health we are forced to look at world patterns of disease and disability.

Furthermore, we shall have to use well-defined and perhaps rather rigid and limited definitions of disease and disability — much more restricted than just the absence of health! Some aspects of disease will be almost completely neglected. This is not because they are unimportant, but because reliable information is not available from enough places to allow meaningful comparisons. In general, diseases involving major physical sickness with well-defined symptoms and signs, or disabilities such as blindness or limb loss, are easier to 'count' in different communities than are, for example, mental illness or more minor physiological disturbances.

Even if we select only certain diseases or disease states to study, there are several different measures that we might use to assess the magnitude of the disease problem in a given community. Measures that are commonly used include the disease incidence, prevalence, disability and severity. Severity is difficult to measure objectively, sometimes being assessed by the amount of (physical) disability or discomfort caused by the disease, and at other times by the **case-fatality rate** — the proportion of all cases of the disease that result in death. These measures are each useful for different purposes but even these are not generally available for many countries.

The major concern of this chapter is to compare the health of populations in different countries, particularly in developing and developed countries. Health data from many developing countries are very limited and so this chapter concentrates on mortality. But you should bear in mind that there are many diseases that kill only a small proportion of the persons they afflict. Chronically disabling diseases such as polio and leprosy in developing countries or arthritis in developed countries are good examples. Nevertheless, in general it is reasonable to assume that communities in which the death rate is high are those in which rates of non-fatal diseases are also high.

2.3   Distribution of the world's population

We begin by reviewing how the world's population is distributed over the globe. In 1999, the total population of the world passed the 6 billion mark (the United Nations designated 12 October 1999 as the 'Day of 6 Billion').

● Before reading on, write down how you would expect this total to be divided between Africa, North America, South America, Asia and Europe.

■ Now compare your estimates with Table 2.1, which shows the population estimates for 1998 published by the United Nations.

Table 2.1   World population estimates, 1950 and 1998, by region.

Region	Population in millions		as a percentage of world	
	1950	1998	1950	1998
Africa	224	779	9	13
North America	172	304	7	5
Central America	37	131	1	2
South America	112	332	4	6
Asia	1 402	3 589	56	61
(of which): China	555	1 255	22	21
India	358	976	14	16
Europe	547	729	22	12
Oceania[1]	13	30	1	0.5
all in developing world	1 711	4 748	68	80
all in developed world	813	1 182	32	20
total	2 523	5 930	100	100

[1] Oceania consists mainly of Australia, New Zealand, Papua New Guinea, Fiji, the Solomon Islands and smaller Pacific islands.

Data from United Nations Population Division, quoted in World Resources Institute (1998), *World Resources 1998–99*, Oxford University Press, Oxford and New York, Table 7.1, p. 244.

Asia alone accounts for over 60 per cent of the world's population. In fact well over a third of all the world's people live in just two countries, China and India. In contrast, only 12 per cent of the world's population live in Europe, including the Russian Federation. Table 2.1 also shows how the world's population was split between the developing regions and the developed regions in 1998, and how this has changed since 1950. Approximately 4 700 million people, or 80 per cent of the world's population, lived in the developing countries in 1998, a substantial increase compared with 68 per cent in 1950.

The growth of the world's population will be examined in more detail in Chapters 4, 5 and 8. It is a simple arithmetical law that population growth occurs when the birth rate exceeds the death rate. However, both the birth rate and the death rate are influenced by the proportional distribution of the population across different age and sex groupings — the population's **age–sex structure**. And the age–sex structure is in turn influenced by the death rate and the birth rate. So if we wish to examine patterns of health and disease in the world as a whole, we must pay close attention to the age and sex structure of the world's population, and how it varies between countries.

2.3.1 The population pyramid

The **age structure** of a population is entirely defined by the rate at which people enter through birth or immigration from another population, and leave through death or by emigration to another population. To simplify things, we shall not be looking in detail at migration, which in most countries has not had an important influence on the overall population structure in recent decades. It should be noted, however, that migration has often had an important influence on differences in the population structure in different regions *within* a country. The **sex structure** of a population simply refers to the proportion of males and females. Usually age and sex structures are combined in official statistics.

A **census** gives a cross-sectional 'snap-shot' of a population at one point in time. A direct and simple way of presenting this snap-shot of the age–sex structure of a population is by means of a **population pyramid**. A population pyramid is drawn in much the same way as a histogram. In effect, it consists of two histograms, one for each sex, arranged horizontally (as opposed to the usual vertical orientation), and set back to back. The bar areas are made proportional to the population in each age–sex group.

Figure 2.1 (overleaf) contains population pyramids for four countries in the 1990s, which show strikingly the contrast in population structure between countries at different levels of development. The four countries are:

- Sweden: a high-income country which is fully industrialised and has been so for a long time.
- The Russian Federation: with a large industrial sector and predominantly urban, but in social and economic turmoil at the beginning of the twenty-first century.
- China: a low-income country undergoing rapid social and economic change, with a large rural sector but relatively well-developed health and social services.
- South Africa: a middle-income country with major income and health disparities between the white and rapidly growing black populations.

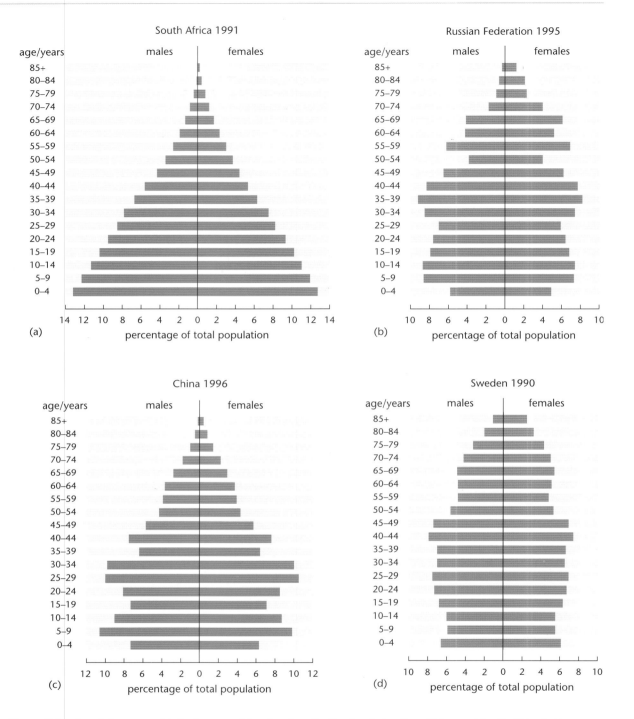

Figure 2.1 *Population pyramids for four countries: Sweden, the Russian Federation, China and South Africa in the 1990s. (Data from United Nations (1999a)* Demographic Yearbook 1997, *UN, New York, Table 7)*

● Describe the pyramid for South Africa (Figure 2.1a), commenting on the distribution by age and sex and noting any obvious differences for males and females.

■ The pyramid is strikingly true to its name, with a broad base, narrowing upwards so as to give a triangular picture. The largest age-groups are the youngest; around 36 per cent of the population is aged under 15 years in South Africa, while middle-aged and old people are relatively few; the percentage of the population over 64 years is less than 5 per cent, with more females than males.

If mortality rates have been high for all ages, the numbers in each age-group will tend to decrease with advancing age. The broad base of the South African pyramid suggests this pattern: because mortality is high, fewer people progress to the next age-band, and so the pyramid narrows.

Another factor leads towards the triangular shape. Throughout most of history, human societies have normally experienced a demographic pattern of high birth rates and high rates of infant and child mortality, and this pattern still prevails in most low-income countries. If these mortality rates fall, then the number of female children who reach childbearing age in each successive generation will increase and the birth rate will rise (so the base of the pyramid widens). This is one of a number of factors that may create an increasing population. Mortality rates are now falling in many low-income countries, and although fertility rates are also falling in many countries (as you will see in Chapters 4 and 8), there are still more births than deaths, over a period of time. This is a major reason for the triangular shape of the population pyramid of a typical low-income country. Generally, therefore, populations with the triangular shape have high birth rates and high mortality rates, and sustain substantial rates of increase in overall population size.

● Now describe the pyramid for the Russian Federation (Figure 2.1b).

■ The Russian Federation exhibits a very different shape compared with South Africa: the base of the pyramid is pinched in, then there is little tapering until the age-bands beyond 45. There is also a marked 'waist' in the 50–54 age-group, and in the oldest age-groups a noticeable excess of females over males.

● How might you go about trying to explain this 'waist' and the excess of females?

■ An obvious starting point would be to look for some event that particularly affected that cohort of the Russian population, for example when it was born. The 50–54 age-group was born between 1940 and 1945, during World War II, and it is likely that the birth rate dropped substantially during this period and that the infant mortality rate increased, thus reducing the size of the cohort. The effect of troop losses in the war and the Stalinist purges also explains the striking excess of females over males, particularly amongst those aged over 65.

Now look at the population pyramid in Figure 2.1c for China. The bottom of the pyramid is quite pinched, then there are bulges in the 5–9 and 25–34 age-groups, and finally a long tapering-off with advancing age with a relatively small proportion of people aged 65 or over.

● How might you explain the narrow base of the Chinese pyramid and the bulges at ages 5–9 and among young adults?

■   The most likely explanation is that the birth rate has been falling substantially in recent decades, thus pinching in the bottom of the pyramid. (Indeed in 1979 China announced a stringent policy of limiting family size to one child in most urban and rural areas, and this contributed to a subsequent fall in the birth rate.) The bulge at age 5–9 is probably an 'echo' of the bulge at ages 25–34, as this large cohort passed through child-bearing age.

The pyramid for China is fairly typical of countries that have experienced a falling death rate and rapidly increasing life expectancy, followed by a falling birth rate. As the generations currently at the bottom of the pyramid get older, so the pyramid will evolve a structure more similar to that in Sweden (Figure 2.1d) or other industrialised countries.

If you look more closely at the Chinese pyramid, you can see a number of irregularities. In particular, there is a curious 'waist' caused by the 35–39 age-group being smaller than the groups on either side of it. Again, a good way of exploring this would be to look for some experience that had a particular effect on that cohort of the Chinese population. In fact, we now know that between 1959 and 1961, when this group were born or were young children, parts of China were racked by a famine that may have killed around 15 million people. Famines, and the disproportionate effect that they have on very young children, will be examined in Chapters 7 and 11 of this book, but clearly this particular famine is one very plausible explanation for the irregular shape of China's present demographic structure. The irregularities in the Chinese pyramid may also reflect the difficulties of conducting censuses of population with limited resources in the world's most populous country, and of determining ages with accuracy. This is a problem in most developing countries, where many people may have little documentary evidence of their date of birth, and are entirely reliant on their own and their parents' memories.

The picture for Sweden (Figure 2.1d) is again quite different. In Sweden, the most numerous age-groups are between 25 years and 49 years. The tapering-off with advancing age, seen so strikingly in the data for South Africa (Figure 2.1a), is only evident in the pyramid for Sweden for ages above 65–69 years. There is a far higher proportion of older people in Sweden and there are rather more elderly females than males. In contrast, the percentage under 15 years of age is well under 20 per cent, much lower than in South Africa.

●   In most Western countries, there was a 'baby boom' after World War II. Can you see the effect of this in the Swedish population pyramid?

■   This is reflected by the 'bulge' in the pyramid in the 40–44 year age-group, whose members were born in the period immediately after the war.

You have seen that a triangular pyramid is typical of the population of a low-income country. It was also typical, in the past, of the countries that are now industrialised, such as England and Wales and the USA. Figure 2.2 shows the population of the USA in 1900 and in 1995. The general resemblance of the American population structure in 1900 to, for example, that of present-day South Africa is quite strong. This has led some people to suggest that as a country undergoes a transition to fully industrialised development, so the population structure also changes, and they refer to this as the **demographic transition**. This is clearly an important concept with wide implications, and we shall return to it in Chapter 6 when we consider the process of industrialisation and development from an historical perspective.

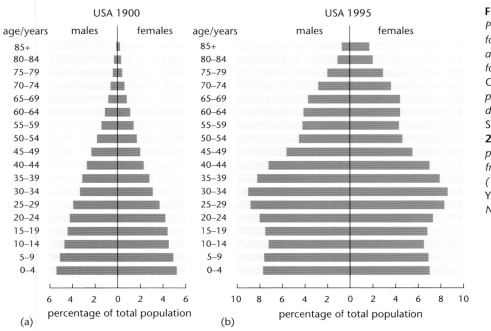

Figure 2.2
*Population pyramids
for the USA in 1900
and in 1995. (Data
for 1900 from Westoff,
C. F. (1974) The
populations of the
developed countries,*
Scientific American,
231 (3), *September,
p. 114; for 1995
from United Nations
(1999a) Demographic
Yearbook 1997, UN,
New York, Table 7)*

2.4 Measuring mortality

From the evidence of population structures, we have already concluded that death rates are in general higher in low-income countries than in the high-income countries. Let us now look at these variations in more detail.

Various measures are employed to compare mortality in the populations of different countries. The crude death rate, infant mortality rate and expectation of life at birth (defined later in this section) are all widely used for this purpose. Table 2.2 (overleaf) shows estimates of these measures for a sample of countries from each continent. These countries were chosen to illustrate the range of variation in mortality both within and between continents.

2.4.1 Death rates

Consider first the **crude death rates** for a number of selected countries shown in Table 2.2. The crude death rate is the total number of deaths in a population in a year, expressed as a rate per 1 000 population.

● Run your eye down the second data column of the table and pick out the highest crude death rates, and the lowest. Did anything surprise you?

■ Looking at the table, you will see that the highest rates among the countries listed were recorded in Mali (17 per 1 000) and the Central African Republic (16 per 1 000), both of which are amongst the world's lowest income countries. Closely behind come Zimbabwe and the Russian Federation. The rates in the high-income countries of Europe and North America were generally lower, at between 9 and 11 per 1 000. You may have been surprised however, to see that the lowest rates in the table, of 6 to 8 per 1 000, were recorded in Sri Lanka, Brazil, Guatemala, China, South Africa and Japan, and of these only Japan would be classified as a high-income country.

Table 2.2   Estimates of crude death rate, infant mortality rate and expectation of life at birth for selected countries, 1998 or nearest date.

Country	Population / millions	Crude death rate (per 1 000 population per year)	Infant mortality rate (per 1 000 live births)	Expectation of life at birth/years	
				male	female
Africa					
Central African Republic	4	16	96	43	47
South Africa	44	8	48	62	68
Mali	12	17	149	49	52
Zimbabwe	12	15	68	51	54
Americas					
Brazil	165	7	42	63	71
Guatemala	12	7	40	61	67
USA	274	9	7	73	79
Europe					
Poland	39	11	13	69	77
Portugal	10	11	8	71	79
Russian Federation	147	15	19	61	73
Sweden	9	11	5	77	82
UK	58	11	6	75	80
Asia					
Bangladesh	124	10	78	58	58
China	1 255	7	38	68	71
India	976	9	72	62	64
Japan	126	8	4	77	83
Sri Lanka	18	6	15	71	75

Data from United Nations Population Division, quoted in World Resources Institute (1998), *World Resources 1998–99*, Oxford University Press, Oxford and New York, Tables 7.1, 7.2 and 8.2.

In general, there is an inverse relationship between expectation of life at birth in a country and the crude death rate for that country, that is, high life expectancy is associated with a low crude death rate. However, this relationship is quite tenuous. For example, Brazil has a lower crude death rate than Sweden, but the life expectancy of both men and women is lower in Brazil. One set of figures appears to indicate that, on average, people live longer in Brazil than in Sweden; the other flatly denies that this is so. How do we reconcile these data? The answer lies in the population pyramids of the two populations. Put simply, Sweden has a higher *crude* death rate than Brazil because it has a higher proportion of old people. If the age distributions of different countries are similar, then crude death rates may be a reasonable basis on which to compare levels of mortality. However, if age distributions differ (and you have already seen in Figure 2.1 how different they can be), the use of crude death rates to compare levels of mortality is likely to be misleading. It would be preferable to calculate **age-standardised death rates** or, if possible, to compare the **age-specific death rates** of the two countries. (Age-specific and sex-specific death rates refer to deaths in a particular age or sex group of a population, expressed as a rate per 1 000 people in that population group.)

To illustrate this, consider a comparison of Sweden and Tajikistan (a low-income central Asian country formerly in the Soviet Union). In 1996, the crude death rate for females of all ages was 6.9 per 1 000 in Tajikistan compared with 10.5 per 1 000 in Sweden. This comparison might suggest the unexpected conclusion that the health of the Swedish population was generally worse than health in Tajikistan. However, Figure 2.3 shows details of the age-specific death rates for both countries.

⬤   What are the main differences between the two age-specific death rate curves?

◼   Figure 2.3 reveals that in every age-group, the death rate is higher in Tajikistan than in Sweden. The most important differences are in the first years of life, when death rates are substantially higher in Tajikistan than in Sweden.

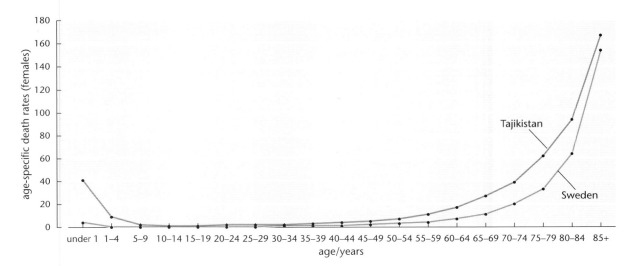

Figure 2.3   *Age-specific death rates of females in Tajikistan and Sweden per 1 000 population in that age group, 1996 or nearest date. (Data from United Nations (1999a)* United Nations Demographic Yearbook (1997) *UN, New York, Table 20)*

⬤   Why is the crude death rate higher in Sweden than in Tajikistan when the age-specific death rates are lower in Sweden?

◼   The two countries must have very different age structures.

If the population of Tajikistan had the *same* age distribution as that of Sweden, the death rate for all females would be 17.4 per 1 000 compared with 10 per 1 000 in Sweden, because the death rates in every age-group are higher in Tajikistan than in Sweden. However, Tajikistan has a much higher proportion of its population than Sweden in the teen and young adult age-groups, which tend to experience relatively low mortality. As a result, its crude death rate unadjusted for age is *lower* than Sweden's. Taking the very different age structures of Tajikistan and Sweden into account *reverses* the result of the comparison of the unstandardised crude mortality rates in the two countries.

As you saw above, low-income countries are characterised by having populations which are, on average, considerably younger than those of industrialised countries.

This very different age structure is the reason why the crude death rate is an unsatisfactory index for comparing mortality in different parts of the world.

The crude death rate is also unsatisfactory for another reason: in many countries it is estimated very inaccurately. In order to calculate the crude death rate, it is necessary to know two things — the number of deaths occurring in a given year and the total population in the middle of that year — and information on both items may be faulty. National censuses are conducted at regular intervals in most countries and often provide a reasonable estimate of the total population, but they can sometimes be misleading. For example, in 1992 a detailed international study of the population of Nigeria, using the most advanced techniques available, concluded that the actual population was up to 20 million less than the official census figure of 110 million. The main reason for this was thought to be a tendency among some regions to exaggerate their size, both as a matter of pride and to obtain more national resources. However, in other countries undercounting is thought to be a problem.

Obtaining a reliable estimate of the number of deaths in a given year is even more difficult. In the majority of industrialised countries this is done by means of a national system of death registration, but in most developing countries either such a system is lacking or else registration is very incomplete. And in such circumstances it is even less likely that accurate breakdowns of the age structure of the population will be available, making age-specific death rates even more difficult to estimate reliably.

2.4.2 Infant mortality rates

You have seen that the crude death rate can be an unsatisfactory index for mortality comparisons, because it may be difficult to estimate and is hard to interpret when countries have very different age structures. Another measure, the **infant mortality rate (IMR)**, is often used as one of the key indicators of socio-economic development. You might think it rather odd to focus on the IMR (the number of deaths in the first year of life per 1 000 live births) when we are really interested in the overall health of a community. It is, however, a very useful index of health for several reasons.

First, the infant mortality rate is relatively easy to measure. In industrialised countries it is calculated by using data on births and infant deaths collected through routine birth and death registration systems. This cannot be done in most developing countries because of the incompleteness of registration systems, but 'indirect' methods of estimating the IMR have been developed by demographers. These methods generally rely on questioning samples of women of reproductive age about the number of children they have had, and the number that have died. By using this information, obtained either from special surveys or from censuses, demographers have derived fairly reliable estimates of IMR for most countries.

A second strength of the infant mortality measure is that it is quite strongly correlated with adult mortality: if infant mortality is high, then adult mortality is likely to be high.

Third, in countries with high overall mortality, policies to reduce mortality are often directed principally at young children. This is because a high proportion of child deaths in such countries is due to infective and parasitic diseases that could be avoided through simple preventive or curative public health measures. When such measures are implemented, the IMR is likely to change much more dramatically than the crude death rate, making the IMR a useful indicator of the impact of such health measures.

● Returning to Table 2.2, identify the three countries with the highest IMR per 1 000 live births and the three countries with the lowest IMR.

■ The three highest IMRs are found in Mali, the Central African Republic and Bangladesh. The three lowest IMRs are in Japan, Sweden and the United Kingdom.

Even allowing for some inaccuracy in the estimates, it is clear that there are dramatic differences in the IMR between countries. An IMR in the Central African Republic of 96 per 1 000 live births means that around one child in ten dies before its first birthday, compared to one child in 250 in Japan. Going beyond the sample of countries in Table 2.2, the general pattern is that the IMR is below 10 per 1 000 live births in most of the world's richest countries, but exceeds 100 in many of the poorest countries. We will consider whether this gap is closing shortly. However, you can see that there is also substantial variation within these broad groupings, even between countries in the same region. There are also important exceptions to the general pattern, for example Sri Lanka has a reported IMR of 15 per 1 000 live births, which is very low for a poor country. Some of these exceptions will be discussed further in Chapter 8.

2.4.3 Expectation of life

Another index of mortality is the **expectation of life at birth**. This can be estimated from a 'life table' of the population. In industrialised countries, life tables are produced using age-specific death rates determined through censuses and death registration. Once again this approach is not possible in many developing countries, and although indirect estimation techniques have been suggested, they are not as reliable as those used to estimate the IMR. Thus, some of the estimates of the expectation of life in Table 2.2 should be regarded as approximations only. We shall return to these expectations of life, and in particular to male/female differences, in the next chapter.

Like the crude death rate, the expectation of life is an index reflecting both childhood and adult mortality. It has the advantage that its interpretation is not complicated by differences in the age structures of populations: an expectation of life must always be related to people at a particular age, usually those who have just been born. However, life expectancy is influenced particularly heavily by childhood mortality, as the following exercise makes clear.

● Suppose that 20 per cent of 1 000 newborn children die in the first five years of life (near the truth in some countries), and that the rest survive until an average age of 60 years. What is the expectation of life at birth, and at age 5? To keep things simple, assume that the 200 children who die in the first five years of life have an average lifetime of 2.5 years.

■ The 800 who do not die in the first five years live on average for 60 years. It follows that the total number of years of life lived by the entire 1 000 is (200 × 2.5 years) plus (800 × 60 years) = 48 500. Thus the average — the expectation of life at birth — is 48.5 years per person. At five years of age the expectation is much greater — 55 years.

This sharp increase in the expectation of life during early childhood is typical of countries with high childhood mortality. To illustrate this, Table 2.3 shows the expectation of (remaining) life at selected ages, for Bangladesh and the United Kingdom.

Table 2.3 Expectation of life (years) at various ages, in Bangladesh and the United Kingdom, 1996 or nearest date.

Sex	Country	Expectation of life at age/years						
		0	1	5	10	30	50	70
male	Bangladesh	59	63	61	57	40	22	9
	UK	74	74	70	65	45	27	12
female	Bangladesh	59	62	60	57	38	22	9
	UK	79	79	75	70	50	31	15

Data from United Nations (1999a) *United Nations Demographic Yearbook 1997*, UN, New York, Table 22.

The first thing to notice is that a boy born in the United Kingdom in 1996 can expect to live for 74 years on average, 15 years longer than his counterpart in Bangladesh. A girl born in the United Kingdom has a life expectancy of 79 years, which is 20 years longer than her counterpart in Bangladesh. Note also that, whereas in the United Kingdom (and in most other countries in Table 2.2) females have a greater life expectancy than do males, in Bangladesh this was not the case in 1996. As mentioned earlier, we will return to these male/female differences in the next chapter. Next, notice how in Bangladesh the expectation of life increases considerably between birth and the age of one year. Once infancy has been survived, the gap between Bangladesh and the United Kingdom is much narrower. Thus a man aged 30 years in Bangladesh can expect to live to around 70 years of age (30 + 40), whereas a 30-year-old man in the United Kingdom can expect to live to about 75 years (30 + 45) which is a relatively small difference.

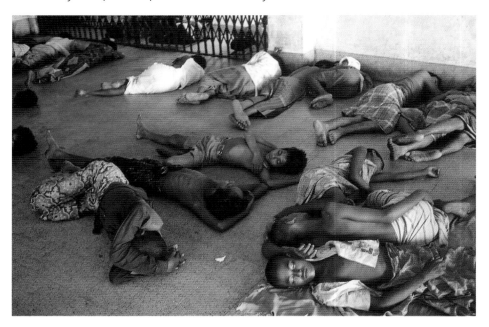

These street-dwelling children in Dhaka, Bangladesh, have survived infancy but their lives are still threatened by considerable risks to health. Expectation of life at birth in Bangladesh is 15 or 20 years less than in the UK. (Photo: Shehzad Noorani/Still Pictures)

Turning back to Table 2.2, you can see that expectation of life at birth in the selected countries ranges from 43 to 77 years for men and 47 to 83 years for women: that is, a female born in Japan can now expect on average to live for 83 years. Life expectancy appears to be closely related to the IMR, with people in countries having high IMRs tending to have a low expectation of life. One way of examining the relationship between the IMR and expectation of life, is to use the information in Table 2.2 to plot a scatter diagram showing the relationship between the two.

● Figure 2.4 has been designed so that you can create such a scatter diagram from the data in Table 2.2. For each country, plot the IMR along the *x*-axis (horizontal) and the expectation of life for females up the *y*-axis (vertical), then place a dot or cross in the graph. What does the completed scattergram reveal? (A completed version of the graph (Figure 2.9) is given at the end of the chapter.)

■ The graph reveals a clear negative relationship between the IMR and expectation of life. This is just what we would expect in view of the strong influence of infant mortality on expectation of life, which has already been noted.

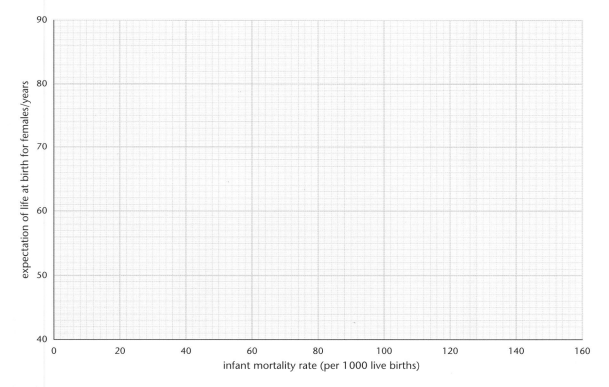

Figure 2.4   *Grid on which to plot data from Table 2.2 (p. 22) on the expectation of life of females and infant mortality rates: selected countries. (The completed version appears as Figure 2.9 on p. 33.)*

2.4.4 Height-for-age

Finally, although this chapter is concerned primarily with differences in *mortality* between developing and developed countries, it is important to note that other systematic differences related to health exist. For example, **anthropometric data** (data based on measurement of the human body) reveal large differences between countries in the average height and weight of populations. One of the most

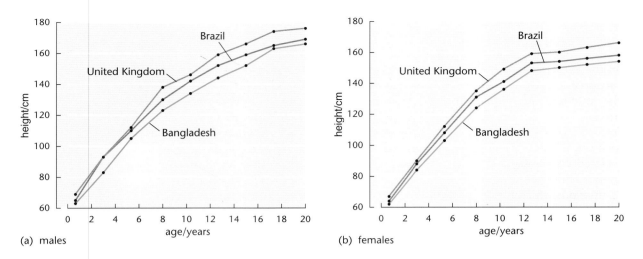

Figure 2.5 *Height-for-age measurements in the United Kingdom, Brazil and Bangladesh, 1987. (Data from James, W. P. T. and Schofield, C. (1990)* Human Energy Requirements: a Manual for Planners and Nutritionists, *Oxford Medical Publications, Oxford)*

commonly used anthropometric measures is **height-for-age**, which is often regarded as a guide to infections in early childhood and past nutritional status. Low height-for-age, referred to as 'stunting', is often taken as an indication that at some point in a person's early life they suffered repeated infections and their food intake may have been chronically inadequate. Figure 2.5 shows height-for-age for males and females in three countries. The interpretation of such data is complex, and we will return to the whole issue of nutrition and health in Chapter 11. For the moment, however, the key point is that systematic anthropometric differences exist alongside mortality differences.

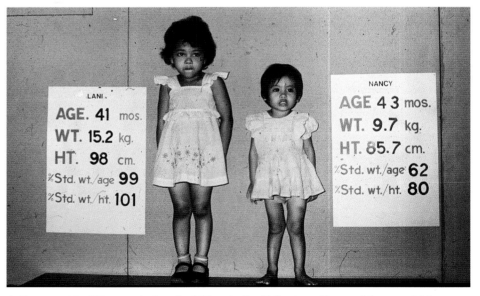

Anthropometric differences in female children in the Philippines. The small-for-age child demonstrates the effects on growth of an adverse early environment, but it is impossible to deduce how much of the 'stunting' has been due to repeated illness and how much to lack of food. (Photo courtesy of Teaching Aids at Low Cost (TALC), P.O. Box 49, St Albans, Herts, AL1 5TX. Details of TALC materials sent free on request.)

2.5   Recent changes and projected trends in mortality rates

All the evidence considered so far leads to the same conclusion: mortality rates vary greatly between different parts of the world. As noted earlier, however, we are also interested in finding out whether these differences are becoming greater or smaller, and to do this we have to look at trends over time in these mortality rates. For the reasons discussed earlier, the infant mortality rate is a particularly useful measure for this purpose. Table 2.4 shows changes in infant mortality rates for selected countries over the period from 1950 to 2000. Note that the IMRs are shown as the average of five-year periods. This removes some of the year-to-year fluctuations which are inevitable in such statistics.

Table 2.4   Infant mortality rates (per 1 000 live births), selected periods 1950–55 to 1995–2000, selected countries.

Country	1950–55	1965–70	1975–80	1985–90	1995–2000
Africa					
Central African Republic	197	160	145	132	96
South Africa	96	83	72	62	48
Americas					
Brazil	135	100	79	63	42
Jamaica	85	45	25	18	12
Europe					
Sweden	20	13	8	6	5
UK	24	19	14	9	6
Asia					
Bangladesh	180	140	137	119	78
China	195	81	52	50	38
India	190	145	129	99	72
all in more developed world	**56**	**26**	**19**	**15**	**9**
all in less developed world	**180**	**117**	**97**	**79**	**62**

Data from United Nations (1999a) *United Nations Demographic Yearbook 1997*, UN, New York, Table 7.

● Describe the main features of the data in Table 2.4, concentrating in particular on similarities and differences between the countries. You may find it helpful to begin by sketching a rough graph in the margin of this page, choosing two or three countries that seem to have different trends.

■ The countries show a similar pattern in that IMRs have decreased steadily between 1950–55 and 1995–2000 for all countries. However, they are different in two main respects: the absolute values of the IMRs vary tremendously between countries in any period, and the rates of decline over time are also very different. To illustrate the last point, the IMRs of India and China were similar in 1950–55, but by 1995–2000 the Indian rate was almost double that of China.

There are several ways of comparing the changes in the infant mortality rates, which will be illustrated by contrasting the IMRs of South Africa and the United Kingdom. One method is to calculate the **absolute difference** in IMRs. In 1950–55, the IMR was 96 in South Africa and 24 in the United Kingdom, an absolute difference of 72 deaths per 1 000 live births. In 1995–2000 this difference was 42 (48 – 6), suggesting a narrowing of the difference. However, an alternative, and perhaps more appropriate, measure is to assess the *relative* chance of an infant dying by expressing the two IMRs in the form of a ratio. In 1950–55 the ratio of the IMR in South Africa to that in the United Kingdom was 96 divided by 24, which is a ratio of close to 4:1. That is, the IMR was 4 times higher in South Africa than in the United Kingdom. This **relative difference** can be compared with 1995–2000, when the ratio was 8:1 (48/6). So although the IMRs in *both* countries had dropped considerably between 1950–55 and 1995–2000, the chance of an infant dying in South Africa relative to the chance of death of a UK infant had actually *doubled*.

It is possible to generalise from the example given above, and consider whether the gap between infant mortality rates in developing and developed countries is closing or widening over time. Figure 2.6 shows the changes in both (a) the absolute difference and (b) the relative difference in IMRs between six countries, and the average for the more developed countries.

In absolute terms (Figure 2.6a), the difference between the IMRs for the six selected countries and the average IMR for the more developed countries as a group has in all cases decreased. A different picture emerges, however, from a comparison of the relative differences in IMRs (Figure 2.6b), with considerable variation from country to country. For example, in 1950–55 a baby born in Jamaica was 1.5 times

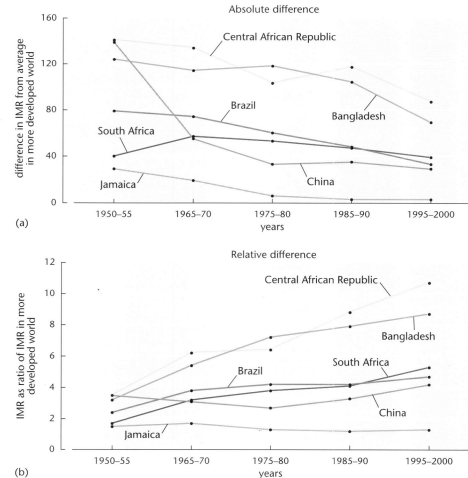

Figure 2.6
(a) Absolute and (b) relative differences in IMR in selected developing countries compared with the average IMR for the more developed world, 1950–2000. (Data from Table 2.4)

more likely to die before its first birthday than one born in the more developed world. This difference increased to 1.7 times in 1965–70 but has since been decreasing, and by 1995–2000 it was down to 1.3. Thus in Jamaica there was a period of relative deterioration followed by a relative improvement.

● In which countries shown in Figure 2.6b have relative differences widened?

■ They all widened over the whole period, except for Jamaica (as noted above) and China, which improved its relative position until about 1980, when the trend reversed.

In summary, although the infant mortality rate has been steadily decreasing in almost all developing countries, in many it has fallen at a much slower rate than in the more developed countries; thus the relative chance of an infant in a developing country dying *increased* in the second half of the twentieth century. The lesson is that even when the IMR is falling everywhere, the gap between countries can still be widening. Even in 50 years time the projected rates for many developing countries are predicted to be considerably higher than those currently experienced in developed countries. This is one example of a growing '**health divide**'.

Another measure of mortality examined earlier was life expectancy at birth, and Figure 2.7 shows how this has changed in major areas of the world, and also how it is predicted to change over the next 15 or so years.

● What general trends in life expectancy at birth are shown by Figure 2.7?

■ Figure 2.7 shows some narrowing of differences over time, and a generally increasing life expectancy in every major area of the world, but it also indicates that the less developed countries, and particularly the least developed countries, will continue to lag some way behind. Even by the period 2010–15, average life expectancy at birth in the less developed countries is predicted to be no higher than it was in the more developed countries in 1950, and will still be around 10 years short of the 77 or 78 years that are likely to be the norm by then in the more developed countries.

The most significant absolute changes are occurring where the IMR is falling most rapidly. As you have already seen, infant mortality has a profound effect on expectation of life at birth.

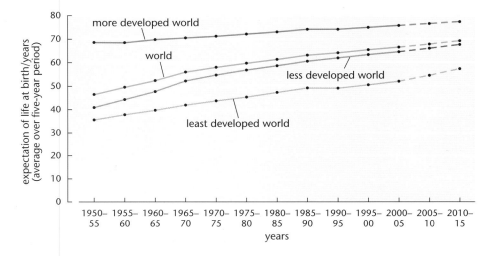

Figure 2.7 *Trends in life expectancy at birth, both sexes, by region, 1950–2015. (Data from United Nations, 1998,* World Population Prospects 1998, *UN, New York)*

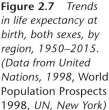

In this chapter you have seen that the mortality patterns of people living in low- and middle-income countries are systematically different from those of people in high-income countries. Death rates are higher at all ages, but particularly in the first few years of life, and expectation of life is lower. Moreover, some of these differences do not appear to be decreasing in relative terms, even when they are tracked over several decades or predictions are made well into the twenty-first century.

However, just as average statistics for groups of countries can disguise variations between countries, so mortality statistics for a country as a whole fail to tell us anything about variations that might exist *within* countries. The general patterns established in this chapter are overlaid by variations between and within countries, and these variations raise many intriguing questions about the origins and determinants of such patterns of health and disease. The next step, therefore, is to examine in more detail the main causes of death and types of disease. These are the themes of the next chapter.

OBJECTIVES FOR CHAPTER 2

When you have studied this chapter you should be able to:

2.1 Define and use, or recognise definitions and applications of, each of the terms printed in **bold** in the text.

2.2 Demonstrate an understanding of how a population pyramid depicts the age–sex structure of a population, and how population structures tend to differ systematically between developing and developed countries.

2.3 Discuss the advantages and disadvantages of the following three measures of mortality: crude death rate, infant mortality rate and expectation of life at birth.

2.4 Use different measures of mortality to describe the main differences between developed and developing countries, and give examples of ways in which relative and absolute measures of mortality can suggest different conclusions about changes over time.

QUESTIONS FOR CHAPTER 2

1   (*Objective 2.2*)

    (a) Using the data in Figure 2.1(b), make an approximate estimate of the percentage of the female Russian Federation population that, in 1995, was 65 years or older.

    (b) Figure 2.8 shows population pyramids for two countries in the late 1990s.

        (i) What are their main features and what kind of societies do they suggest to you?

        (ii) What difference might you expect to find in comparing crude death rates and age-standardised death rates for these two populations?

    (c) Is it possible to predict accurately the life expectancy of a newborn boy or girl from the contemporary population pyramid for the country where he or she was born?

2   (*Objective 2.3*)

    Why is it often more useful to use the infant mortality rate rather than the crude death rate as a measure of the health status of different populations?

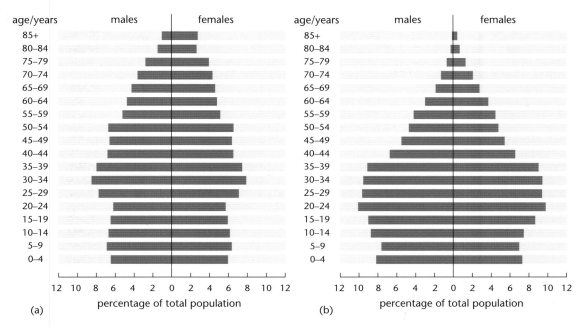

Figure 2.8 *Population pyramids for two countries in 1997; for use with Question 1b.*

3 (*Objective 2.4*)

Look back at Figure 2.6. What conclusions can you draw about the change in the IMR in Brazil, compared with the average for the more developed world, between 1950–55 and 1995–2000?

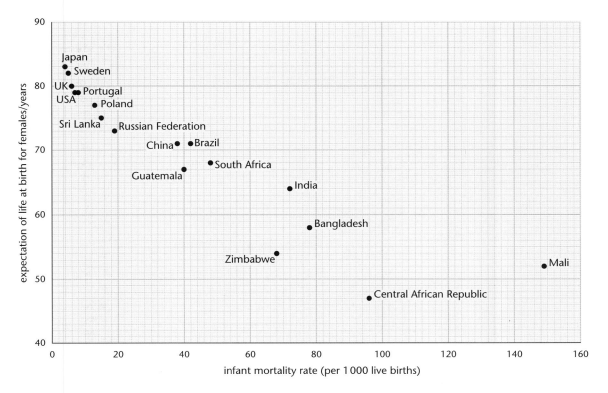

Figure 2.9 *Completed scatter diagram for comparison with your version on Figure 2.4, showing the relationship between infant mortality rate and female expectation of life at birth for selected countries, 1998 or nearest date. (Data from Table 2.2)*

C H A P T E R   3

Mortality and morbidity: causes and determinants

Study notes for OU students

There is a video associated with this chapter, 'South Africa: Health at the crossroads', and an audiotape called 'Smoking: A global health problem'. Details of both can be found in the Audiovisual Media Guide. While studying Section 3.6 of this chapter, you will be asked to read an article in *Health and Disease: A Reader* (Open University Press, second edition 1995; third edition 2001) 'The global eradication of smallpox', by Marc Strassburg.

3.1   Introduction

In the previous chapter you saw that roughly 80 per cent of the world's population live in developing countries, that their population structure is very different from that of developed countries, and that their overall health experience as measured by mortality is generally much poorer than that of the populations of developed countries, especially among children. In this chapter we further explore these differences, by first considering the main causes of death and morbidity (disease or disability), and then looking for some of the factors influencing these patterns. As a first step, we look at the main causes of death in different parts of the world.

3.2   Causes of death

In order to compare patterns of death caused by disease or injury around the world, we need to have some method of measuring the relative importance of different causes. One method of doing this would be to examine the percentages of total deaths that are attributable to different causes; another would be to compare the mortality rates for specific causes, and a third method would be to look at years of life lost from different causes.

3.2.1   Distribution of deaths by cause

Figure 3.1 illustrates the first of these methods, by comparing the **proportional mortality** (percentage distribution of deaths) in different groups of countries and for major causes of death. These data are taken from the World Health Organisation's (WHO) Global Burden of Disease study, an ambitious attempt to produce the first comprehensive estimates of deaths and disease for every country in the world. The first full set of data from this enormous programme of work related to the year 1990, but some aspects are being continuously updated, and most of the data used here relate to 1998.

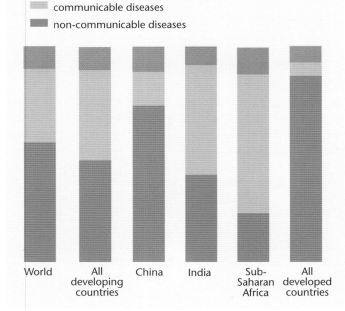

Figure 3.1 *Main causes of mortality by region, 1998 (per cent of total in that region). (Data from World Health Organisation (1999) World Health Report 1999: Making a Difference, Annex Table 2)*

A major cause of death in developing countries is the communicable (infectious and parasitic) **diseases**, maternal and perinatal conditions and nutritional deficiencies: indeed, in Africa these accounted for almost two-thirds of all deaths in 1998. The **communicable diseases** are caused mainly by micro-organisms such as bacteria, viruses, fungi and single-celled parasites, and partly by multicellular parasites such as worms (although for every death caused by parasites there are likely to be six or seven caused by bacteria or viruses). In the developed countries, these communicable diseases accounted for only 6 per cent of all deaths in 1998.

This stark contrast between the developing and developed countries exists largely as a consequence of the profound changes that have taken place in industrialised countries over the last century. One major change has been the virtual disappearance, as major killers, of the acute infectious diseases that remain so prevalent in today's developing countries. In their place other diseases, which were relatively unimportant in the past, have become major causes of public health concern in industrialised countries. These changes will be discussed in detail in Chapter 6 in the context of the United Kingdom, but Table 3.1 shows the twelve leading causes of death in the developed and developing countries in 1998, with the percentage of deaths and the total number of deaths attributable to each.

- How much similarity was there in the top twelve causes of death in the developed and developing countries in 1998? What are the major differences?

■ Six out of twelve causes of death appeared in both lists, but their ranking and relative importance are different. In the developed world, the **degenerative diseases** are to the fore, with ischaemic heart disease and cerebrovascular disease alone accounting for well over one-third of all deaths, and with the remainder of the list dominated by a range of cancers and other chronic and degenerative conditions. (In fact, almost three-quarters of all deaths in developed countries are caused by these degenerative diseases.) In the developing countries, ischaemic heart disease and cerebrovascular disease have also become major causes of death, but lower respiratory infections, HIV/AIDS, diarrhoeal diseases, childhood diseases (such as measles) and tuberculosis also exact a high toll. Childbirth (conditions arising during the perinatal period) is also identified as a highly hazardous event.

Viruses such as influenza are mainly responsible for the respiratory infections, and present a severe threat to health and life, especially among infants and young children in developing countries.

Diarrhoeal diseases are caused by a wide variety of different bacteria and parasites, and a few types of virus, which infect the gut and irritate the cells lining its surface. When irritated, these cells secrete large amounts of water and dissolved salts into the gut, which stimulate the muscular gut walls to contract and expel the watery, infected waste. However, if the infection persists and the diarrhoea is prolonged and severe, so much water and essential salts are lost that dehydration and disruption of body chemistry results. At the least, prolonged diarrhoea causes a failure to absorb nutrients effectively and an increased vulnerability to other infections, which in turn exacerbates the effects of malnutrition. A vicious circle is set up, which acts as a serious check to growth and development among millions of children in low-income countries. Certain diarrhoeal diseases, such as cholera, have high fatality rates because the infectious organism produces a toxin, which stimulates the gut wall to secrete exceptionally large amounts of fluid. In as many as 50 per cent of untreated cases of cholera, death occurs within 48 hours. Treatment of diarrhoeal

Table 3.1 Top twelve causes of death by region, 1998, as per cent of total deaths and in actual numbers of deaths (thousands).

Developing world (population = 4 977 million)			Developed world (population = 907 million)		
Cause of death	% of deaths	No. of deaths /thousands	Cause of death	% of deaths	No. of deaths /thousands
1 ischaemic heart disease	12.0	5 492	1 ischaemic heart disease	23.5	1 884
2 cerebrovascular disease	9.2	4 213	2 cerebrovascular disease	11.1	893
3 lower respiratory infections	6.9	3 146	3 cancers of trachea, bronchus and lung	5.3	422
4 HIV/AIDS	4.9	2 253	4 lower respiratory infections	3.8	306
5 diarrhoeal diseases	4.8	2 212	5 chronic obstructive pulmonary disease (COPD)	3.5	280
6 conditions arising during the perinatal period	4.6	2 102	6 colon and rectum cancers	3.0	243
7 chronic obstructive pulmonary disease (COPD)	4.3	1 969	7 diabetes mellitus	2.0	161
8 childhood diseases	3.6	1 640	8 breast cancer	2.0	160
9 tuberculosis	3.2	1 480	9 stomach cancer	1.8	143
10 homicide, violence and war	2.8	1 282	10 road traffic accidents	1.8	142
11 malaria	2.4	1 100	11 self-inflicted injuries	1.6	130
12 road traffic accidents	2.2	1 029	12 liver cirrhosis	1.5	122
all causes	100.0	45 897	all causes	100.0	8 033

Data from World Health Organisation (1999) *World Health Report 1999: Making a Difference*, Annex, Table 2.

The causes of death, disease and disability in one country that incorporates *both* these patterns is explored in a video for Open University students, 'South Africa: Health at the crossroads'; students should view it before starting Chapter 4.

diseases consists of replenishing the lost water and salts, and giving glucose as an energy source, until the infection subsides. This **oral rehydration therapy (ORT)** is simple, cheap and effective and could save many thousands more lives each year if it was more widely used.[1]

Measles, a viral infection, is certainly not a 'tropical' disease, and why it causes so many deaths in low-income regions of the world is not fully understood. Few diseases occur in isolation in children in low-income countries, and the reason that so many die of measles may be that the infection hits hardest those whose defences are already weakened by malnutrition or malaria and other parasitic or infectious diseases. Measles may also cause so many deaths in low-income countries because it frequently occurs at very young ages, often before the age of one year when the body is less able to cope with such an infection, and often before the age when immunisation would normally be given. In developed countries, even before vaccination programmes, measles was predominantly a disease of later childhood, at least in the recent past.

A look at the actual numbers of deaths by cause in Table 3.1 reveals something else of interest: because there are far more people and far more deaths in total in the developing countries, there are actually more deaths there each year from the 'Western' degenerative diseases than in the developed countries. For example, there were just under 3 million deaths in 1998 in the developed world from ischaemic heart disease and cerebrovascular disease, but almost 10 million deaths that year from these causes in the developing countries.

Since the list shown in Table 3.1 was compiled (using data for 1998), **AIDS (Acquired Immune Deficiency Syndrome)** — caused by infection with the human immunodeficiency virus (HIV) — has continued to increase in importance as a cause of death. This virus is transmitted primarily via sexual contact or infected blood, and the period between infection and onset of illness is often very long — as much as eight or more years in many cases. Consequently, it is extremely hard to know the scale of the epidemic. However, by the end of 1999 it was estimated that 33.6 million people globally were infected with HIV/AIDS, and a cumulative total of 16.3 million had died of the disease — 2.6 million in 1999 alone. At first, the country with most reported cases of AIDS was the USA, which contained two-thirds of AIDS patients in 1990. But by 1999 over 90 per cent of all people living with HIV/AIDS were in the developing countries, particularly in Sub-Saharan Africa (with 23.3 million people affected) and Asia (6.9 million). In Chapter 8 we will look at the possible future impact of HIV/AIDS on population change in countries most affected by this disease.

The spread of HIV/AIDS, along with poorly managed control programmes and the increasing movement of people, has also been a major factor in the global increase in tuberculosis (TB). HIV/AIDS weakens the immune system, greatly increasing the risk that someone who is HIV-positive and infected with TB becomes sick. Indeed, TB is the leading cause of death among people who are HIV-positive, accounting for almost one-third of AIDS deaths worldwide. The emergence of drug-resistant strains of TB is another factor. In 1993, the World Health Organization became so concerned about this modern TB epidemic that it declared TB a global emergency.[2]

---

[1] Attempts to promote oral rehydration therapy in developing countries are discussed in *Caring for Health: History and Diversity* (Open University Press, 2nd edn 1993; 3rd edn 2001), Chapter 8.

[2] The history of tuberculosis from the Middle-ages to the new millennium is discussed in another book in this series, *Medical Knowledge: Doubt and Certainty* (Open University Press, 2nd edn 1994; colour-enhanced 2nd edn 2001), Chapter 4.

It is estimated that between 2000 and 2020, nearly one billion people will be newly infected, 200 million people will get sick, and 35 million will die from TB, unless control is strengthened.

Some of the diseases that predominate in developed countries are purely modern epidemics and their emergence has been closely related to changes in patterns of living — the epidemic of lung cancer that followed the adoption of tobacco smoking on a widespread basis is an example of such a disease, which is now declining in developed countries but increasing rapidly in developing countries such as China.[3] But other diseases have become important not because the causes of the diseases have become more prevalent, but because the population has 'aged'. Many diseases are more common in elderly people and, as infectious diseases that killed children and young adults in previous centuries have been conquered, increasing numbers of people have survived long enough to be at risk of death from the diseases of older ages, such as cancers and heart disease.[4]

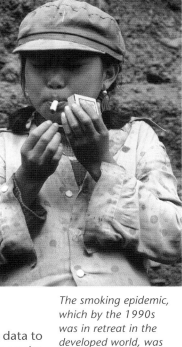

- Given the association between age and degenerative diseases such as cancers, what would it be advisable to do when comparing cause-specific death rates between countries or regions?

- As discussed in Chapter 2, it would be advisable to age-standardise the data to take into account differences in the age structures of the populations under comparison.

The smoking epidemic, which by the 1990s was in retreat in the developed world, was rapidly spreading in developing countries, particularly among boys and young men: Sichuan Province, China. (Photo: Gang Feng Wang/Panos Pictures)

3.2.2 Years of life lost

Comparisons between countries based on the type of mortality data discussed above give only a partial view of the health patterns. For example, numbers of deaths from specific diseases fail to acknowledge that a disease or injury that kills young adults may represent a greater *economic* loss to a country (and create social problems such as orphaned children) than one that causes the death of elderly people. One modification to mortality rates which attempts to take such problems into account is to calculate the **years of potential life lost** due to death from different causes. This method offers an alternative perspective when assessing the relative importance of each cause. For example, if a disease kills a person at age 50 years in a country in which they might otherwise have expected to live to 70 years, they have 'lost' 20 years of potential life. Thus, by looking at the ages at which people die from specific causes and their expectation of life at those ages, it is possible to compute the total years of potential life lost by all persons dying from that cause. Causes of death can then be ranked according to the years of life that each 'costs' the community. Years of life lost are often calculated by using life expectancy in developed countries as the standard. Consequently, if someone dies aged 5 from measles in Zimbabwe, the years of life lost are estimated as the remaining life expectancy at the age of 5 in developed countries, not the remaining life expectancy in Zimbabwe.

[3] An audiotape 'Smoking: A global health problem' is associated with study of this chapter by Open University students, who should listen to it before starting Chapter 4.

[4] The biological and sociological dimensions of old age are discussed in two other books in this series: *Human Biology and Health: An Evolutionary Approach* (Open University Press, 2nd edn 1994; 3rd edn 2001) and *Birth to Old Age: Health in Transition* (Open University Press, 2nd edn 1995; colour-enhanced 2nd edn 2001).

In general, there is a broad correspondence between years of life lost and percentages of deaths as measures of disease burden, but there are some striking exceptions. For example, in the developed countries, as you saw in Table 3.1, road traffic accidents cause around 1.8 per cent of all deaths. However, they are responsible for over 6 per cent of all years of potential life lost.

● Why do you think that road traffic accidents in developed countries cause a far higher proportion of years of potential life lost than of deaths?

■ This method of assessing disease importance gives more weight to those causes of death diseases that kill at younger ages and thus result in a greater loss of years of life. Accident rates are highest in the young and thus are given greater weight.

In contrast, ischaemic heart disease occurs mainly in older age groups, and so, while it is responsible for 24 per cent of all deaths in developed countries, it accounts for 16 per cent of potential years of life lost.

● Which conditions would you expect to see high on the list of causes of death in developing countries *and* on 'years of life lost' tables?

■ Communicable diseases dominate both methods of evaluating mortality in developing countries, since babies and children are more susceptible to infection than are adults.

3.2.3 Morbidity

The different methods examined above of assessing the relative importance of different causes of death using mortality data each have their merits. However, they share the important limitation that they only provide information about lethal diseases and injuries, giving no indication of the **morbidity** (illness) and disability from these or other causes. The measurement of morbidity is fraught with difficulties. Definitions of illness are to some extent subjective, and illnesses vary greatly in severity and duration. Population surveys are expensive and difficult to conduct, whereas measures based on, for example, visits to hospitals or doctors are likely to be influenced by the numbers of doctors and hospitals and their ease of access. So estimating the number of cases of different types of disease on a world-wide basis is a daunting task and is liable to be error-prone.

A good illustration of these problems is malaria. This parasitic disease has been resurgent around the world since the 1970s, and, as you saw in Table 3.1, was responsible for around 1.1 million deaths in 1998 in the developing countries. It probably poses the severest health problem in Sub-Saharan Africa, where the majority of the cases reported world-wide occur, but it is also widespread through Asia and Latin America. The 1.1 million deaths each year make malaria the most serious tropical parasitic disease, killing more people than any other communicable disease except tuberculosis. However, the number of deaths each year is dwarfed by the annual number of *clinical episodes*, which have been estimated at between 300 million and 500 million. Children under five years of age are chronic victims of malaria, suffering an average of six bouts a year, and so their physical and intellectual development are severely impaired. In the most affected countries, as many as 3 in 10 hospital beds are occupied by victims of malaria. We'll come back to malaria in Section 3.3.2.

Another aspect of the morbidity caused by diseases such as malaria in low-income countries is that it causes a disproportionate amount of economic damage. For example, each bout of malaria amongst adults has been estimated as costing the equivalent of 10 working days. This is especially a problem in Africa, where malaria reaches a peak at harvest time. In 1997 it was estimated that the costs of malaria in Sub-Saharan Africa exceeded $2 billion, including costs for control and lost work days, equivalent to between 1 per cent and 5 per cent of the national income of affected countries. The **World Bank** is an international agency founded in 1944 with the aim of assisting member states in reconstruction and development. A World Bank study in the early 1990s collated information on the average number of days of sickness and days off work in a variety of countries. Some of the results are shown in Table 3.2. The countries are ranked in order of their average Gross National Product (GNP)[5] per person in 1989, with the poorest (Ghana) at the top.

Table 3.2 The economic burden of adult illness, 1989 or nearest year.

Country (ranked according to GNP per person 1989)	Average days ill in last month	Work days absent in last month	Per cent of normal earnings lost through illness
Ghana (1988)	3.6	1.3	6.4
Mauritania (1988)	2.1	1.6	6.5
Côte d'Ivoire (1988)	2.6	1.3	6.4
Bolivia (1990)	not known	1.2	4.4
Peru (1985)	4.5	0.9	3.1
Jamaica (1989)	1.2	0.5	2.1
USA (1988)	not known	0.3	1.5

Data derived from World Bank (1991) *World Development Report 1991*, Oxford University Press, Oxford and New York, Table 3.1.

● What does Table 3.2 reveal?

■ The poorer the country, the more frequent are days of sickness and days off work, and the greater is the loss of income from illness. Thus workers in the poorest countries listed lost around one and a half days of work each month through sickness, whereas in the USA barely a third of a day per month was lost. As a result, the proportion of normal earnings lost through sickness was over four times greater in Ghana than in the USA. (This situation is likely to have been made considerably worse in recent years by the emergence of HIV/AIDS in countries such as Ghana.)

A growing body of research confirms this link between health and the ability of individuals and households to be productive and obtain an income: for example one study of the effect of illness on wages in Côte d'Ivoire and Ghana in the early 1990s found that each day of illness or disability significantly reduced the earnings of the individual affected and so compounded their poverty. Conversely, an experiment in Indonesia demonstrated that men with anaemia, who previously had been 20 per cent less productive than men without anaemia, increased their

[5] GNP = Gross National Product, a measure of the total economic output of a country. We discuss GNP further in Chapter 7 when comparing the 'wealth' of different countries and the proportion of GNP spent on health.

productivity almost to the level of non-anaemic men when treated with a low-cost iron supplement. One message from such studies is that good health is important in its own right, but is also an investment in economic development.

3.2.4   Disability-adjusted life years

Another instrument developed in the 1990s by scientists at Harvard University and WHO to capture both morbidity and mortality in a single measure is the **Disability-Adjusted Life Year** or **DALY**. DALYs seek to combine years of life lost from premature death (that is, the difference between actual age at death and life-expectancy at that age in a low-mortality population) with loss of healthy life resulting from disability. For example, if a 20-year-old woman in a low-income country develops meningitis which leaves her permanently deaf, and she subsequently dies at the age of 35, the burden of disease in terms of disability-adjusted life years would be the loss of healthy life for the 15 years during which she had these disabilities, plus the life-expectancy that a female aged 35 in a low-mortality country might expect — around 48 more years. The DALY approach attaches a weight to different disability states, so that, for example, one year in a state of deafness is equivalent to 40 per cent less than a year in full health. Therefore in this simplified example 15 years of deafness would equate to a loss of $(15 \times 0.4) = 6$ years, and premature mortality would equate to a loss of 48 years, giving a total loss of approximately 54 DALYs. So, DALYs express years of life lost to premature death *and* years lived with a disability, so that each DALY is equivalent to one lost year of healthy life.

Some other adjustments are made when calculating DALYs that have proved controversial. First, future events are *discounted*, or given less weight than present events, so that a life lost in 30 years' time is accorded less importance than a life lost this year. Second, weights are also attached to different age groups, so that a year without sight in old age is accorded less importance than a year without sight for a young adult. Debate on these and other aspects of DALYs has ranged across ethical, methodological and empirical issues, and meanwhile the measure is still evolving. However, the results generated by the DALY approach do highlight some features of the global burden of disease and disability that other measures fail to capture. Table 3.3 shows the global burden of disease measured in terms of DALYs, with corresponding information on the proportional distribution of deaths.

Table 3.3   The global burden of disease measured in terms of disability-adjusted life years (DALYs), 1998.

Disease groups	All the world		Developing world		Developed world	
	% of DALYs	% of deaths	% of DALYs	% of deaths	% of DALYs	% of deaths
communicable diseases, maternal and perinatal conditions, nutritional deficiencies (combined)	40.9	30.5	43.8	34.7	7.2	6.3
all non-communicable conditions	43.1	58.8	39.8	53.8	81.0	87.4
e.g. malignant neoplasms (cancers)	*5.8*	13.4	5.1	11.3	15.0	25.1
neuropsychiatric disorders	*11.5*	1.3	10.5	1.1	23.5	2.8
cardiovascular diseases	*10.3*	30.9	9.7	28.5	18.0	44.7
injuries	16.0	10.7	16.4	11.5	11.8	6.2

Data from World Health Organisation (1999) *World Health Report 1999: Making a Difference*, Annex, Table 3.

⬤ What patterns emerge from Table 3.3 when you compare the distribution of DALYs between various causes with the distribution of deaths? Look first at conditions which have a greater impact on DALYs than on deaths, and then at conditions which have the opposite effect.

◼ In all parts of the world, communicable diseases (with maternal, perinatal and nutritional problems) impose a higher proportional burden when measured in DALYs than in deaths, and so do injuries. The neuropsychiatric disorders (including depression, psychoses, and dementia) become *much* more prominent when measured in DALYs than in deaths. Clearly, time lived with disabilities arising from these neuropsychiatric disorders is a major disease burden that has previously been under-recognised. Conversely, cancers and cardiovascular diseases have a lower impact on DALYS than on deaths, suggesting that they tend to involve a shorter period of disabling illness but are more often fatal, particularly in developed countries.

More generally, the DALY approach indicates that:

• lower respiratory infections and diarrhoeal diseases (both are communicable diseases) are the top two causes globally of DALYs;

• that children under 15 account for almost one-half of all DALYs globally;

• and that the burden of disease and disability measured in terms of DALYs lost per 1 000 population, is almost five times more in Sub-Saharan Africa than in the more developed countries.

In summary, therefore, communicable diseases are the biggest killers and the biggest causes of morbidity and disability in low-income countries, but the many exotic-sounding 'tropical' diseases do not top the list. In the next section we consider why it is that infectious organisms have such a big impact, by considering some of the main influences on mortality and morbidity in developing countries.

3.3 Influences on mortality and morbidity within developing countries

The occurrence of disease and disability is part of a complex interaction between humans and their social and physical environment. Health is not possible without various prerequisites, such as safe water and sanitation, and at least a basic minimum of nutrition. Human biology exerts its influence in various ways such as via genetic inheritance, which may confer a measure of resistance or susceptibility to a specific disease. Different diseases and disabilities predominate in different environmental conditions, which include variations in climate, in the prevalence of certain animals and insects, in levels and types of pollution, and in circumstances in the workplace and home. Mass events such as natural disasters or warfare create displaced populations and welfare camps where diseases can thrive, in addition to the immediate deaths and injuries (as Table 3.1 showed, violence and war are leading causes of death in the developing countries). Health care, ranging from immunisation programmes to curative interventions, can affect different aspects of health. In addition, human behaviour and lifestyle, such as drug abuse or smoking, create their own health consequences, as does education via its influence on behaviour and lifestyle. The relationships between these factors are complex; as one set of factors diminishes in importance, others become more pressing.

Here, we will be concerned primarily with environmental factors such as climate, ecological zones, place of residence, and sanitation and clean water; demographic factors such as sex and gender, and intervals between births; and a broad group of social and economic factors, including education and social class.[6]

3.3.1 Environment and health

As is emphasised elsewhere in this chapter, developing countries are a very heterogeneous group and this is particularly clear with respect to patterns of disease. Even within the same continent or country, the disease patterns may be very different from one region to another, and this variation is related in part to differences in the natural environment.

The natural environment of a locality can influence human health in a number of ways. First, the chemical make-up of the soil can affect humans through drinking water and food. For example, in mountainous areas such as the Pyrenees, Himalayas and Andes, where iodine has been leached from the soil, the iodine-deficiency disease of goitre has been found to be endemic. Similarly, an absence of fluorine in drinking water can be reflected in high rates of dental caries, whereas an excess of fluorine — as found, for example, in parts of Uttar Pradesh in India — has been associated with severe skeletal abnormalities.

Second, various aspects of climate such as humidity, temperature and exposure to sunlight can have direct effects on human health. For instance, insufficient sunlight may contribute to diseases associated with a deficiency of vitamin D (e.g. rickets), whereas excessive sunlight may increase skin cancers.

Next, the physical and climatic conditions together exert a powerful influence over the micro-organisms, plants, and animals and insects that are able to exist in a local environment, and these in turn can have a major impact on human health. A wide range of diseases can be transmitted to humans by organisms that thrive in water contaminated by human faeces; these diarrhoeal diseases include typhoid, dysentery, cholera and gastroenteritis. Another group of diseases, called zoonoses (or **zoonotic diseases**), are diseases which are shared by humans and other species and can be transmitted to humans from the disease reservoir in these species. Almost two hundred such diseases have been identified, including brucellosis, rabies, plague, tuberculosis, gastroenteritis and typhus. Some of these diseases can be transmitted directly: for example, rabies by a dog bite. Others are transmitted by some intermediary insect or animal, called a **disease vector**. For example, yellow fever is found in monkeys and rodents, but is transmitted to humans by certain kinds of mosquito: it is therefore a **vector-borne disease**.

All living things require certain environmental conditions in order to survive, and so all the organisms and zoonotic and vector-borne diseases mentioned above have particular geographic distributions. If the combination of physical and climatic environment is not favourable to the species that harbour a zoonotic disease, or to the disease organism itself, that locality will pose less of a disease threat to humans. Thus people living at low altitude in areas of high relative humidity may be exposed to diseases transmitted by mosquitoes, whereas those at higher altitudes or in areas of low humidity escape because mosquitoes cannot exist there.

---

[6] An account of the genetic and other biological influences on health and disease is given in *Human Biology and Health: An Evolutionary Approach,* (Open University Press, 2nd edn 1994; 3rd edn 2001). The impact of health care on health is fully covered in *Caring for Health: History and Diversity* (Open University Press, 2nd edn 1993; 3rd edn 2001).

Low-income countries are mostly located in tropical areas whose warmth and humidity do promote the transmission of water-borne and air-borne infectious diseases. However, it would be misleading to explain many of the current differences in mortality and morbidity between more developed and developing countries simply in terms of physical or climatic conditions. Many of the water-borne diseases that cause deaths from diarrhoea in developing countries are not due exclusively to 'tropical' environmental conditions, and were prevalent in countries such as the United Kingdom until the late nineteenth century, as you will see in Chapter 6. Similarly, the respiratory diseases that kill in the developing countries — including pneumonia, bronchitis, whooping cough, influenza, measles, tuberculosis and diphtheria — can and do occur in industrialised countries. Other diseases such as malaria and cholera have all in the past been prevalent in Europe and North America. So, environment is an important factor in human health, but mainly in combination with other factors. This can be illustrated by the examples of malaria and sickle-cell disease.

3.3.2 Malaria — the influence of environment

An example of how the distribution of a disease is affected by a whole range of environmental factors is malaria, which is transmitted by certain kinds of mosquitoes, which in turn require particular conditions for their survival. As you saw earlier, it is responsible for around 1.1 million deaths each year and 300–500 million clinical episodes.

Malaria is caused by a single-celled parasite, of which there are four species with different patterns of geographic distribution and severity of symptoms. They all invade red blood cells, causing distortion and malfunction of the cell, anaemia, damage to organs in which large numbers of infected red blood cells accumulate, and the fevers, nausea, headache and muscle pain associated with the immune response to persistently high levels of infection. The most fatal species, (Latin name, *Plasmodium falciparum*) has a tendency to accumulate in the brain, eventually causing coma and death, but kidney failure and water in the lungs are other common complications. The parasites are usually transmitted from person to person by a certain species of mosquito (*Anopheles*). In the 1950s and 1960s, mosquito eradication programmes were given priority by the World Health Organisation and malaria was driven out of Europe, North America and parts of Asia. But it remains endemic in the poorer tropical countries and numbers of cases have risen steadily since the early 1970s.

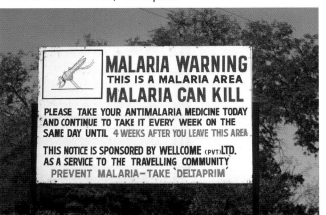

Figure 3.2 (overleaf) shows the complex life cycle of the malarial parasite, involving passage between humans and mosquitoes. Among the factors contributing to the transmission of malaria are: the behaviour, species and biology of the mosquito; environmental conditions such as ground water or the design of houses; the temperature and humidity of the climate; and the degree of human immunity including the presence of high-risk groups such as recent immigrants or refugees with no immunity.

Warning sign on the edge of a forest in Zimbabwe, emphasising threats from mosquitoes as the disease vectors of malaria, and advertising preventative drugs manufactured by the company sponsoring the sign. (Photo: David Read/Panos Pictures)

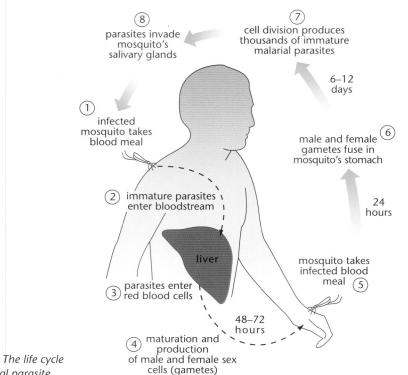

Figure 3.2 *The life cycle of the malarial parasite.*

Although malaria used to be endemic to the United States and Europe, it never presented the health problems there that it does in Africa, Asia and South America because of less favourable environmental conditions for the transmission of the parasite. Moreover, in many of the malarial regions, changing environmental circumstances have encouraged the spread of the disease. Indiscriminate and inefficient use of antimalarial drugs and insecticides has created resistant strains of mosquito; population movements caused by civil wars or growth of human numbers have propelled non-immune people into infected areas and infected people to malaria-free areas; and the spread of irrigation, deforestation and building activity has created many more breeding sites.

●   What effect do you predict global warming could have on the distribution of malaria?

■   Global warming is increasing the risk of disease by expanding the breeding range of mosquitoes. The disease has now spread to highland areas of Africa, for example.

Many other areas of the world have experienced dramatic increases in the incidence of malaria during extreme weather events correlated with climatic changes, including Bolivia, Columbia, Ecuador, Peru and Venezuela in South America, Rwanda in Africa, and Pakistan and Sri Lanka in Asia. Finally, increasing numbers of international travellers have created the phenomenon of 'airport malaria', where air travellers import the disease from affected areas. In 1997, for example, 2 364 cases of malaria were registered in the United Kingdom, all of them imported by travellers. As a result of these factors, attempts to break the mosquito's life cycle in Africa have been undermined and signs of success in the 1970s and 1980s have since been reversed.

3.3.3 Sickle-cell disease: genes and environment

To illustrate further how difficult it is to attribute disease to any single factor, let us now consider the example of **sickle-cell disease**, which is an important cause of years of life lost in parts of Sub-Saharan Africa. Sickle-cell disease is a group of genetically determined conditions (inherited rather than acquired from the environment) in which there is an abnormality in the structure of haemoglobin (the oxygen-carrying molecule in red blood cells). This distorts the cell and makes it fragile and liable to collapse (Figure 3.3). When large numbers of red blood cells collapse, in 'sickle-cell crises', huge numbers of damaged red blood cells accumulate in small blood vessels, blocking them and potentially obstructing vital organs and causing chronic pain. The crisis can subside as new red blood cells replace the collapsing ones, but it can also prove fatal.

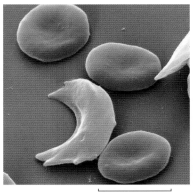

8μm

Figure 3.3 *Normal red blood cells have a regular disc shape and are easily distinguished from the elongated and irregular sickle cells, which characterise sickle-cell disease. (Photo: Eye of Science/Science Photo Library)*

About 1 in 400 Africans and people of African descent inherit two sickle-cell genes (one from each parent) and are affected by sickle-cell disease. However, about 1 in 10 carry only one sickle-cell gene; these people are said to carry the **sickle-cell trait**. The single defective gene can only be detected by special blood tests and rarely causes any ill effects. An interesting feature of this trait is that it confers a degree of resistance to malaria, perhaps because the slightly altered haemoglobin in affected people makes their red blood cells less susceptible to infection by malarial parasites. It has been assumed that the high prevalence of sickle-cell disease in African populations has come about because those with the single defective gene (trait) have a survival advantage in terms of resistance to malaria, compared with people with two 'normal' genes. At the population level, this more than compensates for the increased risk of death among those with the two defective genes (sickle-cell disease). Thus environment and genetic inheritance may both be important factors in its distribution.

3.3.4 Water and sanitation

Earlier in this chapter, it was noted that a wide range of diseases can be transmitted to humans by organisms that thrive in water contaminated by human faeces. Diarrhoeal diseases, for example, spread by both bacteria and viruses through contaminated food and water, are one of the biggest health problems in the contemporary world. The importance of water supplies and sanitation on disease patterns can be illustrated by the example of **schistosomiasis** (also known as bilharzia), common in many tropical countries. It is a disease caused by a tiny worm (*Schistosoma*) that invades many organs in the body and produces huge numbers of eggs (about 5 million per female worm). The eggs and immature larval stages of the developing worms are particularly damaging as they accumulate in tissues and blood vessels.

Schistosomiasis is a particularly striking example of the need to consider morbidity data as well as mortality. In 1998, approximately 7 000 deaths were recorded world-wide as being caused by schistosomiasis, although at least 20 000 deaths annually are estimated to be directly associated with the disease, mostly due to bladder cancer or kidney failure associated with larval infestation. However, it is estimated that in 1998 more than 200 million people in rural agricultural and semi-urban areas of the 74 developing countries where the disease is endemic were infested with *Schistosoma*. Of these, 20 million suffer severe consequences from the disease and 120 million experience some symptoms. Consequently, it is estimated that in

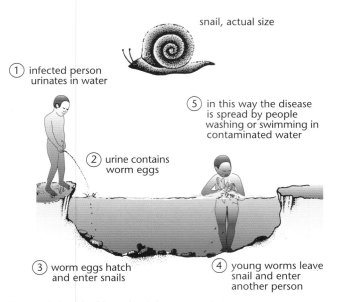

snail, actual size

① infected person urinates in water

⑤ in this way the disease is spread by people washing or swimming in contaminated water

② urine contains worm eggs

③ worm eggs hatch and enter snails

④ young worms leave snail and enter another person

Figure 3.4 *The life cycle of the worms that cause schistosomiasis (also known as bilharzia).*

1998 approximately 1.7 million DALYs were attributable to schistosomiasis, a figure approximately equivalent to the global burden from prostate cancer or ovarian cancer.

The parasite is transmitted from person to person when the eggs are excreted in the urine or faeces, but first it must pass through an 'intermediate host' — in this instance certain kinds of snails — in which parasites develop and emerge in a form that can reinfect people. Thus there must be faecal or urinary contamination of the water in which people bathe or work (for example on irrigated land), and that water must also contain certain kinds of snail. This cycle is illustrated in Figure 3.4. If the snails are not present, or if the water ceases to be contaminated, or if people stop bathing or working in contaminated water, then schistosomiasis cannot persist. Thus the disease is confined to areas in which all elements exist for the life cycle of the parasites to continue. This is true not only of schistosomiasis and malaria, but also of other parasitic diseases. For example, Chagas disease, a serious parasitic infestation which often involves damage to the muscles of the heart, is confined to South America; sleeping sickness, transmitted by the tsetse fly, does not occur outside Africa.

The impact of the lack of adequate sanitation and clean water can also be seen in the high prevalence of parasitic worm infestations, many of which are water-borne. At least a hundred different species of worm can produce disease in humans and it is estimated that about a billion people are infested with these adaptable parasites. They range from the largest tapeworm, over two metres in length, to worms such as the *Schistosoma* species, which are barely visible to the naked eye. Other types of worm that cause significant morbidity in developing countries include the filarial worms, which cause fevers, elephantiasis and river blindness; the hookworms, which suck blood from the gut and cause anaemia and loss of protein; the ascarid worms, which interfere with digestion and stunt the growth of millions of children in developing countries; and the guinea worms, which erupt from the skin through disabling and painful swellings, usually on the legs and feet. Studies in Sri Lanka, Bangladesh and Venezuela have found that over 90 per cent of six-year-old children were infested with intestinal parasitic worms, the commonest being hookworm and ascarid worms, which together account for about 12 000 deaths and 4 million DALYs each year.

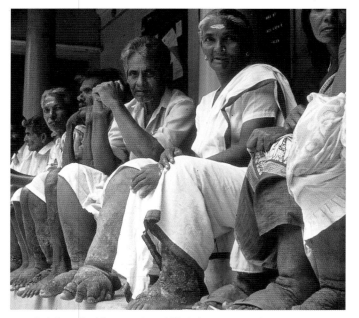

People infested with a species of filarial worm wait for treatment at a clinic near Pondicherry, India. The infestation has caused severe tissue damage in the legs, the appearance of which provides the name 'elephantiasis'. (Photo: R. Umesh Chandra/TDR, WHO/Science Photo Library)

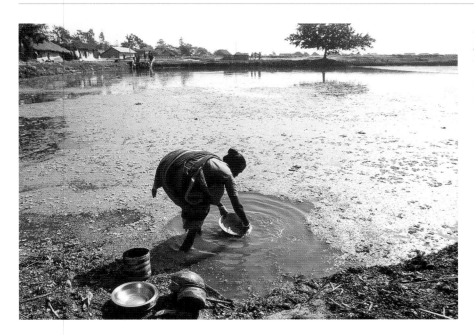

Around 25 per cent of the population of many Asian and African countries do not have access to a safe water supply, as in this village in rural Bangladesh. (Photo: Kim Naylor/Christian Aid/Still Pictures)

In developing countries, the prevalence of mortality and morbidity associated with water-borne diseases, clearly indicates that many people do not have access to safe drinking water or satisfactory sanitation. The United Nations Development Programme has estimated that, by 1995, around 25 per cent of the population of low and middle income countries did not have access to safe water supplies, and approximately 45 per cent were without some form of sanitation.

Resources that did go into improving water supplies and sanitation barely kept pace with growing populations during the 1990s, and in some countries the situation deteriorated. In Brazil, for example, the proportion of the population with access to safe water actually fell from 75 per cent in 1982 to 69 per cent by 1995. One serious consequence has been the resurgence during the 1990s of cholera, which is spread by contact with food or water contaminated with human waste containing cholera bacteria. Between 1991 and 1995 over 1 million people were contaminated and 11 000 died in South America, from where it had disappeared almost a century earlier. Poor water treatment, unhygienic food preparation, irrigation with waste water, and possibly environmental changes such as global warming affecting sea temperatures, have all been implicated.

Safe drinking water and proper sanitation, therefore, are prerequisites for good health, but they are very far from being universally available and it will be a major challenge to expand access to them.

3.3.5 Place of residence

Yet another environmental influence on patterns of mortality and morbidity is **place of residence**. Urban and rural dwellers may be exposed to quite different risks: for example, as you saw above, people in towns generally have more access to safe water and adequate sanitation. Though few developing countries publish mortality data classified by place of residence, some data are available on mortality rates for urban and for rural areas. Table 3.4 (overleaf) gives data for a sample of countries.

● Although Table 3.4 shows that mortality rates are higher in rural populations, can you think of any reasons why these data should be interpreted cautiously?

Table 3.4 Mortality rates classified by rural and urban residence for selected countries, 1997 or nearest date.

Country	Infant mortality rate (per 1 000 live births)		Crude death rate (per 1 000 population per year)	
	Rural	Urban	Rural	Urban
Chile	16	11	6	5.4
Cuba	9.8	8.3	5.1	7.8
India	80	52	10.1	6.7
Japan	4	3.7	9.1	6.8
Russian Federation	19.9	17.4	16.2	14.4

Data from United Nations (1999a) *United Nations Demographic Yearbook 1997*, UN, New York, Tables 15 and 18.

■   There are several reasons.

First, definitions of 'rural' and 'urban' vary from place to place. (You might like to think how you would define them. How large would a town have to be before it would be regarded as urban?)

Second, the crude death rates reported in the table may be misleading if there are differences between urban and rural areas in the demographic structures of their populations.

Third, where rates are calculated using a death registration system, registration will often be more complete in urban than in rural areas, so in some instances the rural rates may be artificially low.

Fourth, in some countries rural dwellers may travel to the nearest urban area to seek hospital treatment for their illness. If any die in an urban hospital, their deaths may artificially reduce the death rate for rural areas. (This would depend on whether care is taken to record the place of usual residence on the death register.)

Finally, it might well be that those people migrating from rural to urban areas, or labour migrants taking jobs far from home, perhaps in another country, tend to be the youngest and healthiest members of the rural population, and those staying behind are the least healthy. In this instance, the death rates for urban areas may be held down and those for rural areas pushed up.

Despite these difficulties, Table 3.4 shows a clear advantage for urban over rural dwellers in almost every country, and there are many reasons why this might be expected. People in urban areas generally have advantages that include higher incomes, better educational opportunities and greater access to preventive and curative health services. On the other hand, some features of urban living may lead to increased mortality. Accidents and violence are often more common in urban settlements, and overcrowding may enhance the transmission of communicable diseases. In some countries, people living in the slums or shanty towns of the cities may be in a much worse position than peasant farmers in the countryside. Air pollution from traffic, heating fuel or industry can often be worse: in Chinese cities, which are heavily reliant on coal for energy, lung cancer is between four and seven times higher than the national average. And, finally, 'megacities' are growing in developing countries, of a size far beyond all previous human experience: by the year 2015, Lagos is expected to contain 24 million inhabitants, Mumbai (Bombay) 26 million, and Mexico City and São Paulo 20 million each. The health consequences of such urbanisation can only be guessed, but a look back at Figure 1.1 of this book may indicate some of them.

3.4 Demographic influences on mortality

You have already seen that mortality rates vary dramatically with age. This is one reason why crude death rates can be difficult to interpret. But other factors must also be taken into account in trying to explain the variations in mortality within developing countries, including sex and gender, and family structure. (As Chapter 9 will show, the same factors are also important influences on mortality rates in an industrialised country such as the United Kingdom.) We will look at each of these in turn.

3.4.1 Sex and gender

Health differences between males and females may arise for a variety of reasons, including sex, defined by biological characteristics, and gender, defined by differences in role, status, and other culturally determined characteristics. It is important to keep in mind the distinction between sex and gender as you study the following material, not least because gender differences are much more likely to vary over time and between different countries and cultures than are genuine sex differences.

● Look back again at Table 2.2 in the previous chapter, in which the expectation of life is shown separately for men and women in different countries. Do men or women tend to live longer?

■ The expectation of life at birth is greater for females than for males in 16 out of the 17 countries in the table, and equal in the other (Bangladesh).

● However, the difference between the sexes is not uniform. See if you can find any pattern in the figures shown in Table 2.2.

■ In the industrialised countries, the expectation of life is consistently higher for females by between 5 and 10 years. The differences in developing countries are generally smaller — between 2 and 6 years.

The data from industrialised countries have generally been taken to imply that, given favourable living conditions and health care, women have a sex-specific biological advantage in terms of longevity. If this interpretation is correct, the smaller differences between the sexes in some developing countries suggest that women there are at some special disadvantage. Since there is no reason to suppose that they are biologically different to women elsewhere, we must consider gender-specific cultural explanations. Childbirth is one important factor. In developing countries, women tend to experience more pregnancies than their counterparts in industrialised countries, and the risk associated with each pregnancy is considerably higher. Many of the deaths of females aged 15–49 in developing countries are due to complications of pregnancy. This interpretation also fits the information shown earlier in Table 2.3, which shows expectation of life at various ages in Bangladesh for males and females: the female disadvantage is greatest around the age of 30.

However, in addition to the hazards of childbirth, women may be disadvantaged by their position in society. For example, a number of studies have demonstrated that women in Asia and North Africa receive less health care and medical attention in comparison with men. Similar evidence has been compiled in relation to education, nutrition and other factors that may influence health. Cumulatively, such disadvantages can produce startling consequences. For example, Table 3.5 shows the results of an exercise to estimate how many women were 'missing' in a group of Asian and North African countries.

The first data column in the table shows the *actual ratio* of males to females in each country. It can be seen that in each country there is a substantial excess of men over women, ranging from around 1.05 males per female (or 105 males per 100 females) in Egypt and Nepal up to almost 111 males per 100 females in Pakistan. The table then shows the *expected ratio* if there were no 'excess' female mortality and if a male : female ratio similar to that in Europe, North America and Japan prevailed. The third column then shows the actual number of females. The demographer Ansley Coale used these data (and others) to make the estimates shown in the last two columns: the percentage and number of females in the Asian and North African countries who were 'missing'. Coale concluded that there were almost 60 million 'missing females' in the countries studied at the dates shown in Table 3.5. Other estimates, for example by the economist Amartya Sen (who focused public attention on this issue through a series of articles), have suggested that the number of missing females in these same countries may be in excess of 100 million.

Of course, gender differences in access to health care, education, occupational stress, nutrition and so on, will vary substantially in different societies and cultures. Indeed, there is no evidence of excess female mortality in Sub-Saharan Africa, South-East Asia, or other major regions of the world: areas where women are more likely to have employment outside the home, and therefore may be more independent and less vulnerable to discrimination. This suggests that gender roles in all societies have an important bearing on health patterns, and require closer examination. Later chapters of this book will return to this issue.

Table 3.5   The number of 'missing females' in Asia and North Africa.

Country	Ratio of males to females		Number of females /millions	Estimated percentage of females missing	Estimated number of missing females /millions
	Actual ratio	Expected ratio			
China, 1990	1.066	1.010	548.7	5.3	29.1
India, 1991	1.077	1.020	406.3	5.6	22.8
Pakistan, 1981	1.105	1.025	40.0	7.8	3.1
Bangladesh, 1981	1.064	1.025	42.2	3.8	1.6
Nepal, 1981	1.050	1.025	7.3	2.4	0.2
West Asia, 1985	1.060	1.030	55.0	3.0	1.7
Egypt, 1986	1.047	1.020	23.5	2.6	0.6

Data from Coale, A. J. (1991) Excess female mortality and the balance of the sexes in the population: an estimate of the number of 'missing females', *Population and Development Review*, **17** (3), pp. 514–24, Table 1, p. 522.

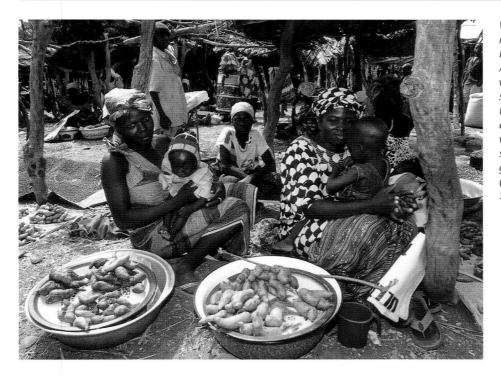

Women running a street market in Burkino Faso, Kalsake village, West Africa. In this region, women dominate market selling and trading, and therefore have some economic autonomy, which may give them some protection from gender discrimination. (Photo: Mark Edwards/ Still Pictures)

3.4.2 Family structure

Family structure is another factor that appears to be associated with childhood mortality, and the spacing of births seems to be particularly important. Figure 3.5 shows the relationship between **birth spacing** and child mortality in four developing countries around 1990. Mortality rates for babies born 24 to 48 months after the previous child are taken as the baseline; the histograms show percentage increases in infant mortality above this level when birth spacing is between 18 and 24 months, or less than 18 months.

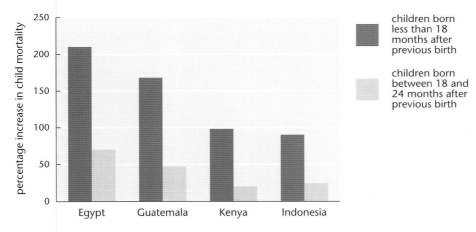

Figure 3.5 *Relationship between birth spacing and child mortality in four countries, 1990 or nearest date: percentage increase in child mortality in relation to children born 24 to 48 months after the previous birth. (Data from: World Bank (1993)* World Development Report 1993: Investing in Health, *Oxford University Press, New York, p. 83)*

● What is the relationship between birth spacing and child mortality in the data from these countries?

■ Short intervals between births are associated with higher child mortality, and the effect is much greater when birth spacing is below 18 months. For example, children in Egypt born less than 18 months after the previous birth had a mortality rate more than 200 per cent greater than the mortality rate in children born at least 24 months after the previous birth.

Short intervals between births can lead to increased infant and childhood mortality for several reasons. First, a rapid succession of pregnancies puts pressure on the mother's health. This can lead to babies with low birthweights, and these are known to be at higher risk of infant death. Second, when the new baby is born, the previous child will no longer be breast-fed, and this may lead to under-nutrition, especially in countries where supplementary foods may be contaminated or inadequate. Third, where there are several young children, the caring resources of the mother are more likely to be stretched. Some researchers have suggested another hypothesis concerning the link between birth spacing and child mortality: that the death of an infant reduces the interval to a subsequent birth. If this is the case — and studies in Senegal and elsewhere provide evidence in support — then it could be inappropriate to aim policies directly at changing the interval between births.

3.5 Socio-economic influences on mortality

A basic difficulty in studying the many socio-economic factors associated with mortality in developing countries — such as education, social class, housing, income and access to health care — is that they may all interact and be hard to disentangle. Here, we focus on three factors in particular: education, ethnicity and economic inequality.

3.5.1 Education

Numerous studies have shown that childhood mortality is associated with the education of the mother and/or father. Table 3.6 shows that childhood mortality is strongly associated with the level of education of the mother: in Morocco, for example, children whose mothers have completed 4–6 years of schooling are 45 per cent less likely to have died by the age of 2 than children whose mothers have received no schooling; when the mother's years of schooling increase to 7 or more, the reduction in the child's risk of dying is even greater: 66 per cent. Research also shows that the father's level of education is similarly related to childhood and infant mortality.

Table 3.6 Percentage reduction in risk of death by the age of two years in relation to mother's years of schooling (compared to no schooling), 1990.

Country	4–6 years of schooling	7 or more years of schooling
Kenya	32	51
Indonesia	36	67
Peru	39	71
Morocco	45	66

Data from: World Bank (1993) *World Development Report 1993: Investing in Health*, Oxford University Press, New York, p. 43.

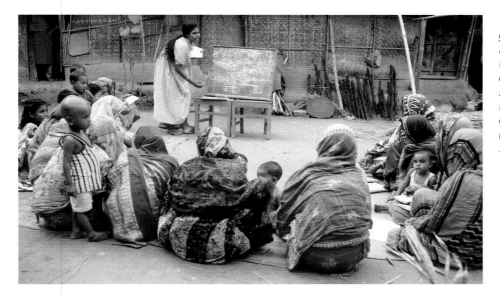

Women's literacy group in Raipur area, Bangladesh. Throughout the developing world, childhood mortality is strongly associated with the level of education of the mother. (Photo: Jorgen Schytte/ Still Pictures)

What factors explain these associations? First, higher levels of parental education are likely to be linked to occupations with higher incomes and hence better social conditions and better access to health care, making it difficult to assess the separate contribution of each of these factors to childhood mortality. Nevertheless, some Latin American studies have shown that the relationship between mortality and parents' education remains strong, even after allowing for the effect of income, suggesting that more education creates a better awareness and use of appropriate health practices.

3.5.2 Ethnicity

The association between ethnicity and health is complex, involving the interaction of social, cultural and economic factors and genetic variation. Where high-quality statistics are available, as in the USA, it is possible to observe quite striking differences in health between different ethnic groups. For example, Figure 3.6 overleaf shows various measures of mortality and life expectancy in the USA in 1997, by ethnicity and by origin of mother. The overall infant mortality rate ('All' in Figure 3.6a) was 7.2 infant deaths per 1 000 births, but black infants died at over twice the rate of white infants. Disorders related to low birthweight were particularly important reasons for this excess mortality. Puerto Rican infants also had a higher rate of infant mortality than the national average, but some other groups, such as infants whose mothers were of Cuban origin, had lower than average infant mortality rates.

● What do Figures 3.6b and c suggest about the effect of ethnicity on health?

■ Similar patterns to those seen for infant mortality are observed in age-standardised death rates, which are substantially higher than average in the black population, but lower than average in some groups such those of Cuban origin. Finally, the black population's life expectancy is significantly lower than in the white population, and the difference is especially marked amongst males.

We would need much more information on causes of death, on factors such as education and income, and on other characteristics of these ethnic groups to explain

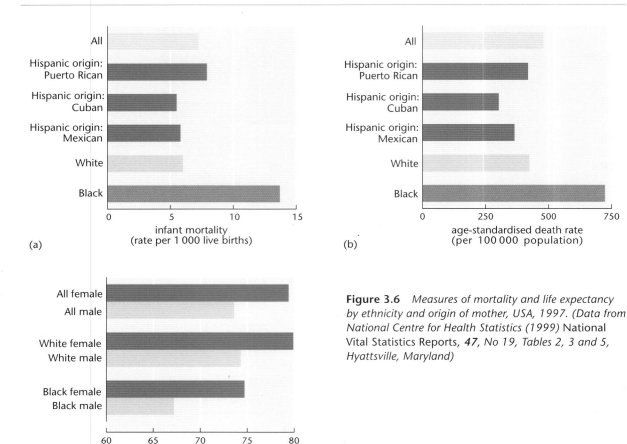

Figure 3.6 *Measures of mortality and life expectancy by ethnicity and origin of mother, USA, 1997. (Data from National Centre for Health Statistics (1999)* National Vital Statistics Reports, *47, No 19, Tables 2, 3 and 5, Hyattsville, Maryland)*

the differences fully. For example, the American population of Cuban origin is generally from a higher social class than the American population of Puerto Rican origin, which partly explains their better health record. But even when factors such as education are taken into account, differences remain: for example, the infant mortality rate is 4.1 for babies with white mothers who have over 16 years of educational attainment, but 10.7 for babies with black mothers with the same level of educational attainment.

Similar patterns of ethnic mortality differences have been found in many other countries, including those in Sub-Saharan Africa. Closer study of these patterns suggests that ethnicity is closely linked to deep-rooted social and economic inequalities, and that these are as marked in poor countries as in high income countries such as the USA.

3.5.3 Economic inequality

Evidence of large health differences within as well as between countries also emerges when we consider the association between economic advantage or disadvantage and health. Table 3.7 shows, for a selection of developing countries, the probability of death between birth and age 5 for those who are categorised as 'non-poor' (that is, who have an income of at least US$1 per day), and then shows how much higher is the probability of death of those who are in absolute poverty (that is, who have an income of less than US$1 per day). Separate figures are given for males and females.

Table 3.7 Health status of the poor *versus* the non-poor in selected countries, around 1990.

| Country | Percentage of the population in absolute poverty | Probability of dying between birth and age 5 (death rate per 1 000 in that age group) | | | |
| | | Males | | Females | |
		non-poor	poor/non-poor ratio	non-poor	poor/non-poor ratio
South Africa	24	47	4.7	31	5.3
Brazil	24	26	6.5	23	5
Chile	15	10	7.1	7	8.3
India	53	33	4.5	40	4.3
China	22	23	5.9	28	6.6

'Absolute poverty' = income less than US$1 per day; 'non-poor' have an income of at least US$1 per day. Data from World Health Organisation (1999) *World Health Report 1999: Making a Difference*, Annex, Table 7.

The table also shows what proportion of the total population in each country is estimated to be in absolute poverty. The data relate to the period around 1990.

The table shows, for example, that 22 per cent of the population of China were estimated to live on an income of less than US$1 per day in 1990. For non-poor females the death rate between birth and the age of 5 was 28 per 1 000, but the death rate amongst females in absolute poverty was 6.6 times higher. A consistent pattern is shown across all the countries in Table 3.7, and for males and females, and similar patterns exist for the probability of dying in older age groups, and for other measures of ill-health. The burden of disease is concentrated in poorer countries, but within these countries it also bears down disproportionately on the poorest sections of the population.

3.6   Prospects for the control of disease

Despite the high mortality rates experienced in developing countries, there have been improvements in health and further improvement is expected, as you saw in Chapter 2. Around one-half of the fall in mortality rates that has occurred over the last few decades has been due to a decline in the number of deaths from malaria, smallpox, tuberculosis and measles (although declines have not been sustained in all these diseases, as you have seen). A further one-third of the fall in mortality in developing countries since 1930 is thought to have resulted from a decline in deaths from the respiratory diseases — influenza, pneumonia, and bronchitis. But a smaller fall was due to a reduction in deaths from diarrhoeal diseases; in other words, one of the commonest causes of illness and death in developing countries remains one of the most intractable.

The decline in deaths from **smallpox** was the consequence of a campaign led by the WHO, which succeeded in eradicating this disease globally. This campaign is described in an article in *Health and Disease: A Reader* (Open University Press, 2nd edn 1994; 3rd edn 2001) by Marc Strassburg entitled, 'The global eradication of smallpox'. (Open University students should read this now.)

● It took almost 200 years from the discovery of an effective vaccine to the eradication of smallpox. What reasons does Strassburg offer for this long delay?

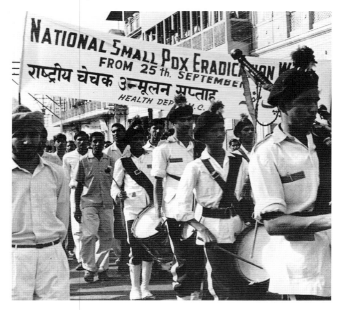

A parade in New Delhi, India, in the 1960s, urges people to get smallpox vaccination. (Source: Popperfoto)

■ First, to be usable in hot climates, the vaccine had to be heat-stable: this was not achieved until the 1950s. Second, the design of needles used in vaccination was greatly improved in the 1960s. Finally, many developing countries had too few resources to run effective vaccination campaigns without assistance.

The WHO campaign began in 1967, at which point it was estimated that there were around 10 million cases of smallpox concentrated in 30 countries. Using an eradication strategy based on surveillance and containment rather than relying solely on mass vaccination, the disease was gradually eliminated from country after country, until the last naturally occurring case was diagnosed in Somalia in 1977.

● In what ways did the natural history of smallpox facilitate this eradication strategy?

■ Smallpox spread fairly slowly, tended to cluster, and had no animal reservoir other than humans; there was no carrier state in which humans could pass on the disease without displaying symptoms; and vaccination conferred long-lasting immunity. Thus case-finding, source-tracing and containment were effective.

● What does Strassburg conclude about the likelihood of eradicating other infectious diseases, and why?

■ That many other major infectious diseases would be much more difficult to eradicate, either because not enough is known of their natural history, or because they are zoonotic diseases and the reservoirs of infection are difficult to control, or because the costs of eradication would be so high. However, measles shares certain characteristics with smallpox and might be susceptible to a similar eradication campaign.

There have been attempts to eradicate a number of other diseases prevalent in developing countries, including hookworm, yellow fever and malaria. The most successful campaign concerned poliomyelitis, which is scheduled to be eradicated by 2005. However, it was partly a disillusionment with the eradication approach that led the WHO in 1978 to turn to a much broader strategy of comprehensive primary health care, including

> ... education concerning prevailing health problems and the methods of preventing and controlling them; promotion of food supply and proper nutrition; an adequate supply of safe water and basic sanitation; maternal and child health care, including family planning; immunisation against the major infectious diseases; prevention and control of locally endemic diseases; appropriate treatment of common diseases and injuries; and provision of essential drugs. (The Declaration of Alma Ata, World Health Organisation, 1978)

This WHO strategy of 'Health for All by the Year 2000' had a strong influence on health policies in the latter decades of the twentieth century.[7] However, it clearly failed to achieve its ambitious goal. One line of argument is that it was too diffuse, too ambitious and too costly to succeed, that all health problems cannot be tackled at the same time, and that a better strategy would be to set realistic and attainable priorities based on the morbidity and mortality caused by particular diseases, and the feasibility and cost of controlling them.

During the 1980s, this more targeted approach led to a massive effort by a group of international agencies to immunise children against a group of vaccine-preventable diseases including tuberculosis, diphtheria, polio, tetanus, whooping cough and measles. This initiative did succeed in increasing the proportion of the world's children who were immunised from around 20 per cent in 1984 to around 75 per cent by 1990; by 1997, 88 per cent of all one-year-olds in developing countries were immunised against tuberculosis, and 79 per cent were immunised against measles. However, by the late 1990s there was evidence that immunisation rates seemed to have peaked at around 80 per cent , with around 2 million children each year still dying from vaccine-preventable diseases. In response, an international alliance of charities, governments, the leading vaccine manufacturing pharmaceutical companies and international agencies announced in 1999 the formation of the **Global Alliance for Vaccines and Immunisations (GAVI)**. With financial support mainly from the Bill and Belinda Gates Foundation, GAVI offered the hope of increasing access to vaccines. It also stated an intention to invest in research and development for new vaccines, particularly for malaria, tuberculosis and AIDS.

Also during the 1990s, the World Bank and others promoted the concept of an essential national package of health services, based on the measured burden of diseases and the cost-effectiveness of interventions available to deal with them. For example, in all developing countries around 70 per cent of childhood deaths and a higher proportion of DALYs are attributable to just five diseases: diarrhoea, pneumonia, measles, malaria and malnutrition. One way of controlling them is by an approach called the **Integrated Management of the Sick Child**, in which children seeking health care are assessed for specified signs and symptoms, and then referred, treated or given advice according to guidelines. It is estimated that this would cost around US$9 per recipient and about $30 to $50 for every DALY saved. By comparison, the expanded programme of immunization is known to control diseases that account for about 10 per cent of all DALYs lost, and costs around $15 per recipient and $12 to $20 for every DALY saved.

By assembling comparative information in this way, an essential package of health interventions can be identified, with the objective of obtaining maximum health improvement with the available resources. Table 3.8 overleaf gives more detail about this kind of approach, and shows that such a package of health services could cost as little as $12 per head of population per year. However, even this expenditure would exceed the amount spent on health services in some of the world's poorest countries.

Another approach to the health problems of developing countries is to argue that the root cause of infectious disease is poverty, which manifests itself in unsatisfactory water supplies and sanitation, insufficient food, poor education and inadequate health care. From this perspective, the industrialised world has largely rid itself of

[7] Strategies adopted by the 'Health for All by the Year 2000' programme are discussed in more detail in *Caring for Health: History and Diversity* (Open University Press, 2nd edn 1993; 3rd edn 2001), Chapter 8.

Table 3.8 Annual cost of an essential minimum package of health services in a low-income country.

Intervention	Cost per beneficiary (US$)	Cost per capita (US$)	Cost per DALY (US$)
public health services:			
expanded programme of immunization	14.6	0.5	12–17
school health programme	3.6	0.3	20–25
tobacco and alcohol control programme	0.3	0.3	35–55
AIDS prevention programme	112.2	1.7	3–5
other public health interventions	2.4	1.4	
sub-total		*$4.2*	
clinical services:			
chemotherapy against tuberculosis	500.0	0.6	3–5
integrated management of the sick child	9.0	1.6	30–50
family planning	12.0	0.9	20–30
sexually transmitted diseases treatment	11.0	0.2	1–3
prenatal and delivery care	90.0	3.8	30–50
limited acute care services	6.0	0.7	200–300
sub-total		*$7.8*	
total cost		**$12**	

Source: Bobadilla, J. L., Cowley, P., Musgrove, P. and Saxienian, H. (1994) Design, content and financing of an essential national package of health services, Table 2, p. 175, in Murray, C. J. L. and Lopez, A. D. (eds) *Global comparative assessments in the health sector: Disease burden, expenditures and intervention packages*, WHO, Geneva.

infectious diseases through social and economic development. Consequently, some have argued that the over-riding priority in developing countries is to follow the same path and industrialise. However, the precise ways in which the infectious diseases receded in the industrialised world, the extent to which the present developing countries can learn from this historical experience, and indeed the implications of global industrialisation for the future health of humanity, are all fiercely contested questions to which much of the remainder of this book is devoted. Before turning to some of these issues, the next chapter concludes this initial survey of world health and disease with a case study in which we aim to give you some sense of the experience of health and disease in a developing country, not at the level of national or regional statistics, but at that of individuals and localities.

OBJECTIVES FOR CHAPTER 3

When you have studied this chapter, you should be able to:

3.1 Define and use, or recognise definitions and applications of, each of the terms printed in **bold** in the text.

3.2 Compare the important causes of death in developing and developed countries.

3.3 Describe the uses and advantages of the 'years of potential life lost' calculation and the 'disability-adjusted life year' calculation as ways of comparing the relative importance of different causes of disease or disability.

3.4 Discuss the links between morbidity and the economy in developing countries.

3.5 Set out the main ways in which environment may influence health, using examples of specific diseases to illustrate the interaction between factors.

3.6 Describe how mortality rates in developing countries differ between males and females, between different ethnic groups, and in relation to economic inequality, and offer possible explanations for these patterns.

3.7 Discuss methods of deciding which health services to provide in low-income countries.

QUESTIONS FOR CHAPTER 3

1   (*Objective 3.2*)

To what extent are the patterns of mortality in developing countries a result of diseases peculiar to these countries?

2   (*Objective 3.3*)

Given what has been said about causes of death in developing and industrialised countries, why might the 'years of potential life lost' or 'disability-adjusted life years' measures be good ways of emphasising differences in mortality patterns in these two regions?

3   (*Objective 3.4*)

What arguments might be used to persuade the Finance Ministry of a developing country to increase investment in health care?

4   (*Objective 3.5*)

Explain, giving examples, what is meant by zoonotic diseases and why they may be difficult to control.

5   (*Objective 3.6*)

Making use of material from this and the previous chapter, answer the following:

(a) What is the gender difference in expectation of life at birth in Bangladesh and in the United Kingdom?

(b) Does the advantage in terms of life expectancy of one sex over the other persist in both countries?

(c) What is one consequence of these gender differences in Bangladesh on the country's population structure?

6   (*Objective 3.7*)

During a discussion of what to include in a minimum package of health services in a very low income country, it is suggested that AIDS prevention should be left out because it costs $112 per person receiving care, whereas some acute services should be included as they only cost $6 per person who would benefit. What approach would you recommend in order to decide what to include?

CHAPTER 4

Livelihood and survival: a case study of Bangladesh

Study notes for OU students

This chapter is written in a rather different style to any other in the book. It illustrates the 'case study' approach to investigating health and disease by focusing on a single developing country — Bangladesh. It refers back to data on Bangladesh, which you have already studied in Chapters 2 and 3.

Case studies are essentially multi-disciplinary in character. As you will see, the Bangladesh case study draws on research methods from across the range you have already learnt about in *Studying Health and Disease* (second edition 1994; colour-enhanced second edition 2001; Open University Press).

4.1   Introduction: 'A Quiet Violence'

We saw why early travellers to the region spoke of its fertility in glowing terms. From the windows of buses and the decks of ferry boats, we looked over a lush green landscape. Rice paddies carpeted the earth and gigantic squash vines climbed over the roofs of the village houses. The rich alluvial soil, the plentiful water and the hot humid climate made us feel as if we had entered a natural greenhouse. In autumn, as the ripening rice turned gold, we understood why in song and verse the Bengalis call their land 'sonar bangla', 'golden Bengal' ... As we travelled through the countryside, trying at once to comprehend the lush beauty of the land and the destitution of so many people, we sensed that we had entered a strange battleground. All around us, beneath the surface calm, silent struggles were being waged, struggles in which the losers met slow bloodless deaths. We began to learn about the quiet violence which rages in Bangladesh, a violence of which the famine victims were only the most visible casualties. (Hartmann and Boyce, 1983, pp. 11 and 17)

This is how the anthropologists Betsy Hartmann and James Boyce, in their book *A Quiet Violence*, tell of their first impressions of rural Bangladesh (Figure 4.1). We have reproduced this quotation here to set the scene for a different way of looking at and understanding how illness and the threat of hunger still dominate and shape the lives of many people living today. Up to this point, we have been making broad general comparisons between the populations of industrialised and developing countries. For the most part, these have used *quantitative* measures, such as the rates at which disease or death strike in a population and the numbers and ages of those affected. Now we shall develop a **case study** approach to health and disease by looking in more depth at the lives of people living in a specific developing country — Bangladesh.

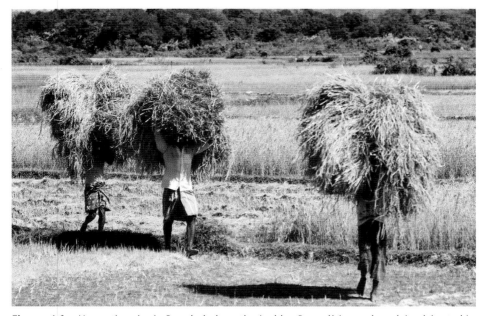

Figure 4.1   *Harvesting rice in Bangladesh — the 'golden Bengal' (sonar bangla) celebrated in songs and verses. (Photo: Jorgen Schytte/ Still Pictures)*

4.2   The general scene and the particular case

Case studies combine two methods of gathering information: they build on numerical data to describe the average levels of health and disease and the social and economic conditions of the population as a whole, and they make use of descriptive accounts — or **narrative profiles** — obtained quite literally by asking people to tell the stories of their lives. In this chapter we shall show how a narrative profile of the life of a single Bangladeshi family can typify the conditions of people living in that predominantly rural country.

We begin with a discussion of the advantages of using case studies that include narrative profiles of this kind and also some of the dangers. We may know from objectively verifiable sources, such as records of hospital admissions, or land sales, that people frequently suffer from a particular infectious disease, that children die of malnutrition, or that small farming families often have to sell up. We may also know in general terms *why* this is so: specific organisms cause the diseases; people live in poverty; sometimes the food supply collapses. But that is not the whole story — case studies can fill in some of the blanks.

- What do you think is the main advantage of case studies as a method of researching health problems?

- ■ The great strength of the case study approach is that it allows us to gain insights into the *processes* by which people's health or even their lives are threatened, and how these processes are influenced by the circumstances of their everyday lives.

For example, a case study approach can help us to explain why certain diseases occur so often in a particular location, or in people dependent on a particular means of livelihood. It may reveal common sequences of events that culminate in the break-up of a family following the death of a productive member. It might identify what the people in villages of type 'A' do for each other to sustain themselves through famines, while the poorest members of villages of type 'B' die.

4.2.1   How do we know what is typical?

Potentially offsetting the advantages of the case study approach is the temptation to draw general conclusions on the basis of too few examples about what kinds of processes usually take place. There is a danger of relying perhaps on a single case, which might later turn out either to be unique (i.e. to be the only member of a class of one), or not be sufficiently typical to justify drawing general conclusions about the nature of the causal processes involved. Clearly, it is important to develop a case study that may be partly historical and partly situational, combining descriptive information from narrative profiles with statistical sources of data so that one illuminates the other.

The systematic approach to developing a case study starts from an investigation of the *general* situation, then focuses down on a *particular* group, individual or situation as a source of ideas about what processes are taking place, and goes back again to the general picture to see if those ideas are consistent with it. If so, the number of specific cases can be extended and their content broadened and so on, in a repeating cycle: the general to the particular to the general. Case studies, therefore, use descriptive, qualitative data to enrich and inform the available quantitative data, which in turn suggests new areas on which to focus further investigation.

The use of descriptive material raises another problem. Suppose we were just interested in getting reliable quantitative measurements of average income, or family size. Statisticians have rules that can be used to estimate the smallest number of cases from which to calculate an average, which could then be extrapolated to the larger population at a given degree of accuracy. If our purpose however, is not just to derive quantitative estimates of some variable, but to use qualitative information to gain insights into *processes,* then it is impossible to apply these conventional statistical rules. There are no mathematical guidelines that will help us to decide how many similar case studies have to be collected and how these should be combined with statistical data, in order to be confident that a 'typical' pattern has been established. This means that if they are to be valid, case studies must be the result of the exercise of judgement. Furthermore, that judgement must be formed not only from a knowledge of the statistical data, but by a combination of the information contained in both observation and measurement. In general, this task requires the qualitative descriptive skills and concepts of anthropology and sociology, together with the quantitative and interpretative skills of epidemiology, demography and statistics[1].

Good case studies have practical applications. They can be used to inform planners and politicians about the circumstances and processes in the lives of individuals, families and communities that place them at risk of illness. Such profiles can then provide the basis for the selection and design of programmes and policies that might be effective in reducing those risks. Against this background, we turn now to Bangladesh.

Our case study begins with a review of the current demographic and epidemiological situation of Bangladesh and of its people as a whole. Except where other references are cited below, the principal sources of statistical data come from the Bangladesh Bureau of Statistics, 1995; the Asian Development Bank, 1997; and the World Resources Institute, 1998. The case study continues with a narrative profile of the condition and life experiences of a single family. This is not the story of an actual family, but combines features which have been taken from the life histories of several families and of many individuals. Thus, the case study draws upon many different sources of numerical data, surveys and measurements on samples of the population, to give body sizes, ages, food consumption, farm size, etc., which are representative of a particular class of rural people, and it uses the accounts of anthropologists and social scientists who have investigated the daily lives of people belonging to that class.

4.3   Bangladesh: the national setting

Bangladesh had a troubled political history in the twentieth century. As East Bengal, it was under British colonial rule as a province of India prior to partition in 1947, when it became East Pakistan. The independent state of Bangladesh (Figure 4.2 overleaf) was created after a war of liberation from Pakistan in 1971. The population is predominantly Muslim, with about 15 per cent from other faiths.

4.3.1   Population growth and fertility decline

When it seceded from Pakistan in 1971, Bangladesh had a population of about 73 million. By the beginning of the twenty-first century, this had grown to an estimated 125 million. Moreover, with an average of 860 people per square kilometre, it has become the most densely populated country in the world, but is also one of the

[1] These methods and their combination in multidisciplinary research are extensively discussed in *Studying Health and Disease,* 2nd edn 1994; colour-enhanced 2nd edn 2001; Open University Press.

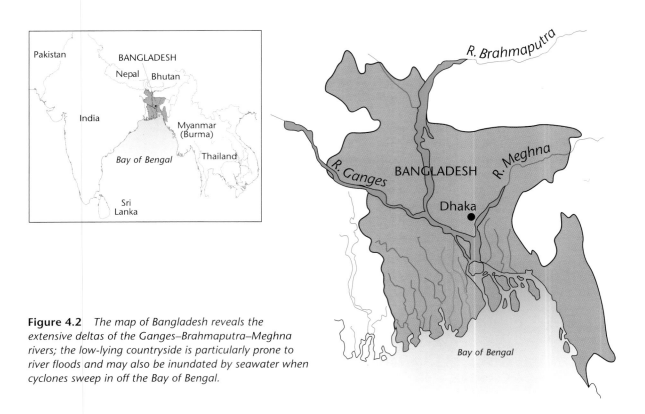

Figure 4.2   *The map of Bangladesh reveals the extensive deltas of the Ganges–Brahmaputra–Meghna rivers; the low-lying countryside is particularly prone to river floods and may also be inundated by seawater when cyclones sweep in off the Bay of Bengal.*

least industrialised and least urbanised in Asia. 100 million (80 per cent) of its people still find their livelihoods in the 'golden' countryside. Of these, 60 million belong to families that are either landless, or own such small plots of land that they cannot achieve self-sufficiency for food (Figure 4.3). They are wholly or partly dependent on wages earned either by working for richer peasants, or in tiny enterprises related to agriculture or rural commerce, such as duck farming or making kapok mattresses.

The urban population has seen one of the fastest growth rates of any developing country in recent years, from about 5.2 million living in towns and cities in 1962, to around 25 million in the year 2000 — over half of whom live in the 'mega' capital city, Dhaka. (The frontispiece photograph, Figure 1.1, in this book gives an insight into urban congestion in Dhaka.)

However, Bangladesh is achieving a remarkable slowing down in the rate of growth of the population. Evidence for this trend began to emerge in the 1990s and it is now clear that it had begun at least 20 years earlier. Before the 1970s, the population was increasing at a rate of 2.6 per cent per year, but by 1996 the rate had fallen to 1.8 per cent (Asian Development Bank, 1997). The underlying cause of this decline has been a fall in the **total fertility rate**, that is, the average number of children born to each woman in her lifetime. Starting from levels of about 7 children born to each woman in the population, fertility began to fall rapidly from the early 1970s, reaching just under 4 children per woman in 1993 and further falling to 3.3 in 1996 (Adnan, 1998). However, you should keep in mind that although this decline in fertility is unprecedented, the population of Bangladesh will continue to grow until fertility has fallen much further, to the 'replacement rate' of about 2.2 children per woman. Even on present trends, the population is predicted to reach 250 million before it stabilises in about 2045.

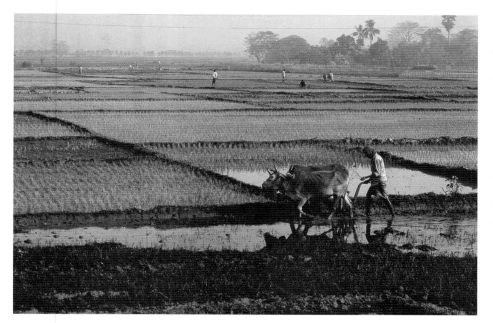

Figure 4.3 *Most of the farmland of Bangladesh is divided into small fields, usually only a fraction of an acre in size. Even when several of these fields are owned or rented by an individual family, the yields of rice, wheat and vegetables from the combined holding are often insufficient to meet their food needs. (Photo: Shoeb Faruquie/DRIK)*

4.3.2 Food, floods and famines

Before the twentieth century, the size of the population was limited by the high mortality caused by the combined effects of infectious diseases such as malaria and smallpox, together with limited and insecure food supply. In addition, deaths from famines resulting from droughts and floods went largely uncontrolled. (Checks on population growth are discussed further in Chapter 5.) However, since the end of British colonial rule in 1947, the impact of acute failure of food supply has been lessened through the availability of food aid provided from the agricultural surpluses of the developed countries. Freedom from colonialism has in some ways been replaced by a different kind of economic and political dependence. For example, in 1974 the USA abruptly suspended food aid shipments to Bangladesh in retaliation for Bangladeshi jute exports to Cuba. The effect of food aid has been to underpin national food security year on year, at a level sufficient to provide relief supplies and to counter the impact of floods or droughts on agricultural production. Thus, Bangladesh has avoided the worst excesses of famines (with deaths numbered in millions) that were recurrent in the region before World War II.

Until the early 1970s, growth of food production in Bangladesh depended largely upon expansion of the area of land under cultivation, almost up to the limits of what was available. Since that time, further growth in food production has been mainly through conversion of traditional rice varieties to high-yielding varieties. However, the increased yields from these newer varieties are only achievable given greater use of chemical fertilisers, pesticides and herbicides, together with (in some areas and at some times of the year) more water for irrigation. All of this has required additional investment, either from landowners wealthy enough to do so in their own right, or by those smaller farmers whose credit rating was sufficient to secure loans. Since the 1980s, this 'green revolution' in food production has broadly kept pace with the growth of population. As you will see in Chapter 11, in other parts of the developing world, some choice still remains between further extension of land area under cultivation, or alternatively of increased intensity of cultivation giving higher yields per acre. However, Bangladesh now has little option but to pursue the latter strategy, since it has barely any unexploited land to cultivate.

Against these signs of progress must be set the relatively slow growth of industrial development, which has resulted in low wage rates in both urban and rural sectors. This, in combination with the high rate of population growth, has produced a continuous rise in the proportion of the rural population living in absolute poverty. Many of these are landless people or own less than half an acre of land. Their numbers are increasing not only because of sub-division of land among the growing numbers of descendants, but also due to forced sales following indebtedness.

The rate at which families fall into destitution is regularly accelerated by disasters. The low-lying countryside is particularly prone to flooding along the extensive deltas of the Ganges–Brahmaputra–Meghna rivers and cyclones sweep in off the Bay of Bengal. Within recent history, the cyclone of 1970 probably killed more than 300 000 people who were swept away from coastal islands. There was a major famine in 1974–5; a 'near famine' in 1979, following severe drought in 1978; flooding and heavy loss of rice crops in 1984; a drought and rural unemployment in 1982; floods leading to the loss of 1 657 lives and 1.5 million tons of rice in 1987; even worse floods in 1988 with 2 400 deaths; cyclonic flooding of off-shore islands and coastal land in 1991, which killed 140 000 people, and further serious floods in both 1996 and 1997. In 1998, Bangladesh experienced the most extensive floods of the twentieth century (Figure 4.4); 34 000 square miles were flooded for two months, making over 23 million people homeless and killing over 1 000.

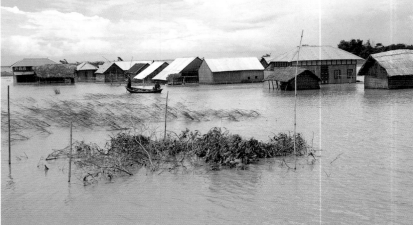

Figure 4.4 *In 1998, Bangladesh experienced the worst floods of the twentieth century; 34 000 acres were under water for two months. (Photo: Fred Hoogervorst/ Panos Pictures)*

In addition to the immediate death and destruction caused by flooding rivers and cyclonic inundations of seawater, great numbers of people have their future liveli-hoods destroyed. This happens through immediate loss of crops and possessions and also the water-logging of land. In the case of seawater, soil from low-lying fields may either be washed away, or rendered uncultivable by salination (impregnation with salt water). Even temporary displacement, or the loss of part of a crop, can spell disaster for people with no reserves to fall back on. Such crises commonly lead to loss of jobs and possessions and the break-up of families. Men and increasingly single women or women supporting children, migrate to the urban slums in search of work (Figure 4.5). A survey of such migrants by the nutritionist Jane Pryer in 1986 found that nearly 50 per cent gave poverty and lack of employment as the reason for leaving their villages. Another 16 per cent gave loss of land due either to flooding, or to legal problems following a death, disputes over title deeds, or family quarrels. This steady process of impoverishment, accompanied by the 'squeezing out' of people from their traditional livelihoods by sheer growth of numbers, has now brought to Bangladesh one of the fastest rates of urban population growth in the world.

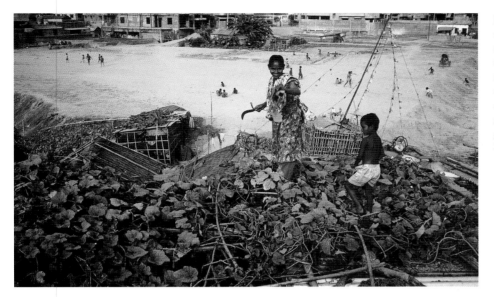

Figure 4.5 *A woman collects fruit from the squash vines growing over her makeshift home in an urban squatter camp; throughout Bangladesh, squash grown in this way provide additional food and shade. (Photo: Gil Moti/Still Pictures)*

4.3.3 International aid

The numbers of deaths resulting from natural disasters in Bangladesh are very large by comparison with those in developed countries. But they are much smaller than they would have been before independence, because of better preparedness and much prompter and more extensive rescue and relief services, both national and international. At the start of the twenty-first century, Bangladesh has in continuous operation over 1 300 **Non-Governmental Organisations (NGOs**, for example Oxfam, Save the Children and many other much less well-known organisations, some with very specific areas of activity such as housing or education) engaged in emergency assistance and relief, and in supporting social and economic development programmes — more than any other country in the world. Many of these NGOs receive funds from outside the country and together they provide US$300 million per annum of development assistance, in addition to that provided by Bangladesh itself.

Several of these NGOs have been in the forefront of the move towards participatory approaches to initiating social development. They are founded on the idea that the people who are the potential beneficiaries of services or assistance programmes should themselves be agents of change — deciding, implementing and managing programmes, rather than remaining passive recipients. Probably the best known example of this in Bangladesh has been the Grameen Bank initiative, which pioneered the idea of recycling loan money at low interest rates amongst groups of participants, devolving the responsibility both for assessing credit status of recipients and for securing repayment onto the group members themselves.[2]

In relation to agricultural development, there is a down-side to this 'cornucopia' of assistance agencies. Consortia formed from groups of donor agencies sharing common ideological approaches to rural change, have vied with each other for dominance in the competition for influence on the government over the direction of Bangladesh's agricultural policies. Moreover, critics have argued that in some instances these ideologies have coincided with the interests of the dominant rural classes, shifting income distribution in the direction of larger land and water owners and increasing the impoverishment of the rural poor (Rogaly *et al.*, 1999).

[2] The role of NGOs in raising the health status of people in developing countries is further discussed in another book in this series, *Caring for Health: History and Diversity* (Open University Press, 2nd edn 1993; 3rd edn 2001), Chapter 8.

4.3.4 Threats to health

Infectious disease

In many ways, health has held its own balance sheet of good and bad for the first generations since partition from India and the end of British colonial rule. In 1947, as well as reducing the working efficiency of the population through illness, *malaria* caused many deaths in infants, children and adults. The introduction of the insecticides DDT and Dieldrin led first to control and then the virtual eradication of the malaria-carrying mosquitoes by about the early 1960s. Like some other infections, malaria is believed to increase the rate of spontaneous abortion. In regions where it is **endemic** (always present; numerous outbreaks occur every year), it is a major contributor to deaths in early childhood. One immediate and dramatic effect of the malaria control programme was an increase in live births and in the rate of population growth in the 1960s.

In Bangladesh, as in many other countries, malaria has returned in recent years and again has the potential to become a significant threat. Parasites are being carried across the borders of neighbouring India and Myanmar (formerly Burma), not only by mosquitoes but by humans. Air travel is an increasing mode of re-infection involving both infected people and mosquitoes taken onto planes in clothing and luggage. In addition, growing insecticide resistance of the mosquitoes, and drug resistance in the parasites, threaten to make the re-emerging disease more difficult to control. Even more serious is that the type of parasite *Plasmodium falciparum*, which is associated with more violent symptoms (including cerebral malaria), has increased in proportion to the milder *Plasmodium vivax*, which was formerly the dominant type. This means that if the disease does once again become endemic, a larger proportion of infected people will die before they acquire any natural immunity.

Tuberculosis (TB) is an even more serious endemic health problem in Bangladesh. In 1997, a global survey of TB estimated that 46 per cent of the population were 'carriers' of the bacteria, 620 000 of whom had actively infectious TB. 300 000 new cases developed that year and 68 000 people died (Dye *et al.*, 1999). Only three countries in the world (India, China and Indonesia) had higher absolute numbers of new cases (incidence) and people with active TB (prevalence). But although the prevalence of TB rose in Bangladesh in the 1990s, as it did throughout the developing world, the cure rate also improved as new treatment strategies were adopted. In the DOTS programme — Directly Observed Treatment Short-course — patients are observed taking their daily medication for at least the first two months of a six-month course. A further encouraging sign is that the prevalence of multiple-drug resistant strains of TB in Bangladesh remains low.[3]

Another positive aspect of the health profile in Bangladesh is the relatively low level of HIV infection, despite the country's proximity to areas of high infection in neighbouring India and Myanmar. By the end of 1998, only 102 people in a country of 125 million had tested HIV-positive and seven had died of AIDS (Hawkes and Azim, 2000). But there is no cause for complacency. Other sexually transmitted diseases are already prevalent in certain sections of the population; 22 per cent of a sample of nearly 4 000 'high-risk' individuals (sex workers, cross-border truck drivers and injecting drug-users) were found to be infected with syphilis. Condom use is very low, and the successful family planning programme is based on the distribution of contraceptive pills or injections to women. The country has a vast

[3] The global rise in tuberculosis in the 1990s, the DOTS programme and multiple-drug resistant strains are discussed in *Medical Knowledge: Doubt and Certainty* (Open University Press, 2nd edn 1994; colour-enhanced 2nd edn 2001), Chapter 4.

migrant workforce, up to one million sex workers, and a growing population of injecting drug-users. Thus, all of the ingredients for the wildfire spread of HIV are present in Bangladesh if the infection takes hold.[4] And if it does so, attempts to bring TB rates under control may be overwhelmed, since people whose immune defences are reduced by HIV become particularly vulnerable to TB.

● Based on your reading of Chapter 3, which other infectious diseases would you expect to be a serious threat to health in Bangladesh?

■ *Measles* and *influenza* are serious public health problems, with *pneumonia* often supervening, causing many deaths. *Tetanus* remains an important cause of death, especially in children, and outbreaks of *typhoid* frequently occur. Of the 'great' epidemic diseases — smallpox, plague and cholera — *smallpox* was eradicated in the late 1970s, and *plague* has almost disappeared, but outbreaks of *cholera* still occur. Cholera is one of many *diarrhoeal diseases,* which inflict a considerable burden in terms of illness and suffering, loss of production, bereavement and orphaning.

Out of every 1 000 children born, 150 die before the age of 5 years. High levels of child mortality persist, despite improvements in the delivery of technical health interventions such as immunisation against the most common childhood diseases, greater availability of essential drugs, and the increasing use of inexpensive techniques for better treatment of diarrhoea such as oral rehydration therapy (ORT) — feeding home-made solutions of sugar and salt to prevent deaths from dehydration.

Arsenic contamination of groundwater

Although not by itself sufficient, it has long been recognised that pro-vision of a supply of bacteriologically safe drinking water is a necessary pre-condition for reducing the incidence of diarrhoeal diseases. To this end, as well as to provide irrigation water for food production, major investments were made in the 1980s and 1990s by international agencies such as UNICEF (United Nations International Children's Emergency Fund) to increase the number of bore-hole water sources. There are now about four million such 'tube-wells', providing drinking water to 95 per cent of the Bangladesh population (Figure 4.6). Tragically, although these sources are much less prone to faecal contamination than the more traditional open wells, it has recently been estimated (British Geological Survey, 2000) that as a result, about 21 million people are now exposed to an entirely new hazard: poisoning from drinking water containing up to 100 times the maximum safe level of arsenic. When consumed continually in a water-soluble form, arsenic is both toxic and carcinogenic (cancer-inducing), causing symptoms that take between five and fifteen years to appear and which, if left untreated, are ultimately fatal.

In Bangladesh (and in neighbouring West Bengal) the arsenic is of geo-logical origin: silt consisting of fine iron oxide particles covered with a layer of tightly bound arsenic has, at some time in the distant past, been washed down from the Himalayas by the Ganges, Brahmaputra and Meghna rivers, and has settled out in the delta regions as strata into

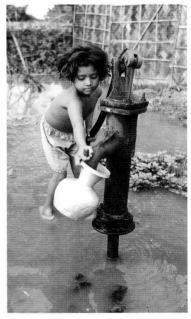

Figure 4.6 *Water being pumped from a shallow tube-well in Mymensingh, Bangladesh. Contamination of groundwater with naturally occurring arsenic presents a growing health hazard in Bangladesh and West Bengal, but the alternative of taking drinking water from surface pools increases exposure to bacteria and parasites. (Photo: Shehzad Noorani/Still Pictures)*

[4] The spread of HIV in developing countries is further discussed in *Caring for Health: History and Diversity* (Open University Press, 2nd edn 1993; 3rd edn 2001), Chapter 8, and *Experiencing and Explaining Disease* (Open University Press, 2nd edn 1996; colour-enhanced 2nd edn 2001), Chapter 4.

which many of the bore-holes have penetrated. Probably as a result of agriculture and the density of the overlying human population, bacterial decay of organic material in the topsoil largely depletes rainwater of any dissolved oxygen before it filters down to these arsenic-bearing deposits. The oxygen-depleted water then reacts with the iron oxide particles of the silt, causing them to release the arsenic which dissolves in the water (Nickson, *et al.*, 2000). Water pumped up from these bore-holes is usually drunk without further treatment.

Whilst there is some hope that high rates of extraction of water for irrigation, sustained over decades, will eventually result in 'washing out' the primary source of the arsenic, there is no short-term solution in sight for a problem which affects at least half a million wells. Replacement of drinking water sources by very deep (more than 200 meters) bore-holes, which are carefully sited and monitored, is clearly essential but also very expensive. An emergency interim solution depends on treatment of drinking water by methods that are simple and cheap enough to be used at village level. These consist of aeration and filtering the water through iron-rich sand, earth or crushed brick, followed by settling out of suspended particles — reversing the process that released arsenic from iron oxide in the first place.

This example illustrates that however successfully already known and understood threats to health are countered and reduced, new and unexpected hazards are always likely to arise which are contingent upon the ever-increasing demands made by human populations on the resources of the natural environment.

Health improvements

The degenerative diseases of the developed world — heart disease, high blood pressure, strokes, diabetes — are emerging as significant threats to health among adults, albeit at a lower level than in neighbouring India. But despite all these problems, the balance at the turn of the millennium seems to be on the positive side. Health statistics show overall improvements in life chances in recent decades. The infant mortality rate (IMR) has almost halved from 144 per 1 000 live births in 1965, to 78 per 1 000 in 1998 (refer back to Table 2.2). As far as adult health is concerned, the picture is of increasing life expectancy, especially for those who survive the dangerous period of early childhood. In 1989, expectation of life at birth in Bangladesh was 57 years for males and 56 years for females; by 1996 it had reached 59 years for both sexes.

● According to data presented in Chapter 2 (Table 2.3), how does current life expectancy in Bangladesh at birth, and further life expectancy at the age of 5 years compare with that in the UK?

■ Table 2.3 reveals that male life expectancy at birth in Bangladesh is 15 years lower than in the UK, and female life expectancy is 20 years lower. Bangladeshi children who survive the hazards of their first 5 years of life can expect to live for 61 more years (males) and 60 years (females); an equivalent figure for the UK population at age 5 would be about 70 more years (males) and 75 more years (females).

4.3.5 Gender inequalities are reducing

The trend towards equalisation of life expectancy for males and females is one of several signs that discrimination against females in terms of access to food and health care has been reducing in recent years, though gender inequalities remain.

Surveys of food consumption have been made at regular intervals over the past two or three decades, using samples of households and of individuals living in them. Some of these surveys have included comparisons of food energy intakes at different times of the year, by the same families, and show a slow decline in average energy consumption of about 10 per cent per decade, paralleling the decline in the purchasing power of the average wage. During the 'hungry' period, just before the main harvest, consumption is about 12 per cent lower than just afterwards. Bangladeshi families do not seem to discriminate against children or against females in terms of food. The nutritionists Abdullah and Wheeler (1985) found that all the individuals within families — men, women, girls and boys — had energy intakes that were in the same proportion to their estimated energy requirements. This 'fair sharing' of hardship was continued even in the 'hungry' season. Similarly, a survey of 4 227 people in 757 households in the two months following the 1998 floods showed that although food consumption fell, it did so equally for both sexes (Smith *et al.*, 2000).

In the early 1980s, government surveys had shown that in children under five-years-old, girls were between two and three times more likely to suffer acute episodes of severe weight-loss than boys (Bangladesh Institute of Nutrition, 1981). However, the proportion of rural Bangladeshi children under five-years-old who are **stunted** (short for their age) declined from 72 per cent in 1975 to 51 per cent in 1996. The proportion who were **wasted** (low in weight for their height) also declined over the same period, from 22 per cent to 17 per cent (Adnan, 1998). In 1996, girls showed only a 3 per cent greater likelihood of being underweight, as compared to boys. These improvements are probably due as much to better control of endemic diseases and better access to primary health-care services as to improvements in nutrition. The same surveys also showed that, notwithstanding the fairness of food sharing, there were important differences in health care exercised by parents for boys and girls. Female children experienced fewer visits to health centres, were less likely to receive immunisation, purchased medicines or oral rehydration, and had less time spent on breast-feeding and hand-feeding.

As you will see in Chapters 10 and 11, differences between the sexes in levels of health at an early age may result in the 'programming' of differences in health and survival chances in later life. As a result, over the population as a whole the ratio of living males to females was 1.064 in 1981 (or 106.4 males to every 100 females; refer back to Table 3.5). If there was no discrimination against females in the provision of food, or in access to health care, this ratio would have been expected to be similar to that in Europe or North America, that is close to 1.025. These data suggest that in Bangladesh at that time, an estimated 1.6 million women may have been 'missing', that is, presumed to have died from causes which might have been preventable. Here again there are signs of change: by 1996, the ratio of males to females in the population had fallen to 1.05.

However, the lives of adult Bangladeshi women remain at considerable risk. Maternal mortality is one of the highest in Asia, with around 500 women dying for every 100 000 live births (Bangladesh Bureau of Statistics, 1995). Suicide has become a relatively common means of escape from the 'quiet violence' of hopeless destitution. A study of the causes of death of 29 000 Bangladeshi women who died aged between ten and fifty years in 1996 and 1997, showed that 23 per cent had died as a result of intentional or unintentional injury. About half of these injury-related deaths were from suicide and 352 of the sample had been murdered (Yusuf *et al.*, 2000).

The more hopeful signs of a gradual trend away from the traditional bias against girls are reflections of a general increase in the economic value placed on females. There is a growing realisation that girl children are as good as boys at earning cash in local employment (making kapok mattresses, small-scale poultry production), and that there are as many opportunities for adult women to migrate to the cities and find significant sources of wages in, for example, the textiles industries, as there are for men. In a society where wages barely cover subsistence, this perception can quickly change a traditional view that the 'completeness' of a family is to be judged entirely in terms of surviving males — towards contentment with not too many of either sex. In fact, by 1996, the average completed family size considered most desirable had fallen to 2.5 children.

Other factors indicate increasing empowerment of women. These include a quadrupling of school attendance and literacy rates in girls since the 1960s — although female literacy is still only about 25 per cent; a large increase in female-headed households following the economic migration of men; and house-to-house delivery of predominantly female contraceptives. Opinion surveys show that women are now much more often involved in making important decisions in the family. All these changes in the roles and status of women have been, if anything, more rapid among the rural poor than in the urban context, and are now recognised as among the most important causal factors in the decline of fertility (Adnan, 1998).

4.3.6 Education

Education, or rather the lack of it, is still a huge problem in Bangladesh. Even on the best estimates, 43 per cent of adults are literate (and some surveys put the figure as low as 35 per cent), compared with a developing-world average of 70 per cent. As you saw earlier, female literacy rates are lower still. Poor parents cannot afford to keep their children at school: even though 70 per cent of primary schools are government funded, parents still have to pay for uniforms and classroom supplies.

● What else is likely to make it hard for parents to send their children to school?

■ They would have to forego the children's contributions to the work of the household and their earned income — which tiny though it will be, could spell the difference between survival and destitution for the family.

Average attendance rates at school are no more than 60 per cent, and around 20 per cent of children do not complete even their first year. A more hopeful sign, which is very much in line with other recent trends in Bangladesh, is that enrolment rates at primary level are now identical for boys and girls (94 per cent). There has also been a dramatic growth in the numbers of 'non formal' schools run by NGOs. Starting in 1992 with government support, there were about 120 of these NGO-run schools; by 1996 there were 52 000 supplementing the 38 000 formal state primary schools.

Against this general background of the national picture, what can we learn from focusing on specific families in Bangladesh? At this point in the case study, we introduce a fictional family constructed from many narrative profiles, to represent some of the important recurring themes of rural life.

4.4 Sonar Bangla? A profile of a typical Bangladeshi peasant family

Our typical poor peasant family consists of a husband Abu, a wife whose maiden name was Sofi but who is now known as 'mother of Anis', and four children: Sharifa, a girl of 10; Anis, a boy of 7; Naila, a girl of 5; and a boy of 2, named Hali. Husband and wife are both illiterate; Anis attends primary school, but only intermittently. They own their house, which is built entirely of palm thatch and has mud floors (Figure 4.7). Their water comes from a tube well shared with thirty other households and there is no means of disposal of excreta or refuse, except for the fields and open rubbish heaps.

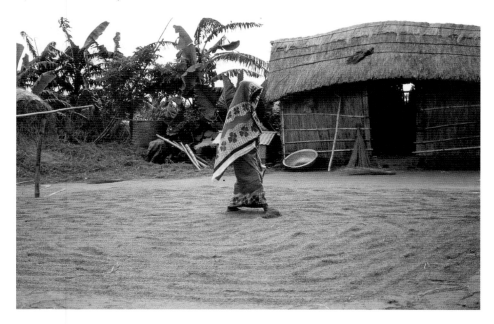

Figure 4.7 *A woman 'treading' rice to remove the husks; the rice is spread on packed earth in front of a typical village house of palm thatch, near the Brahmaputra river, Bangladesh. (Photo: Vanya Kewley/Camera Press)*

All the members of this family are shorter and lighter than the average for European or North American people of the same age and sex. The wife weighs 40 kg and the husband 46 kg.

- How do the body weights of Abu and Sophi compare with those of adult members of the UK population? Think of your own weight and those of other adults in your family.

◼ The average weight of UK adults is around 70 kg for females and 83 kg for males (Health Survey for England, 1997). These rural Bangladeshis only weigh just over half the weight of adults of the same sex in the UK.

The two older children are about 20 cm shorter than the average for children of the same age in the industrialised countries of the developed world, whereas the two younger ones are not only short but are also about 10 per cent lighter than European children of the same height. Several times during her life, Naila has been severely ill, losing at the time an additional 30 per cent of body weight, relative to a healthy European child of the same age. During the past year, she has had an episode of diarrhoea with fever, scabies (a skin inflammation caused by parasites) and an ear infection with bad fever. Because of her worsening condition, Naila was taken first to a paramedic in the nearest town, who gave her just one dose of penicillin. Although trained in the Western tradition, he is well aware that he can care for only perhaps a fifth of the village population and he encourages respect for traditional Ayurvedic (Hindu) and Unani (Islamic) systems of medicine. When the single injection did no good, Naila was taken to a Hindu herbal doctor, who sold the family pills over which he had chanted mantras. Two other children had been born to this family, both of whom died before reaching their second birthdays.

The family's ability to obtain food is derived in part from a quarter of an acre of land that was left to Abu on the death of Sofi's father. From this, in an average year, they get two crops of rice, enough to provide them with one-fifth of their food energy requirements. The rest of their food procurement relies on payment 'in kind' or from cash, earned by working for richer farmers. In past years, the family 'share-cropped' an additional acre, but the owner now finds it more profitable to farm it himself and to hire their labour when he needs it. Husband and wife both work for wages, as do the two older children: father and son at farm work; mother and daughter chopping and carrying firewood, washing clothes and parboiling rice (a hot soaking of unmilled grain preliminary to re-drying and husking).

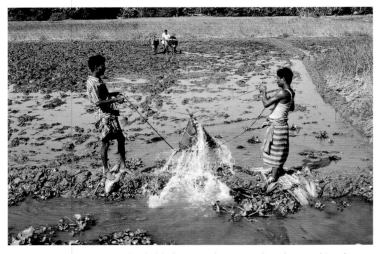

Figure 4.8 *Preparing the fields for rice planting takes the combined labour of all family members (Photo: Jorgen Schytte/Still Pictures)*

Their own piece of land is an essential part of their food procurement and they try to make up for its smallness by the intensity of their labour (Figure 4.8). They plough with a hired ox and meticulously weed and harvest by hand, although this has to be done just at the time when the best wage rates are on offer from the richer peasants. Rice dominates their landscape, their diet and often their thoughts. As the Innuit have many words for snow, so Bangladeshis have many words for rice — each of the dozens of varieties has its name and each of these can be eaten in several different ways: parboiled, double parboiled, puffed, flaked, fried, etc. Although their waking hours are devoted to this work, no one takes a daily meal for granted — neighbours greet each other with the simple question 'have you eaten'?

Of the family earnings, 80 per cent is spent on food: the rest goes on clothing, medicines and other essentials. The average year-round food energy consumption of the family is 10 200 kcal per day, or 1 700 kcal per head.[5] Ninety per cent of this comes from rice (2.9 kg a day), the rest from vegetables, occasionally fish. Even if they did no productive work and only rested quietly all day, the family would still need 7 800 kcal per day, just to stay alive and maintain their present body weights. The 2 400 kcal the family consume over and above this is what is available to them to support their physical activity. This amount of energy has to cover not only what they expend in working their own land and in paid employment, so as to secure their food, but also the energy cost of essential domestic work, carrying water and fuel, cooking and cleaning.

[5] 1 kcal (colloquially a calorie) is the amount of heat energy required to raise 1 kilogram of water through 1°C. The labels on food packaging often give energy values also in kjoules; the joule is the internationally accepted scientific unit of energy and a kjoule (1 000 joules) is equivalent to 4.2 kcal.

The energy budget for the year includes a peak of food availability after the *aman*, the larger of the two rice harvests, and a trough or 'hungry' period just before. The difference between this peak and trough in daily consumption for the whole family is 1 200 kcal, equivalent to about 400 grams of rice per day. They 'share' this seasonal hunger among themselves roughly in proportion to their individual energy needs. That is to say, they each go short by amounts which depend on their body weights and on the amounts of physical work they do: no-one makes extra sacrifices and no one is deprived of food by reason of their sex or age.

The struggle to make do is gradually getting worse with each decade that passes. Although, to the casual observer, the intensively cultivated landscape presents an appearance of pastoral harmony, beneath the surface there is an increasingly desperate competition for land and employment. Abu's greatest worry is that Sofi's brothers have never fully accepted his right to the inherited land from their father. Forgery of land title deeds has become commonplace and people as poor as he cannot afford legal defence. For families in this situation, the continuous grind of poverty is both a background and an underlying cause of more dramatic and usually tragic events — a child dies, a wage-earner gets sick, there are droughts and, more commonly, floods. The initial response to such a crisis is to borrow money and sell household goods and ornaments; later, land and tools have to be sold and finally people themselves, into bonded labour for men and prostitution for women and children. A World Health Organisation survey in 1997 reported that approximately half of the rural population were in absolute poverty (Sen, 1997).

Of course people do survive. There is food aid relief; crises pass, sometimes just through a better than average harvest. But a number of studies of the rural poor have shown that for many people things are never the same again: those who managed to keep their land have an extra burden of debts to bear; those who sold join the ranks of the landless whose numbers are increasing in pace with the rate of growth of the population as a whole (Figure 4.9). One of Sofi's unmarried sisters now works in a textiles factory in Dhaka. It has become commonplace for an adult family member, most often a woman, to migrate for employment in this way. Along with tiny remittances from her sister, come stories of a city life in which physical oppression and murder are increasingly commonplace.

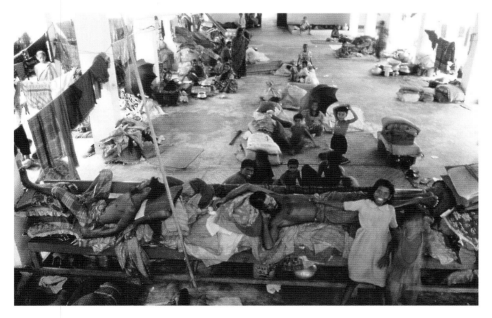

Figure 4.9 *Destitute families, unable to sustain life on the land, migrate to the cities with their few possessions and find shelter wherever they can. (Photo: Abir Abdullah/DRIK)*

4.5 Future prospects

It seems that in Bangladesh, as in most countries, the retreat of several of the major epidemic diseases has had a profound effect upon survival and vitality of the whole population, of all ages, extending even to the rural poor. Similarly, the better control of infectious diseases of childhood, together with the adoption of better child-care methods by those who have access, education and the financial means to do so, has begun to reduce the problem of early child deaths.

- What do you see as the most pressing problems facing Bangladesh in achieving better health for its population? Will these be resolved by delivering more technical health services, better education of the population about health and nutrition, improved living standards, or all of these?

- From now on it will become increasingly hard to sustain further health improvements unless something is done to at least halt the growth of the numbers in absolute destitution. Moreover there has to be some tangible means of helping the very poorest to have both the means of securing the essentials of life and to be better supported in the face of natural disasters. There is little to be gained by 'educating' people in the use of resources they do not possess, or in the use of facilities that are either out of reach or ephemeral.

It is clearly necessary for a country which aims to *maintain* the health of its people, to ensure, as indeed Bangladesh has succeeded in doing, that food production keeps pace with the growth of population. However, as you will see in Chapter 7, this in itself is not sufficient to *improve* health status. To do that it is necessary at the same time to ensure the extension of individual *entitlement* to the essentials for health at all levels in society, not only to adequate amounts of food, but also access to health services and education within the context of a safe environment. In other words, there needs to be a sustained reduction in the numbers of people who have no choice but to live in conditions of absolute poverty, in locations where the risk of natural disaster is so high.

4.5.1 Are there pre-conditions or absolute priorities?

There are many contributory causes of the problem of poverty in Bangladesh. Some of the most important — that of the poor comparative performance of the industrial sector of the economy and the fact that global warming is already making the regular flooding worse — are well beyond the scope of this book. Nonetheless, the case study does help to bring into focus some critically important aspects, chief among them the very positive finding that given adequate family planning services, significant reductions in fertility can be achieved even among the very poor. Moreover, the decline in birth rate began in the early 1970s, at a time when 20 per cent of children were still dying before the age of five. Both these aspects of change are contrary to the predictions of many public health experts, whose view has generally been that high fertility rates are positively sustained by conditions of extreme poverty and in particular by expectations of high child mortality. Reduction of both these factors have therefore been seen as necessary *pre-conditions* for the success of family planning services.

Whilst the reversal of this expectation in Bangladesh is encouraging, it would be equally wrong to assume that success in curbing population growth will, by itself, be a cheap and effective route to achieving all the other aims of development, in particular a good standard of health for all. Family planning in Bangladesh does not come cheap. Although contraception of some kind is now used by about 50 per cent of the population, with a major part of the distribution in the form of delivery to households, it costs US$50 to prevent each avoidable birth. This means that the family planning service currently costs US$93 million per year, half of which comes from donor agencies and half from the Bangladesh government. To put this figure in context, government spending on all aspects of health care and family planning amounts to US$3.50 per head of population. The ultimate goal of a 'replacement' fertility rate of 2.2 children per woman will mean not only extending uptake of contraception to the majority of the population, but also increasing the average period for which contraceptives are used (in 1996, half of new users stopped within 12 months). It is estimated that if the family planning service were to be extended using the current structure, it would increase the annual cost by nearly three times, to an amount comparable with the entire government public health budget (Asian Development Bank, 1997).

Thus, whilst there is now a realistic prospect of just one more doubling of total numbers and then of population stability at 250 million by about 2045, the cost of meeting the level of demand this would imply for family planning services is daunting. The challenge for the future will be to combine the potential resource now being created by the gradual empowerment of women, with a participatory structure of family planning service delivery and perhaps the manufacture of contraceptive supplies within Bangladesh.

4.5.2   A sustainable future?

Given a realistic possibility of a final population size of 250 million, what can be said about the concomitant prospects for **sustainable development** in Bangladesh? Can the stabilisation of population growth and the achievement of food security be sustained long-term and still avoid the total destruction of what remains of the natural environment and its biodiversity? The growth rate of food production in the twenty-first century is just about keeping pace with that of the human population (albeit they remain largely impoverished), but this process has resulted in the erosion of forests, wetlands, natural grazing areas and inland and marine fisheries (mangrove belts). These areas not only constituted the ecological niches and natural habitats of the wildlife of the country; they were formerly common-land property 'reserves' which were appropriated by the rich and powerful (Hughes *et al.*, 1994). By 1996, only 9 per cent of the original tree cover was left and 30 per cent of the mangroves had already been destroyed (Adnan, 1998).

There is no possibility of sustaining food security in Bangladesh through self-sufficient production without a major investment in increased yields, but there is general agreement that current yields per acre are on average no more than 50 per cent of their potential maximum. Intensification of agricultural technology could, in theory, double food production without further encroachment into the habitats of the great diversity of bird and fish life that still remains (Figure 4.10). As in relation to the concerns about

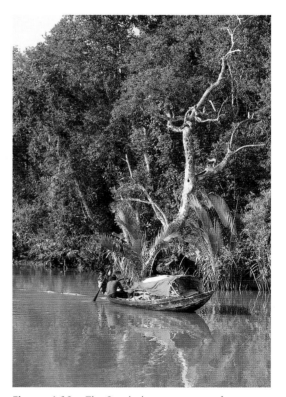

Figure 4.10   *The Sundarbans mangrove forest on the southern edge of the Ganges–Brahmaputra–Meghna delta. Environmental conservation in Bangladesh is now largely reduced to the management of small refuge 'hot spots', which are crucial for the survival of dwindling plant and animal biodiversity. Do scenes like this hold the promise of future reclamation, or will they serve only as a reminder of riches lost forever? Photo: Shehzad Noorani/Still Pictures)*

achieving reasonable levels of self-sufficiency and food security for the human population, the questions about conservation of wildlife are not so much about whether it can be done at all, but will it be done in time?

OBJECTIVES FOR CHAPTER 4

When you have studied this chapter, you should be able to:

4.1 Define and use, or recognise definitions and applications of, each of the terms printed in **bold** in the text.

4.2 Outline the essential features of the case study approach to researching health problems, and illustrate the main advantages and limitations of this method by reference to the Bangladesh case study.

4.3 Describe the main causes of mortality and morbidity in Bangladesh and comment on how and why disease patterns have changed over time.

4.4 Give an account of the way in which economic, social and demographic changes affect the health of the poor in Bangladesh.

4.5 Discuss the threats and opportunities for sustainable development in Bangladesh, with particular reference to population growth rate, food security and preservation of the natural environment.

QUESTIONS FOR CHAPTER 4

1 (*Objective 4.2*)

What did the narrative profile of Abu and Sophi's family situation add to the statistical data on life in Bangladesh? Why must caution be exercised in reading the account of their lives?

2 (*Objective 4.3*)

List the main problems that face Bangladesh in its efforts to maintain and extend control over infectious diseases.

3 (*Objective 4.4*)

Compare and contrast the benefits that a small farming family might experience from: (a) improved access to basic health services and (b) improved security of food procurement.

4 (*Objective 4.5*)

How would you rank the importance for Bangladesh of the need to commit resources to family planning programmes during the next 30 years, as compared to investment towards achieving other development aims?

C H A P T E R 5

The world transformed: population and the rise of industrial society

Study notes for OU students

The interaction of human cultural and biological evolution is introduced here, and discussed at length in another book in this series, *Human Biology and Health: An Evolutionary Approach* (Open University Press, second edition 1994; third edition 2001). During this chapter you will be asked to read two extracts contained in *Health and Disease: A Reader* (Open University Press, third edition 2001*)*, the first entitled 'Agriculture's two-edged sword' by Jared Diamond, and the second entitled 'Health: 1844' by Frederick Engels.

5.1 Introduction

Amid all the various patterns of health and disease that we examined in Chapters 2 to 4 of this book, probably the most obvious fact to emerge was the degree to which good health is not simply something enjoyed by some individuals and not by others, a biological roulette game where everyone starts off more or less equal. In fact, health varies enormously from one society, nation or part of the world to another, such that it is possible to talk about the collective health of different populations: health seems to be a state that is socially shared as much as individually experienced.

Another important aim of Chapters 2 to 4 is to question the widespread assumption that the present differences in health between different parts of the world are narrowing. Of course, it is difficult to generalise over long historical periods, because the further back in time we go the less reliable sources of information become. Nevertheless some of the available measures of health, such as infant mortality rates, indicate a relative widening of differences between a number of developing countries and the industrialised countries.

How did this come about? The period in which these health differences started to become more pronounced — the eighteenth and nineteenth centuries — was also the period when the Industrial Revolution began to transform a small but expanding group of countries. Thus these contemporary international differences in health and disease, and the way in which they have evolved historically, seem to be related to patterns of social and economic development. Broadly, societies that are rich and industrialised also have comparatively high levels of health and relatively stable populations, and societies that are poor have a much poorer health experience and rapidly growing populations. So here, and in the following three chapters, we explore some of the reasons for the differences in health between the developing and developed countries, by looking more systematically at the links between health and disease, social and economic development, and population change.

Figure 5.1 charts these links in a simplified way. The figure indicates that each corner of the central triangle is linked in both directions to the other corners, suggesting that there is no single direction of causality. In addition, the triangle is placed

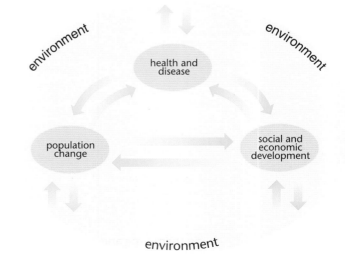

Figure 5.1 *A model of health and disease linkages.*

within an oval representing the environment, with each part of the triangle again linked to the environment both directly and via the other corners of the triangle.

Some of these links have already been discussed. For example, in Chapter 2 you saw how death rates affect population structure and how population structure influences death rates, and in Chapter 3 how the natural environment influences the prevalence of specific diseases. Sometimes these links are very direct, but often they are more complex, indirect and subtle. For example, the following three extracts have been selected in order to illustrate different ways in which health and disease are related to social and economic factors and the wider environment. As you read them, make a note in the wide margin beside each extract of the sequence of events described. Try to define ways in which the sequences differ.

Extract from *Mirage of Health* by René Dubos

The main reservoirs of the plague bacilli [bacteria] in nature are wild rodents which are infected but sufficiently resistant not to suffer from their infection under normal circumstances. They carry the plague bacilli throughout their life, just as so many healthy men and women are infected with tubercle bacilli or with viruses without showing signs of disease. Among the naturally infected animals are the tarabazan (Manchurian marmot), which has long been hunted for its fur. The professional Manchurian hunters carefully avoid any tarabazan which appears to be sick and in fact a religious taboo specifically instructs them in this regard. This taboo is probably related to the fact that the plague bacilli become active in sick tarabazans and therefore can more readily be transmitted to man. Around 1900 there occurred a change in women's fashion in Europe which increased the demand of the fur trade for the pelt of the tarabazan. Attracted by the high prices of the fur, inexperienced Chinese took to tarabazan hunting. Being ignorant of the ancient taboo, they did not hesitate to catch sick animals which proved the easiest prey. Several of the hunters caught plague from the tarabazans and transmitted it to the population of the inns of Manchuria. Thus began the great epidemic of pneumonic plague in Manchuria. (Dubos, 1979, pp. 187–8)

Extract from *Plagues and People* by W. McNeill

Nearly twenty years ago … I was reading about the Spanish conquest of Mexico. As everyone knows, Hernando Cortez, starting off with fewer than six hundred men, conquered the Aztec empire, whose subjects numbered millions. How could such a tiny handful prevail …? A casual remark in one of the accounts of Cortez's conquest … suggested an answer to such questions … For on the night when the Aztecs drove Cortez and his men out of Mexico City, killing many of them, an epidemic of smallpox was raging in the city. The man who had organized the assault on the Spaniards was among those who died on the *nocha triste*, as the Spanish later called it. The paralysing effect of a lethal epidemic goes far to explain why the Aztecs did not pursue the defeated and demoralized Spaniards, giving them time and opportunity to rest and regroup, gather Indian allies and set siege to the city, and so achieve their eventual victory. Moreover, it is worth considering the psychological impact of a disease that killed only Indians and left Spaniards unharmed. Such partiality could only be explained supernaturally, and there could be no doubt about which side of the struggle enjoyed divine favour ... little wonder, then, that the Indians accepted Christianity and submitted to Spanish control so meekly. God had shown himself on their side, and each new out-break of infectious disease imported from Europe (and soon from Africa as well) renewed the lesson. (McNeill, 1976, pp. 1–2)

Extract from *Inside the Third World* by P. Harrison

In a World Bank study in Indonesia, agricultural labourers and rubber tappers with hookworm-induced anaemia were found to be around twenty per cent less productive than their non-anaemic colleagues. Their foreman's views of which workers were 'lazy' or 'weak' were found to correspond closely to the incidence of anaemia. Workers with higher levels of anaemia earned less in incentive payments than their colleagues, and as a result of their lower income they consumed less calories, protein, vitamins, and iron than non-anaemic workers. This poorer nutrition contributed to their poor productivity and lowered their resistance to disease, hence they were more likely to lose time off work. ... Disease may also close up many areas that could be productive: river-blindness and sleeping sickness have emptied the river valleys in West Africa's Sahel region, while the tsetse fly has prevented the development of mixed agriculture in much of Africa. So disease creates poverty, while poverty, continuing the cycle, maintains the conditions that foster disease. (Harrison, 1979, pp. 288–9)

● In the first extract, Dubos mentioned a social/economic event, and a change in the pattern of health. What were they, and how were they related?

■ The event Dubos mentions was a change in fashion in Europe; the health change was an outbreak of pneumonic plague in Asia. Dubos is arguing that the change in fashion set off the change in health.

Even in quite unexpected or indirect ways, social or economic factors can have repercussions on health. In this first extract, the 'cause' of the pneumonic plague epidemic to which Dubos refers seems to have been these social and economic influences as much as the plague bacilli.

● Now consider the second extract. In what way does the sequence of events described by McNeill differ from that outlined by Dubos?

■ One way of interpreting McNeill's argument is as follows; if it had not been for the debilitating effects of disease on the Aztecs, it would have been much more difficult for the Spaniards to impose their cultural and economic domination. In other words, a change in disease pattern strongly influenced the social and economic history, and the population history, of the Americas.

In fact, the sequence of events described by McNeill seems in some way to be in the opposite direction to that in the first extract.

● Finally, how does Harrison's account construct a sequence of events?

■ In the extract from Harrison, the emphasis seems to be placed on interaction and interdependence between health and socio-economic factors. Health conditions are influenced by social and economic factors and the environment, which in turn are influenced by the prevailing pattern of health and disease.

In practice, it is this more complex kind of relationship that is most frequently encountered. To return to the extract from McNeill, for example: the spread of disease assisted the Spanish conquest, but it could be argued that it was the overseas expansion of the Spanish that triggered the spread of disease. It could further be argued that the overseas expansion of Spain would not have been possible without the help of navigational discoveries and new shipbuilding techniques, and so on. In one sense all of these factors caused a change in disease patterns in America, but none was *the* cause.

With this lesson about the complexity of causal relationships in mind, let us now examine in more detail some of the complex ways in which population change is related to changes in health and to economic and social change.

5.2 Population change

The explosive growth in the human population of the world during the period we live in is one of the most dramatic facts of human existence. Figure 5.2 overleaf shows the acceleration in human **population growth**. Humans and their immediate ancestors have been on Earth for only about 2 million years. It took almost this long for humankind to reach its first billion, around the year 1800. It took just 130 more years to add another billion, 30 years to add a third, and 15 years to add a fourth. By the year 2000 the world's population had passed the 6 billion mark, and by 2025 it is likely to have reached almost 8 billion (we will look more closely at such predictions and how they have changed in Chapter 8). Clearly such a radically unstable situation cannot continue for very long, but before looking to the future we must try to understand the past. As a starting point, let us look at population and disease in the pre-industrial world, and try to sketch briefly both the kinds of diseases that are likely to have afflicted our early ancestors, and how these might have changed as human society evolved through different stages of development.

5.2.1 Population and disease in the pre-industrial world

Forty thousand years ago, members of our human species had colonised most of the inhabitable areas of the world. They were food-collectors rather than food-producers, and they lived by hunting other animals and gathering foodstuffs such as fruit, seeds, nuts, roots and honey. The only way we can estimate the numbers of these **hunter–gatherers** is by calculating their food-collecting efficiency in relation to the maximum population sustainable by the environments in which they lived (sometimes referred to as the **carrying capacity** of the environment). On this basis, it is unlikely that there were more than two million of our human ancestors on earth at this time.

The causes of illness and rates of death among these human ancestors are largely a matter of speculation. They would have been subject to mites, fleas, ticks and worms, and invaded by viruses, bacteria, fungi and parasites, although the practice of cooking meat (developed early in human evolution) gave humans a unique degree of protection from food-borne diseases. Through their development and mastery of hunting skills, hunter–gatherers dominated the food chain, and this

Population (millions)

Year

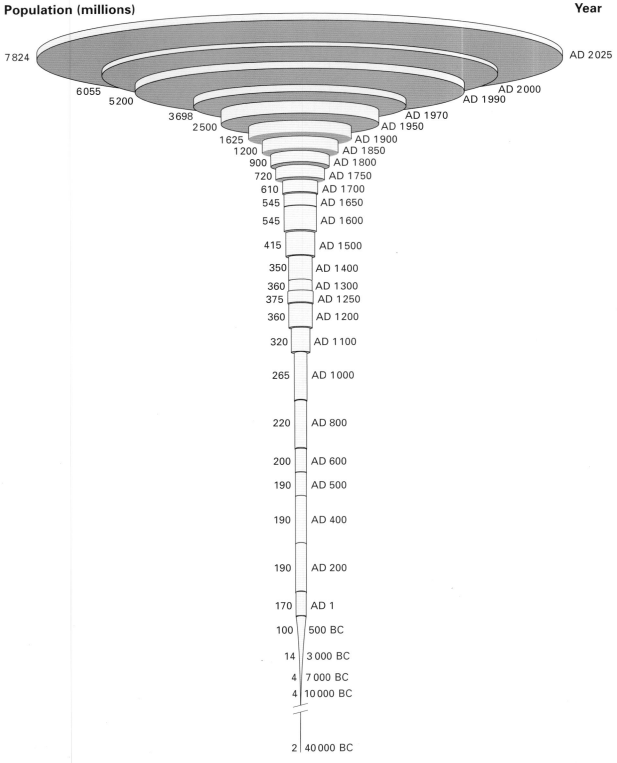

Figure 5.2 *Estimated population of the world. (Data from McEvedy, C. and Jones, R. (1978)* Atlas of World Population History, *Penguin, London, and United Nations (1998)* World Population Prospects 1998, *UN, New York)*

largely removed the threat of being preyed on by other species. However, it posed a new survival risk: slaughter by other humans. Additional stresses would have arisen regularly from food shortages and from changes in climatic conditions, such as the advance and retreat of successive Ice Ages.

In so far as any species can be said to be in equilibrium with its environment, these human societies were close to stability, both in numbers and in age structure. An important element in this stability was likely to have been population control, probably by means of infanticide, abortion, sexual abstinence and protracted breast-feeding (which suppresses ovulation). This would have ensured that these societies did not press too hard against the carrying capacity of their environment, but had some safety margin which allowed them to cope with periods of scarcity, and to recover from periodic disease epidemics or famines.

However, underlying this apparent stability it appears that there was a very slow growth in total population size—perhaps 2 per cent per 1 000 years. By approximately 10 000 BC, human numbers may have doubled to around 4 or 5 million. Over the same period a number of major meat sources, such as mammoths and mastodons, were hunted to extinction. Perhaps both the rising human population and its impact on other species are evidence of a kind of human adaptability and skill. But as the last Ice Age retreated around this time, it seems that growing human numbers, the disappearance of some food sources, and unusually large climatic variations may well have combined to create a slow collision between human populations and their resource base. These were the conditions in which an entirely new phase of human history unfolded, as humanity switched from food collecting to food production, and hunting and gathering gave way to the cultivation of crops and the domestication of animals: the first Agricultural Revolution.

5.3   The first Agricultural Revolution

The switch from food collecting to food production surged forward from around 8000 BC. This is sometimes referred to as the Neolithic period, the last phase of the Stone Age. It was based on the domestication and cultivation of a wide range of plants — cereals such as maize, rice, millet and wheat; roots and tubers such as potatoes and yams; pulses and fruits — and the parallel domestication of many animal species, including sheep, cattle, goats, pigs, camels and chickens. This process was remarkably widespread, and may have commenced independently in a number of regions: the prevailing view at present is that it centred on China, India, the Near East and Central America, from where it advanced into most other regions of the world. As it spread, hunting and gathering was displaced.

This first **Agricultural Revolution** transformed the social organisation of humans. Small, wandering groups who rarely came into contact with one another were replaced by much larger, settled communities in most (though not all) parts of the world. Settled agricultural communities also began to domesticate animals and rear them for meat, milk and hides. There was a greatly increased division of labour and specialisation of tasks. This has been regarded by some commentators as the most significant change humans have ever experienced:

> Of the 50 000 odd generations in the last million years of history, only about 400 have occurred since agriculture was first adopted by one part of the human population. With agriculture came dramatic changes in diet, population density and patterns of daily

life, and the human organism was exposed to stresses that were, in evolutionary terms, novel. It is unlikely that there has been major biological change in man since the Neolithic revolution. Such change is highly improbable with respect to the more recent adoption of urban and advanced industrial patterns of life. (Powles, 1973, p. 4)

The Agricultural Revolution made it possible to produce more food, which in turn allowed a substantial increase in population. From an estimated 4–5 million humans in the world at the beginning of the Agricultural Revolution, numbers increased to perhaps 170 million by the birth of Christ. As regards human disease, the Agricultural Revolution is likely to have led to the rise of infectious diseases as the main cause of illness and death.

●   Why should infections have assumed such importance as a consequence of the social changes of the Agricultural Revolution?

■   The most important effect was the increase in both the total population size and the size of local groups living in close personal contact, not only with each other, but with domesticated livestock.

Many infections require a minimum size of human population if they are to be maintained. Whereas some diseases depend on an animal host (e.g. rats in the case of plague), others, such as measles, are specific to humans, although the measles virus may have evolved from one that infects dogs — an example of a zoonotic infection (Chapter 2). It has been suggested that measles requires a population of about one million to be maintained as an endemic (always present) infection.

Other less important reasons include more numerous intruders such as rats and mice into human habitations, attracted by the stored food that food production necessarily entails. In addition, the switch from the often highly varied diet of the hunter–gatherers to the mono-diets of the early agriculturalists may have had severe health consequences. These have been summarised by the American physiologist Jared Diamond in his book *The Rise and Fall of the Third Chimpanzee* (1992); an extract is included under the title 'Agriculture's two-edged Sword' in *Health and Disease: A Reader* (Open University Press, 3rd edn 2001). Open University students should read it now.

●   What disciplines does Diamond mainly draw from to illustrate his arguments?

■   He makes particular use of evidence assembled by archaeologists and by paleo-pathologists.

●   What effect did the adoption of agriculture have on the height of humans, according to Diamond?

■   He cites evidence that the average height of hunter–gatherers in the areas we now know as Greece and Turkey was around 5 foot 10 inches for men and 5 foot 6 inches for women; that heights were much lower following the adoption of agriculture; and that in modern times inhabitants of these areas have still not regained the heights of their healthy hunter–gatherer ancestors.

● What main reasons are advanced by Diamond for this adverse impact of agriculture on health, at least initially?

■ He argues that the range of foodstuffs was drastically reduced, that infectious disease became more common, and that wide inequalities between social classes appeared.

Although the evidence of paleopathology is accumulating rapidly, much is still unknown concerning the impact of the Agricultural Revolution on human health. What is clear is that, as Diamond notes, the implications of this decisive event in human history are still unfolding. Infections were to remain the predominant threat to human survival for almost 10 000 years (and in many parts of the world are still the leading cause of death and disease). And the 'starvation, warfare and tyranny' that accompanied the adoption of agriculture are still all too evident in many parts of the modern world.

5.4   Scarcity or plenty

These stages of development in human society — from hunter–gatherers to agriculturalists — are of course crude approximations to what was a long, complex and still poorly understood series of changes. However, it seems clear beyond reasonable doubt that major shifts in the experience of health and disease attended these changes. A second point to note is less obvious but equally important: each stage of development was characterised by a particular way of obtaining the means of subsistence, and it was the *balance* between that means of subsistence and the number of people it had to sustain which dictated whether there would be scarcity or plenty. To illustrate the relative nature of these concepts, let us examine the traditional view anthropologists once took of hunter–gatherer societies: that they were characterised by permanent scarcity, meagre resources, hand-to-mouth subsistence, and a life of continual struggle for survival. This seems to be remarkably similar to the famous description of life without social organisation suggested by Thomas Hobbes, the seventeenth-century social theorist, as 'solitary, poor, nasty, brutish and short'.

However, as modern anthropologists began to accumulate evidence on surviving hunter–gatherer societies, it became increasingly difficult to reconcile these views with their irregular and not prolonged hours of labour, the amount of time spent dozing, chatting, playing games or engaged in ceremonies, and the generally low esteem in which many material possessions were held (Figure 5.3). Among the !Kung Bush-people of the Kalahari, for example, researchers found that there seemed to be little or no material pressure in life, and possession of objects conferred no status on individuals. Similarly, among Australian natives in Arnhem Land, work was intermittent and averaged around four hours a day, and dietary intake was more than adequate.

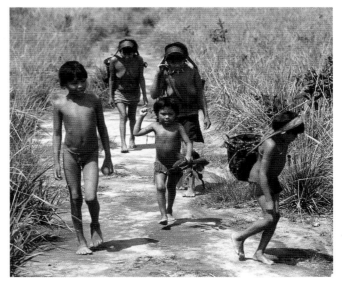

Figure 5.3   *A Yanomani family group foraging for edible plants on the edges of their forest territory in the Serra Parima region of the Orinoco River basin, Venezuala, 1992. (Photo: Mark Edwards/ Still Pictures)*

One possible explanation for this anomaly is that anthropologists began with inappropriate assumptions. Their point of reference was their own industrial societies, where material wants and desires are great. But supposing human material wants were limited, and the technical means to meet them were unchanging but broadly adequate: in these circumstances, it would be possible to have a 'low' standard of living but enjoy material plenty. This hypothesis, and evidence to support it, comes from the work of the American anthropologist Marshall Sahlins (whose recent work has questioned whether Western scholars can ever really 'speak for' non-Western peoples). In the 1970s, Sahlins gathered together a great deal of information on hunter–gatherer societies and economies in a book entitled *Stone Age Economics*. The emergence of modern societies, he argued, created new relationships between members of society, one feature of which is the existence of poverty:

> One third to one half of humanity are said to go to bed hungry every night. In the Old Stone Age the fraction must have been much smaller. This is the era of hunger unprecedented. Now, in the time of the greatest technical power, starvation is an institution … This paradox is my whole point. Hunters and gatherers have by force of circumstances an objectively low standard of living. But … all the people's material wants usually can be easily satisfied. The world's most primitive people have few possessions, but they are not poor. Poverty is not a certain small amount of goods, nor is it just a relation between means and ends; above all, it is a relation between people. Poverty is a social status. As such it is the invention of civilisation. (Sahlins, 1974, pp. 36–7)

According to this view, the Agricultural Revolution depended on a much higher degree of social order than previously existed, and the emergence of social hierarchies or strata inevitably produced inequality, wealth and poverty. **Stratification** is typified by the existence of social class or hierarchy, and is one of the most important aspects of health and disease patterns. But the essential point here is that stratification is not unique to industrialised societies. In fact, it seems that every society that produces more than is immediately consumed, that can accumulate a surplus of food or other wealth, inevitably confronts the question of how that surplus should be used. Out of this develops conflict, and such conflicts are resolved within a hierarchical structure in which power is exercised. The emergence of poverty as an 'invention of civilisation' is therefore one feature of the power relationships between different groups in a hierarchical structure.

Returning briefly to the human population of the world, it seems that growth slowed down during the early Christian era, as the Agricultural Revolution reached the limits of easily cultivable land. From AD 200 to 500, population may have been virtually static. Then another cycle of growth commenced, as a medieval economy emerged bringing new technologies of farming, new towns and settlements, and the clearance of large areas of forest. By 1200 world population may have reached 360 million. But again growth faltered as medieval society appeared to reach some limit of expansion and was stricken in Europe by plague and in Asia by Mongol attack. Not until 1500 did the upward path of population resume, accelerating after 1800 as the Industrial Revolution took hold.

Over this great sweep of time, therefore, we can see in faint outline the links between population size, disease, and the food supply or more generally the economic base. Historians and paleo-anthropologists (who study ancient civilizations and tribal groups) face great difficulties in attempting to assess the degree to which food supplies may have affected the health of populations in the past. No one questions that there must be some connection: if a population is constant in size, or nearly so over a long period, there must be sufficient food to sustain it at that level. Equally, if numbers are continuously growing, food supply must be continuously expanding. The controversy is about the nature of the mechanism that holds the balance between the two.

5.5 Balancing population and resources

Many people have tried to understand and explain the nature of the links between population and resources, but one of the most influential was Thomas Malthus. Let us now see what light his work casts on the pre-industrial world.

5.5.1 Thomas Malthus

The Reverend Thomas Malthus (Figure 5.4) was born near Dorking in Surrey in 1766 and died in 1834. As you will see, the lifetime of 'Population Malthus' (as he was caricatured) covered a key period of history. Like that of Machiavelli, the first great modern political theorist, the name of Malthus has acquired a patina of unpleasantness. It is not always clear whether this is because he has been regarded as having made observations which were untrue, or simply unpleasant; certainly his work has at times been enlisted in support of repressive ideologies.

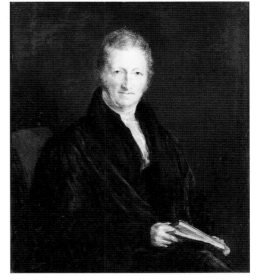

In 1798 Malthus published the first edition of *An Essay on the Principles of Population*, in which he put forward the following views, which we can call the **Malthusian model**.

1   The survival and increase of a population is completely dependent upon the means of subsistence.

Figure 5.4 *Thomas Malthus, 1766–1834, painted by J. Linnel in 1833. (Source: Courtesy of Haileybury and Imperial Service College, Hertfordshire)*

2   The 'passion between the sexes' is so strong and unalterable 'that population, when unchecked, goes on doubling itself every twenty-five years, or increases in a geometrical ratio'.

3   As a general rule, it is simply not possible for the means of subsistence to grow in the same geometrical ratio as population: 'Taking the population of the world at any number, a thousand millions, for instance, the human species would increase in a ratio of: 1, 2, 4, 8, 16, 32, 64, 128, 256, 512, etc., and subsistence as: 1, 2, 3, 4, 5, 6, 7, 8, 9, 10, etc. In two centuries and a quarter, the population would be to the means of subsistence as 512 to 10'. (Malthus, 1970 edition, pp. 25–26)

4   This disequilibrium is prevented from arising by a set of checks, producing 'misery or vice', which are unfortunately to be found 'in ample portion' in 'the cup of human life'. The main checks that he identified were starvation and the outbreak of epidemics of infectious diseases.

●   What strikes you about the kind of checks on population increase that Malthus identified?

■   In this first essay on population, Malthus concentrated on checks which increased *mortality* among the existing population, rather than checks on the number of births.

Malthus labelled these checks on the existing population as **positive checks on population growth**. At this stage, he barely considered the possibility of checks such as *coitus interruptus* and other forms of contraceptive practice which were known and practised, such as abortion, infanticide and — perhaps most important of all — the pattern of marriage. He later styled these as **preventive checks on population growth**.

How can **marriage patterns** influence the birth rate? In most societies childrearing outside marriage carries certain moral, social, legal or economic penalties, which are often strong enough to deter people from having children until they are married. It follows that two key features of marriage patterns can affect the birth rate:

1   The proportion of the population who enter into marriage — referred to by demographers as **nuptiality**;

2   The average *age* of marriage, which influences the potential childbearing years of women. (The importance of marriage patterns in the demographic history of England will be examined in Chapter 6.)

Malthus initially failed to understand the importance of marriage patterns: he took a view similar to that of Dr Johnson: 'It is not from reason and prudence that people marry, but from inclination. A man is poor; he thinks, "I cannot be worse, and so I'll e'en take Peggy".' Later, however, Malthus grasped more fully the importance of marriage patterns and other preventive checks, which he put under the heading of 'moral restraint'.

5.5.2   The Malthusian model in action

The overall scheme of **Malthus' Theory of Population** is shown in Figure 5.5. Looking at this figure, you will see that there are two loops: the upper one deals with the positive checks on populations, and the lower one with the preventive checks.

The centre row of the figure begins by showing a positive association between population size and food prices; that is, a rise in population size leads to a rise in food prices, a fall in population size to a fall in food prices.

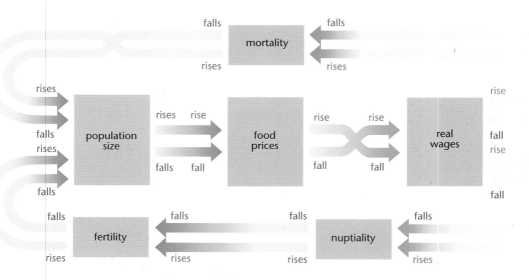

Figure 5.5   *A schematic representation of Malthus' Theory of Population.* Upper loop: 'positive checks' on population size mediated by changes in mortality rates. Lower loop: 'preventive checks' mediated by changes in nuptiality and fertility.

The next part of the figure connects food prices and real wages. Rising food prices mean that the same amount of money buys less food, and so real wages fall. Conversely, if prices were to fall, real wages would rise; in other words, there is an *inverse* relationship between food prices and real wages.

The upper loop shows that as real wages fall so mortality starts to rise through starvation, malnutrition and disease. The rise in mortality is the final positive check on population size, which falls back as 'nature wields her red pencil', and as the population size comes down so food prices start to fall, and so on.

Following the lower loop, the effect of a fall in real wages brought about by population increase is to lower the nuptiality rate and increase the average age of marriage: to paraphrase Dr Johnson, a man becomes poorer, realises things are worse, and postpones taking Peggy. As nuptiality falls, so fertility falls, and thus the population increase is thrown into reverse.

5.5.3 Inventiveness and self-regulation

Malthus was one of the first to suggest that 'positive checks' to the size of human populations might be imposed at some point by an upper limit to food production. In part, his argument was an attempt to counter contemporaries such as the anarchist philosopher William Godwin, who believed in the possibility of constant social progress and improvement. 'Man is perfectible, or in other words susceptible of perpetual improvement', Godwin asserted. Godwin railed against Malthus' insistence that the earth imposed limits on social development, stressing instead the almost boundless inventiveness and creativity of humans: in time, he contended, mankind would have the ability to produce its entire food supply from a solitary flowerpot.

More recently, ecologists and evolutionary biologists have developed another position, which modifies Malthus' view that the 'natural' sizes of populations are determined by the capacity of their environments to support them, and introduces the idea of population **self-regulation**. The numbers of many small-bodied species such as insects and some small mammals and birds fluctuate continuously through phases of 'boom and bust', and the kind of 'positive checks' Malthus identified are strongly in evidence. However, ecologists have now identified many examples of physiological and/or behavioural mechanisms which provide a 'feedback' link, whereby the *current* density of a population influences the *subsequent* reproductive performance of individual members — a process known as **density-dependent reproduction**. The most common way this kind of spacing behaviour happens is through territoriality. Each individual or kinship-related group such as a troop of animals dominates a fixed area. Those unable to find and defend territory of their own are denied access to mates or to breeding sites, and are more vulnerable to predators. This results in populations that regulate themselves at levels which are always somewhat below the maximum that existing food supplies could sustain.

Whether humans have self-regulating characteristics which might have operated to control population size in the distant past is of course impossible to prove, since it would require detailed long-term studies of human groups living in an environment unmodified by the activities of modern people. However, as you saw earlier in this chapter, evidence collected from surviving groups of hunter–gatherers, and everything that is known about the way such groups lived in the past, suggests that they almost certainly exercised population control to keep their numbers somewhat below the carrying capacity of their environment and provide some safety margin for times of scarcity. Moreover, as ecologists Robert Moss and Adam Watson and zoologist John Ollason suggest in their book *Animal Population Dynamics* (1982), most larger-bodied animals — particularly those, like humans, with slow rates of reproduction and systems of co-operative social group organisation — have been shown either to self-regulate their numbers, or at least display characteristics which would produce density-dependent reproduction or other kinds of spacing behaviour.

5.5.4 Natural selection and fitness

Stable characteristics such as spacing behaviour must have evolved over a long time span, appearing first in one individual and, over many generations, spreading through the whole population. According to modern evolutionary theory, characteristics that become shared by every member of the population did so because they conferred some survival advantage on those individuals in which the characteristics originally evolved. When there is competition for resources, **natural selection** of the best adapted individuals ensures that their genes (and hence their characteristics) are passed on to succeeding generations. A characteristic that increases the chance of an individual surviving long enough to reproduce, and for its offspring to reproduce in their turn, is said to increase the individual's reproductive success or **fitness**. But, to return to the theme of biological checks on population growth, spacing behaviour is a characteristic that *reduces* the chance of reproduction.

At first sight it is difficult to understand how evolution could result in characteristics that cause an individual animal to forgo (either consciously, or involuntarily) some part of its own reproductive success in order to promote the fitness of others. This looks like an example of purely altruistic behaviour which (other than that between parents and offspring) could not be expected to evolve, if the only thing that counts is competition for survival and transmission to future generations of sets of genes which are carried by individuals. But many species do display individual behaviour which, translated into human terms, could be described as apparently self-sacrificing. This either involves exposure to immediate risk from predators, or the acceptance of a seemingly reduced chance of procreation.

The clue to understanding this apparent paradox lies in a controversial concept called **inclusive fitness**. In brief, this interpretation of evolutionary processes suggests that the competition for survival and propagation of genes operates *between groups* of related individuals, as well as between the individuals who belong to these groups. Because, through kinship, they share among them some identical pieces of genetic information, individuals will display characteristics which promote the survival of that common information set, even at the cost of a threat to their own survival: hence inclusive fitness. The evolutionary biologist Richard Dawkins argued in his book *The Selfish Gene* (1976), that what looks superficially like a choice of altruistic behaviour by an animal, can alternatively be understood as an act of pure self-interest on the part of the genes that the animal carries in its cells.

On balance, it seems unlikely that humans would have been such a successful species in biological terms, unless they also displayed a capacity for self-regulation of numbers. As both human history and the study of other species shows, this strategy does not prevent the kind of famines which are the result of external or perhaps random processes, such as shifts of climatic zones, unusual sequences of bad weather, warfare with other groups of humans or invasions of territory by other species such as locusts. It does however prevent famines being repeatedly and regularly caused by population outstripping food supply. What is significant for this discussion of the general relationship between food and health, is that it suggests that the prehistoric condition of humanity, although far from paradisiacal, should not be thought of as a more or less permanent state of near starvation. This is the point Sahlins also made in the discussion earlier in this chapter.

5.6   Evidence for the Malthusian model

How do these different views of Malthus, Godwinian optimists and evolutionary biologists compare with what we now know of population history around the time that Malthus was alive? In fact, there is evidence in support of all three positions but, putting qualifications temporarily to one side, it is Malthus' harsh picture of human existence in the centuries preceding 1800 that seems to be closest to the mark. Summarising the available evidence, the economic historian Carlo Cipolla gives the following assessment:

> ... any agricultural society ... tends to adhere to a definite set of patterns in the structure and movements of birth- and death-rates. Crude birth-rates are very high throughout, ranging between 35 and 55 per thousand ... Death-rates are also very high, but normally lower than the birth-rates — ranging generally between 30 and 40 per thousand ... [But] death-rates show a remarkable tendency to recurrent, sudden dramatic peaks that reach levels as high as 150 or 300 or even 500 per thousand. On a few occasions these peaks coincided with wars. But much more frequently they were the result of epidemics and famines that wiped out a good part of the existing population ... The intensity and frequency of the peaks controlled the size of agricultural societies. (Cipolla, 1974, pp. 85–7)

A more detailed picture is provided by the French historian, Fernand Braudel, in *The Structures of Everyday Life* (1981), which is the first volume of a monumental and richly referenced history of civilisation and capitalism from the fifteenth to the eighteenth century. What characterised this period, writes Braudel, was 'a number of deaths roughly equivalent to the number of births; very high infant mortality; famine; chronic undernourishment; and formidable epidemics' (p. 91). It was a precarious battle for existence 'waged on at least two fronts; against the scarcity and inadequacy of the food supply ... and against the many and insidious forms of disease that lay in wait' (p. 90). Famine was ever-present: in France, for example, there were '10 general famines during the tenth century; 26 in the eleventh; 2 in the twelfth; 4 in the fourteenth; 7 in the fifteenth; 13 in the sixteenth; 11 in the seventeenth and 16 in the eighteenth' (p. 74). In the 1696–7 famine in Finland, a quarter or a third of the population perished. 'Things were far worse in Asia, China and India. Famines there seemed like the end of the world ... In 1555 and again in 1596, violent famine throughout north-west India resulted in scenes of cannibalism ...' (p. 76), and on and on.

Moreover, 'famine was never an isolated event. Sooner or later it opened the door to epidemics'. Each fresh disaster, however, was followed by a reassertion of life, as the population bounced back: for example,

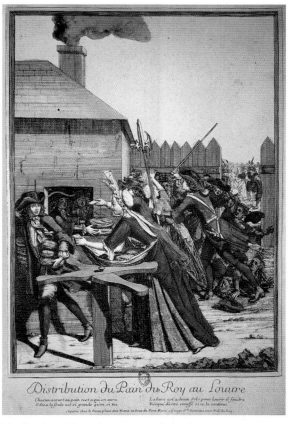

Distribution of bread to the poor in Paris, the Louvre, in the famine of 1662. (Photo: The Art Archive)

when plague mowed down the population of Verona in 1637, '… the soldiers of the garrison, almost all French — many of whom had escaped the plague — married the widows and life gained the upper hand again' (p. 71). Rise and fall is the rhythm of population history and of 'standard of living', each cycle permeating the whole fabric of life: 'trees and wild animals overran fields that had once flourished. But soon the population again increased and had to win back the land taken over by animals and wild plants, clear the stones from the fields and pull up trees and shrubs' (p. 33). What evidence we have suggests that this rhythm stretched across the inhabited world, a procession of 'social massacres' and revivals that seems to confirm the Malthusian model.

However, underlying the increases and decreases was a faint but perceptible longer-term trend, where 'revival ultimately had the last word. The ebb never entirely removed what the preceding tide had brought in' (p. 92), and the population of the world slowly increased, as you saw earlier in this chapter. Second, although famines were widespread and sometimes frequent, they were none the less periodic events with some respite allowed in between. The fact that specific dates of violent famines in north-west India are recorded, for instance, could be interpreted as implying that chronic malnutrition and widespread starvation was *not* the continual norm there. Third, we know from the monuments and relics of the past, that, whatever relationship existed between the mass of population and the means of subsistence, sufficient surplus was provided by the economic system to invest in mammoth schemes of building, often on a scale that might impose severe strains on not only the developing countries of today, but also on some industrialised countries (Figure 5.6).

There are so many gaps in our knowledge of the pre-industrial world that there is ample room for disagreement. We have seen one picture of the world as essentially a procession of 'social massacres', of sweeping epidemics, famines, and 'die-offs' as the population seemed to collide with the subsistence barrier in the way Malthus expected. On the other hand there is evidence, at least in parts of the world, that to be poor did not imply continual misery and uncertainty about where the next meal was to come from. What is certain is that, even as Malthus was writing, a decisive break with his scheme of things was about to occur, caused by the sequence of events and changes known as the 'Industrial Revolution'.

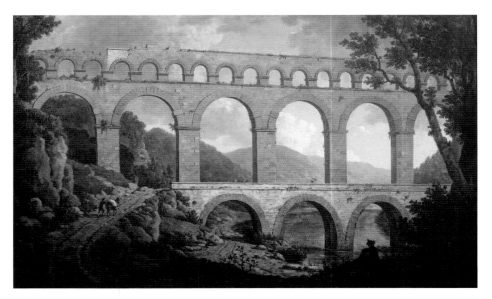

Figure 5.6
Subsistence or surplus? The Roman Pont du Gard aqueduct, Nimes, is typical of the massive building works that pre-industrial societies could produce. From a painting by William Marlow (1740–1813) © Sheffield Galleries and Museums Trust. (Photo: Bridgeman Art Library)

5.7 The Industrial Revolution

5.7.1 England escapes from the Malthusian model

It is paradoxical that the first country in the world for which there is evidence that the Malthusian model no longer applied was the same country in which the theory was formulated: eighteenth-century England. Here it seems that the population was not pressed hard against the basic means of subsistence, that bad harvests could be overcome without too much hardship or hunger, and that the population could slowly grow without causing real wages to slump. For example, one French traveller, the Abbé le Blanc, making his way from the south coast to London in 1747, was 'struck with the beauties of the country, the care taken to improve lands, the richness of the pastures, the numerous flocks that cover them, and the air of plenty and cleanliness that reigns in the smallest villages' (quoted in Hobsbawm, 1969, p. 11).

Figure 5.7 shows changes in the population of England from the sixteenth to the eighteenth century, and changes in real wages over the same period. Some of the problems involved in estimating population size have already been discussed. The problems of estimating the average value of wages over such a long period are in many ways even more difficult to solve. The real wage index for England from 1551 to 1900 shown in Figure 5.7 is based on the work of two population historians, Anthony Wrigley and Roger Schofield who, remarkably, managed to trace the wage rates of builders and the price of various foodstuffs back to the twelfth century! (Phelps, Brown and Hopkins, 1956, reworked by Wrigley and Schofield, 1989).[1]

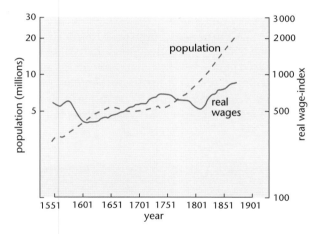

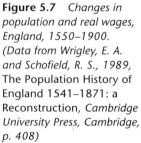

Figure 5.7 *Changes in population and real wages, England, 1550–1900. (Data from Wrigley, E. A. and Schofield, R. S., 1989,* The Population History of England 1541–1871: a Reconstruction, *Cambridge University Press, Cambridge, p. 408)*

● Look carefully at Figure 5.7. What are the main features of it that strike you as important? Does the figure fit the Malthusian model?

■ In the years up to 1600 we can see population increasing and real wages falling, a pattern that broadly fits in with the Malthusian theory. Around 1650 population growth is checked, while real wages are rising. Then from about 1700 to 1750 population starts rising again (and this growth accelerates after 1800). Meanwhile, real wages decline very slowly, but around 1800 they start rising also: a sustained and rapid increase in the population has not set off the system of checks Malthus predicted.

[1] The research methods used by Wrigley and Schofield to construct their population history of England from 1541–1871, are discussed in *Studying Health and Disease* (Open University Press, 2nd edn 1994; colour-enhanced 2nd edn 2001), Chapter 4.

England was the first country in the world to experience this pattern of development. This is why it is important to look closely at what happened in England before returning to a world view. The problem in explaining what happened is that it was a unique event, and cannot be repeated experimentally to increase knowledge of why — or even precisely how — it happened. The first key to understanding what was happening takes us back to Malthus and his geometrical versus arithmetical rates of growth of population and the means of subsistence (agriculture).

In eighteenth-century England, agriculture was undergoing a whole series of changes which allowed it to expand at a rate that at least kept up with the increasing population. This expansion was made possible in part by new techniques such as crop rotation, stock-breeding (Figure 5.8), the famous seed-drilling machine invented by Jethro Tull, and improved drainage and fertilisers. New crops were also introduced: clover and hays (which provided winter feeds so that livestock could be fed over the winter months); root crops (such as carrots and parsnips from the Low Countries); and the potato, introduced in the sixteenth century from America by Walter Raleigh (and first domesticated in Andean America during the first Agricultural Revolution many thousands of years previously). There seems little doubt that the potato was the predominant influence on the growth of population in Ireland, and had a significant effect in Britain from about 1750. Finally, in the eighteenth century, the construction of canals in Britain is thought to have made a major contribution to improving the distribution of the increased amounts of food being produced, as did improvements in coast, river, and road transport.

But these changes in technique and technology were encouraged and widely adopted largely because of other social and economic upheavals that were also taking place. For example, common land was taken over and enclosed by a new class of private landowners. Although this resulted in the size of fields and of farms being rapidly expanded, it also meant that the peasant subsistence farming, which had been based on small plots of land, was completely disrupted and then painfully eliminated. Thus Malthus' view that agricultural production could not increase at more than a slow, 'arithmetical' ratio of growth was made obsolete at the very time that he was developing his theory. Agricultural growth was fast enough to lift the checks on population growth by facilitating both a reduction in mortality and allowing the birth rate to increase.

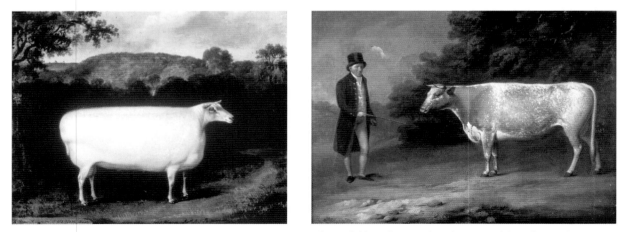

Figure 5.8 *Eighteenth-century agricultural change in England: careful breeding produced improved farm livestock, such as these proudly displayed animals: Four Shear Ram by T. Weaver, 1831 and Shorthorn Cow, 1800 (artist unknown). (Source: © Museum of English Rural Life, University of Reading)*

As we noted earlier, there is no agreement over why the Industrial Revolution commenced in the way, the place and the time that it did. Some theories have laid stress on factors such as climate. For example, it has been suggested that weather conditions in the eighteenth century provided a long series of good harvests in England, and that the surplus produced triggered off wider changes. This argument, however, does not explain why previous runs of good harvests did not produce similar changes. Other theories have focused on the values of the Protestant Reformation, arguing that Protestantism was ideally matched to the innovative and individualistic forces required to alter England's economic and social system. But again, this argument does not explain why Catholic Belgium was quicker to follow England's lead than Protestant Holland. The break-down of the Malthusian model, coupled with major agricultural and demographic changes, were simply part of a much bigger set of changes occurring in England at that time, and attributing such changes to a single factor such as climate or religion ignores the many circumstances and combinations of factors that were undoubtedly present.

5.7.2 Defining the Industrial Revolution

So what do we mean by the **Industrial Revolution**? We commonly think of it in terms of a sudden increase in economic activity, and this is certainly part of it. The last quarter of the eighteenth century in England witnessed a boom in the construction of canals and roads, a flourishing of the cotton and textiles industries, a doubling of imports and exports, and a sudden increase in the size of towns such as Manchester.

However, to reach a definition of the Industrial Revolution that will help us to understand what was happening, we must think not simply in terms of *quantitative* change, of an increase in the amount of economic activity. As the English economic historian Eric Hobsbawm points out, the important point to grasp is that the Industrial Revolution was

> ... not merely an acceleration of economic growth, but an acceleration of growth because of, and through, economic and social transformation [culminating in] ... self-sustained economic growth by means of perpetual technological revolution and social transformation. (Hobsbawm, 1969, p. 20)

This concept of **social transformation**, or changes in the social structures that regulated human life, is the cornerstone of the process of development and social change. This process dramatically altered the everyday life of the population of England, and also altered the nature of the relationship between newly industrialised countries such as England and the rest of the world, with profound consequences for patterns of health and disease.

One example of the changes in social structures occurring during the process of industrialisation in England involved the use of land and of agricultural labour. At the beginning of the eighteenth century, at least half of the agricultural land in Britain was farmed on an open-field system. This system gave equal shares of good and bad land to each farmer in a community, with no physical barrier between the farmed strips, and with each farmer's cattle grazing together on common pasture. But weeds spread easily, as did cattle disease, and there were few incentives to improve or innovate. The economic historian Michael Flinn comments:

> The system, originating almost a thousand years before, was devised to ensure livelihoods for all members of the communities. In protecting the weak, it inevitably hampered the strong and enterprising. (Flinn, 1965, p. 170)

During the second half of the eighteenth century, however, the need to feed England's rapidly rising population placed farmers under intense pressure to expand production, and this open-field system was pushed aside by Acts of Parliament and commercial pressure. The land was enclosed into compact areas of fenced land, and customs of access and use were renounced. In the 34 years up to 1760, a mere 70 000 acres were enclosed, but between 1760 and 1792 the total jumped by half a million, and by 1812 had increased by a further million acres. In consequence, a large number of people no longer had any direct access to the produce of the land, their means of subsistence was cut away, and many became destitute paupers.

It would be impossible to put any figure on the mortality or morbidity that may have resulted from this dislocation, but it is quite plausible to argue that, from being poor but relatively comfortable, large numbers of people became poor and frequently desperate about getting enough to eat. In 25 of the 37 years from 1811 to 1848, for example, the agricultural areas of England witnessed widespread rioting and disorder, and their plight is summed up in the words of a rioter from the Fens in 1816:

> Here I am between Earth and Sky, so help me God. I would sooner lose my life than go home as I am. Bread I want and bread I will have. (quoted in Hobsbawm, 1969, p. 74)

According to this Punch cartoon, agricultural destitution was still an issue in the 1860s. (Punch, 19 September 1863)

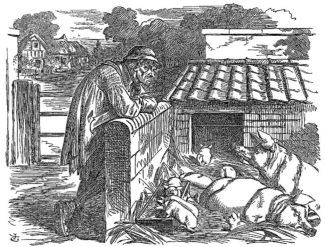

THE PIG AND THE PEASANT.
PEASANT. 'AH! I'D LIKE TO BE CARED VOR HALF AS WELL AS THEE BE!'

5.7.3 Creating an industrial labour force

Accompanying these changes in land ownership and land use, an entirely different kind of labour force was created. In modern industrialised countries such as Britain, the great majority of people make a living for themselves and their dependants by obtaining work from an employer in return for a wage or salary. Such paid employment normally takes place separated from home and family in offices or factories where quite large numbers of people work. In pre-industrial England the contrast is striking. Although wage-labour was not uncommon — even in the sixteenth century perhaps two-thirds of all households earned some part of their living from wages — nevertheless, far fewer households were dependent on wages for all of their living all of the time. Instead, they worked the land tied to the home and exchanged the produce for other necessities. And in the home they carried out 'industrial' activities such as spinning or weaving. Because agricultural work is seasonal, large numbers of people would have spent part of the year looking for other forms of employment, and some would fail to find any and become beggars. But, as the British historian Peter Laslett has observed:

> the trouble then … was not so much unemployment, as under-employment, as it is now called … the comparison is with the countries of Asia in our own century. Too many members of a family were half-busied about an inadequate plot of infertile land; not enough work could be found for the women and children to do around the cottage fire, in some districts none at all, for there was no rural industry in them. (Laslett, 1971, p. 33)

●   What similarities strike you between this description of pre-industrial England and the case study of village life in Bangladesh in Chapter 4?

■   Temporary migration to casual labouring jobs, pavement-dwelling in cities and short-term unskilled employment are features of life for the rural population in Bangladesh and for pre-industrial England.

During the Industrial Revolution in England, therefore, another change in social structures was the transformation of the workforce into much larger groupings of employees dependent on wages. Without this transformation, it would not have been possible to organise production in factories and the industrial towns they gave rise to, or to increase the specialisation of tasks and the division of labour, or to practice the rapid hiring and firing of labour that accompanied technical innovation. A mass of labouring people was created, depending for their livelihood on selling their labour. Only this wage relationship stood between the labourer and destitution, and if jobs were scarce destitution was rife. Even with a job, there was no guarantee that the wage the employer chose to pay would adequately sustain the labourer.

5.7.4 An industrial society

These changes in the position of land and labour would not have been possible without a series of even more profound and subtle social transformations. An economy based on commodity exchange and markets can only operate with the use of *money*, and the role of money had been increasing in English society since at least the Tudor period. Shakespeare frequently mentions the growth in the importance of money, and in *Timon of Athens* he was scathing about the

> … common whore of mankind, that putt'st odds among the rout of nations … Thus much of this will make black, white; foul, fair; wrong, right; base, noble; old, young; coward, valiant … This yellow slave will knit and break religions. (Shakespeare, *Timon of Athens* IV, iii, pp. 28–44)

A final example of the changed social structures that occurred during the Industrial Revolution, is provided by the historian Edward Thompson in a study of changing perceptions of *time*. Thompson begins by noting the way in which clock time was irrelevant and disregarded in any pre-industrial fishing, crafting or farming community

> … whose framework of marketing and administration is minimal, and in which the day's tasks (which might vary from fishing to farming, building, mending of nets, thatching, making a cradle or a coffin) seem to disclose themselves, by the logic of need, before the crofter's eyes (Thompson, 1967).

He perfectly illustrates his point with an observation made by the Irish writer J. M. Synge on a visit to the Aran Islands, off the coast of County Clare:

> The general knowledge of time on the island depends, curiously enough, upon the direction of the wind. Nearly all the cottages are built … with two doors opposite each other, the more sheltered of which lies open all day to give light to the interior. If the wind is northerly the south door is opened, and the shadow of the door-post moving across the kitchen floor indicates the hour; as soon, however, as the wind changes to the south the other door is opened, and the people, who never think of putting up a primitive dial, are at a loss … When the wind is from the north the old woman manages my meals with fair regularity; but on the other days she often makes my tea at three o'clock instead of six. (Quoted in Thompson, 1967, p. 59)

RULES AND REGULATIONS
TO BE OBSERVED BY THE
WORKMEN
EMPLOYED BY
SAMUEL BASTOW,
CLIFF HOUSE IRON WORKS.

I.

The Engagement of each Workman shall be subject to a Fortnight's Notice, such Notice to be given at the Office on the pay day only, except in Cases of Dismissal for misconduct.

II.

Each Workman to enter and leave Work by the Office Door, where he must put his Ticket in the Box in the Morning, and at each Meal-time, or he will not have any time allowed for such neglect, the Box being open Five Minutes for that purpose, previous to the time of commencing Work; and in the Morning Five Minutes after the time for commencing Work.

III.

Any Workman absenting himself from his Employment for a longer period than 2 Working Days, without leave, shall be held to have left his service, and dealt with accordingly.

IV.

Work to commence at 6 o'clock in the Morning, and to end at 6 o'clock at Night, except on Saturdays, when the Days Work shall end at 4 o'clock, and on the Pay Saturday at 2 o'clock, no Dinner hour being allowed.

V.

Meal Hours to be from 8 to ½ past 8 o'clock, for Breakfast; and 12 to 1 o'clock, for Dinner. No Dinner Hour being allowed on Pay Saturdays.

VI.

Time to be kept by the *Hour*.—10 Working Hours to be a day's work.

VII.

The Door shall be closed every Morning when the Bell Rings, at 6 o'clock; but, should any Workman over-sleep himself, he may be admitted at 10 minutes past 6 o'clock, forfeiting ½ an hour.

The new work disciplines of the Industrial Revolution: factory regulations in Hartlepool, 1857. (Source: R. Wood, from Shellard, P. (1970) Factory Life in 1774–1885, Evans Bros)

● Why might such nature-dependent rhythms of life and work be incompatible with life in industrial society?

■ The operation of a large factory using powered machinery and employing several hundred workers, or the running of a railway network or school, requires coordination of time-keeping by everyone concerned.

And so the Industrial Revolution witnessed a complete restructuring of the whole rhythm of life, with clocks and bells, timetables and schedules, set times for eating, sleeping, working and resting, and a sharp distinction between work and the rest of life.

In short, the whole process of industrial development meant much more than a growth in the national product: the kinds of processes outlined above make it clear that development cannot be seen as simply a quantitative increase in economic activity brought about by technological changes. Development did eventually bring massive improvements in health to England, which will be looked at in much more detail in Chapter 6 of this book. However, these were only one facet of a complete social, political, cultural and economic upheaval, which caused massive social dislocation, which did not happen overnight, and which was accompanied for a long period by great hardship and misery among the rural and especially the urban populations before general improvements in the standard of living and levels of health began to appear.

5.7.5 Reactions to the Industrial Revolution

At the time, many people were horrified at the consequences of the Industrial Revolution in England. Some, like the Romantic poets, recoiled from it and wished to reject it completely. Others, like Charles Dickens and his illustrator, Gustave Doré, devoted their lives to exposing its cruelties (Figure 5.9). And some, like the German social revolutionary Frederick Engels, condemned the conditions that the Industrial

Revolution had created as part of a critique of the whole social order. An extract from the book he published in 1845, *The Condition of the Working Class in England*, is included (as 'Health: 1844') in *Health and Disease: A Reader* (Open University Press, 2nd edn 1994; 3rd edn 2001). (Open University students should read it now.)

● In the statistics he quotes, Engels concentrates on two particular aspects of the pattern of health and disease: social class differences and differences between town and country. What findings does he make?

■ Engels notes that scarlet fever, rachitis (rickets) and scrofula were confined largely to the working classes, and did not seriously afflict the middle and upper classes. He also draws on evidence that the mortality rate in lower-class streets was up to twice as high as in upper-class streets. He then observes that the death rate in the industrial cities — at around one in thirty — was substantially higher than in rural districts, where it was around one in forty. (It is interesting to compare this with modern rural : urban mortality rates, which Table 3.5 showed are generally higher in rural areas.)

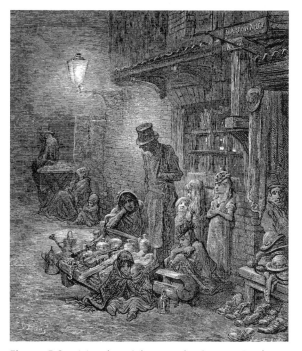

Figure 5.9   *A London night scene by Gustave Doré, 1871. Doré's images were a major influence on the twentieth century's view of the cruelties of the Industrial Revolution. (Source: The Mansell Collection)*

● Within an historical perspective, what other dimension of health and disease patterns not considered in the extract would be of particular interest?

■ Perhaps the most important is some comparison of health and disease patterns around 1844 with patterns before the Industrial Revolution.

Intense controversy surrounds the question of the initial health consequences of the Industrial Revolution. This controversy is part of a wider dispute about trends in the standard of living of the population for, although it is plain that from the 1840s onwards average standards of living were definitely rising, the pattern before then is not at all clear. The fact that there is no obvious answer to this question suggests that there can have been very little if any general improvement for at least half a century.

But, whatever the short-term consequences of the Industrial Revolution in England, a giant break with the past had clearly occurred, involving among many other things, health and disease patterns, populations and food. The next step, therefore, is to look in more detail at the impact of the Industrial Revolution on the health and the population of England.

OBJECTIVES FOR CHAPTER 5

When you have studied this chapter, you should be able to:

5.1 Define and use, or recognise definitions and applications of, each of the terms printed in **bold** in the text.

5.2 Summarise the available information on disease patterns in early human societies up to and including the first Agricultural Revolution.

5.3 Sketch the broad history of human population growth to the mid-nineteenth century.

5.4 Outline the Malthusian population model, and the alternative views of Godwinian optimists and evolutionary biologists. Then assess evidence from the pre-industrial world about the validity of these views of population change.

5.5 Outline the principal features of the Industrial Revolution in England, giving due emphasis to changes both in economic activity and social structures.

5.6 Describe the initial impact of the Industrial Revolution on the living conditions in English cities and among the rural peasantry.

QUESTIONS FOR CHAPTER 5

1 (*Objective 5.2*)

We have almost no hard data on how disease patterns altered during the first Agricultural Revolution. Why is it possible to state fairly confidently that infectious diseases were a much bigger threat *after* this revolution than before?

2 (*Objective 5.3*)

'Stability punctuated by sudden changes.' How accurate is this as a description of human population history in the eighteenth century?

3 (*Objective 5.4*)

In the Malthusian population model, population and real wages are linked in two ways. Describe them briefly.

4 (*Objective 5.5*)

In the eighteenth and nineteenth centuries, many public buildings in England began to display clocks, and there was a big expansion in the manufacture of cheap pocket watches. What does this tell you about changes in English society at the time?

5 (*Objective 5.6*)

According to Engels, life in England's nineteenth-century cities was one of 'toil and wretchedness, rich in suffering and poor in enjoyment'. And yet many people were migrating to the cities from rural areas. How would you account for this?

CHAPTER 6

The decline of infectious diseases: the case of England

Study notes for OU students

During Section 6.5 of this chapter you will be asked to read two extracts contained in *Health and Disease: A Reader* (Open University Press, second edition 1995; third edition 2001). The first is, 'The medical contribution' by Thomas McKeown, taken from his book *The Modern Rise of Populations*. The second is, 'The importance of social intervention in Britain's mortality decline, 1850–1914: a reinterpretation of the role of public health' by Simon Szreter.

6.1 Introduction

The rise of industrial society sketched in the previous chapter has profoundly affected the world in which we live. This chapter looks in more detail at the effects of the Industrial Revolution on health. Focusing on just one country, England, the chapter surveys what is known of changes over time in disease patterns and demographic structure. England makes a good subject for this survey, because it had a pioneering role in the Industrial Revolution and has good records of disease and demography covering a relatively long period of time. (Scotland and Wales, which also made a pioneering contribution to industrial society, have population histories which are equally interesting and display many similar features, but which are less comprehensively documented and researched.) However, just as the introduction to the description of village life in Bangladesh (in Chapter 4) warned of the dangers of generalising from one case study, so the same applies in this chapter. Although England is, in many respects, a typical industrialised country, it is also in other ways unique, not least because it was the first industrial nation.

The chapter is divided into three periods. The first begins with the earliest available quantitative data on population size — the Doomsday Book of 1086 — and stops around 1680. All such historical 'book-marks' are a little artificial, but 1680 is chosen because it is believed that at around this time the population size started to increase rapidly, considerably faster than during the preceding centuries. The end of the seventeenth century also marks the end of the second pandemic of plague (1666). The second period covered in the chapter is from 1680 to 1850, around which date accurate and reliable information on cause of death became widely available. The chapter concludes with the period from 1850 to the beginning of the twenty-first century.

6.2 Infection, famine and mortality crises, 1086–1680

The period from the first agricultural communities to the end of the seventeenth century — a passage of around 10 000 years — is significant for the consistency rather than the changes in the pattern of diseases that affected humans. The main threats to health remained infectious diseases and food shortages. These two, together with violence, both accidental and deliberate (such as warfare), accounted for almost all deaths. Their relative contribution and demographic impact are our main concern when considering this period.

Much of our knowledge is speculative, based on a variety of different sources: from archaeology, diaries, chronicles and other texts, parish registers of births and deaths since the sixteenth century, and Bills of Mortality from the following century. Most of the information on disease tends to be limited to records of mortality: the ages at which people died; the numbers dying at a particular time; and the causes of their deaths. This is a problem you have already encountered in earlier chapters, that our picture of the spectrum of disease is biased towards the more lethal diseases. In addition, because of the even greater limitations of epidemiological information on mental illness, throughout this chapter the emphasis will be on physical (often termed 'somatic') illness.

6.2.1 Population 1086–1680

England is especially interesting to students of historical demography because records of its population are so detailed: parish registers of births, marriages and deaths were introduced in 1538, and form a set of records that begins earlier and is wider in coverage than in any other country. Estimates of population before this date are much less reliable, although sources such as the Doomsday Book of 1086 and the poll-tax returns of 1377 are very useful. From figures recorded in the Doomsday Book, the population of England has been estimated as numbering about 1.75 million in 1086, and that is taken as the starting point for Figure 6.1, which shows estimates of changes in the size of the population of England from 1100 to 1820.

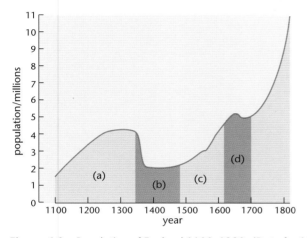

Figure 6.1 *Population of England 1100–1820. (Data for 1100–1540 from Chambers, I. D., 1972,* Population, Economy and Society in Pre-Industrial England, *Oxford University Press, Oxford, Figure 1; for 1540–1820 from Wrigley, E. A. and Schofield, R. S., 1989,* The Population History of England 1541–1871: a Reconstruction, *Cambridge University Press, Cambridge, Table A3.1)*

● Consider Figure 6.1 and describe the features of population change during the years (a) 1100–1348, (b) 1348–1480, (c) 1480–1620, and (d) 1620–1700.

■ You should have noted that: (a) from 1100 to 1348 the population appears to have trebled in size; (b) from 1348 to 1480 there was an overall decline in size, including a possible 50 per cent reduction between about 1348 and 1375; (c) from 1480 to 1620 there was a rapid expansion of population; and (d) that 1620–1700 was a period in which population expansion came almost to a halt.

Although the population figures shown in Figure 6.1 probably represent the current view of most historians, it should be noted that some estimates of the population during the fourteenth century — before the Black Death caused the collapse shown in (b) above — range as high as 5 to 7 million.

Figure 6.2 overleaf shows some other aspects of English population during the period from 1541 right up to the present: the crude birth and death rates and the average annual rate of population growth. From 1541 to 1871 these data are based on estimates from a detailed analysis of many thousands of parish registers, a vast project from which the historians Wrigley and Schofield have reconstructed the history of England's population since 1541.

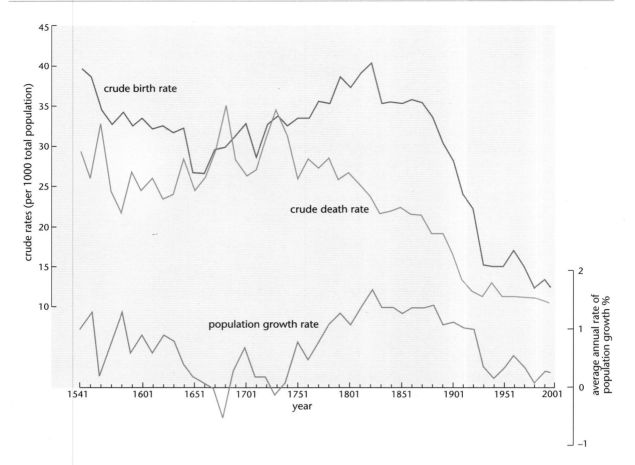

Figure 6.2 *Crude birth rate, crude death rate and average annual rate of population growth, England 1541–1998.*
(Data up to 1871 from Wrigley, E. A. and Schofield, R. S., 1989, The Population History of England 1541–1871:
a Reconstruction, *Cambridge University Press, Cambridge, Table A3.1; from 1871, Registrar General, various years,*
Annual Abstracts of Statistics, *HMSO, London)*

The figure shows that over the period 1541 to about 1631, the birth rate generally exceeded the death rate by a substantial margin, so the rate of population growth was fairly rapid: around 1 per cent per annum on average. But from 1641 to around 1741 birth and death rates are almost in line, so that population growth almost comes to a halt and for a period is reversed (the population growth rate dips below zero between about 1665 and 1685).

● What other feature of the birth and death rates in Figure 6.2 strikes you?

■ They seem to be constantly fluctuating from one decade to another.

These fluctuations become even more marked when annual rates are considered, and the reasons for these fluctuations, especially in the death rate, have attracted a great deal of interest. Let us now look in more detail at these mortality crises.

6.2.2 Mortality crises: frequency and cause

Mortality crises are events where there is a sudden increase in the mortality rate for a fairly short duration. The definition adopted by Wrigley and Schofield is any year in which the crude death rate was at least 10 per cent above the average for the 25 years around that date.

Using this definition, Wrigley and Schofield identified 31 years between 1541 and 1701 in which a mortality crisis occurred in England, or roughly once every 5 years. After 1701 the frequency of such crises fell to once every 13 years on average, although they could be equally severe when they did occur.

● What limitations of the definition of mortality crises used above can you think of?

■ Because it is annual, this definition may miss sudden surges in mortality that last only a month or two. Also, because it is national it may miss local mortality crises.

Using monthly mortality rates from hundreds of parishes, Wrigley and Schofield have been able to throw some light on these *local* mortality crises. They found that in every year around 2 or 3 per cent of all parishes experienced a mortality crisis, but that in years of *national* crisis this rose to between 15 and 20 per cent. However, even in the very worst national crises no more than 40 per cent of parishes were involved. On average a parish might be affected by a mortality crisis six times every century. It would last on average for just over two months, and during it there would be five times the usual number of deaths. Some parishes appeared to be more prone to these crises than others, but less than 1 per cent managed to avoid them completely. Crises were more likely in parishes with a large population, and less likely in parishes that were remote from market towns.

An obvious question posed by these crises is: what caused them? One useful piece of evidence would be to discover whether specific diseases were responsible, and if so, which particular diseases. However, death certificates were not introduced until the nineteenth century, and parish registers seldom entered a cause of death. Therefore, discovering the diseases responsible requires a study of the *demographic features* of each crisis:

• the seasonal pattern of deaths;
• the ages and the social background of the victims;
• the duration of the crisis;
• the size of the geographical area affected.

For example, diarrhoeal diseases such as dysentery are most likely to occur in late summer and early autumn. A crisis that spreads rapidly and widely suggests an airborne infection such as influenza. Deaths of more adults than children would suggest typhus, whereas deaths occurring only among children suggest a smallpox epidemic in an area where smallpox was endemic (i.e. adults would have built up some resistance to the disease).

However, knowledge of the main causes of death from disease during a mortality crisis goes only part way to answering the question of what caused the mortality crisis in the first place: in particular, in trying to establish whether it was related to a shortage of food or a fall in real wages, or simply resulted from an infectious disease that reached epidemic proportions and then died down. The occurrence of mortality crises at times of *adequate* food supplies would lend support to the notion of **autonomous infectious epidemics** (sometimes called **exogenous epidemics**). By this is meant an infectious disease that strikes down large numbers of people *independently* of other factors internal to that society that render the population more vulnerable or trigger the epidemic. By contrast, **endogenous epidemics** are related to social factors such as famine, warfare or **crises of subsistence** (a collapse of the ability to procure food and shelter).

● What evidence on the social backgrounds of the victims of a mortality crisis would suggest autonomous infections as the cause of a mortality crisis, rather than (say) a shortage of food?

■ Deaths occurring in all social sections of the population and not just the poorest and weakest would point to an autonomous infectious epidemic, such as the plague.

In a few cases it is not possible to distinguish autonomous infection from food shortage as being primarily responsible: sometimes they simply coincided — a likely event given the frequency with which they both occurred; or a crisis of subsistence may have stoked an existing outbreak of an infectious disease, particularly if famine and starvation caused an increased number of people to move from rural to urban areas, thus favouring the spread of an infection. Similarly, if the population was weakened by an epidemic infection, this could lead to, or at least exacerbate, a failure to produce sufficient food. However, in most cases it appears that mortality crises were not related to harvest failures or more generally to falling real wages, but were indeed due to autonomous infectious epidemics. It has also been estimated that the mortality rate in a crisis resulting from a lack of food tended to be about three to four times the 'normal' rate, whereas that resulting from an infectious disease outbreak was up to a twelve-fold increase.

6.2.3   The 'Golden Age of Bacteria'

Infectious diseases are caused by micro-organisms such as bacteria and viruses. Although information is limited, we do know something about those diseases responsible for the epidemics during the five or six hundred years up to 1680; about earlier times, however, we can only speculate. One of the most dramatic causes of mortality was plague. Although many recorded cases attributed to plague were almost certainly not due to infection with the plague bacterium (*Yersinia pestis*), this organism *was* responsible for many of the most devastating mortality crises between 1348 and 1666 in Britain.

The first hundred years of that period (1348–1448) is sometimes referred to as the **'Golden Age of Bacteria'** in recognition of the repeated infectious epidemics that held back any growth in population. It should, however, be noted that not all such infections were caused by bacteria — some (such as smallpox) were the result of viruses. Between 1348 and 1375 the population may have been reduced by half, as successive local epidemics occurred. Apart from plague, the other main causes are thought to have been smallpox, typhus and dysentery. There is considerable difficulty in recognising the true nature of past epidemics. Moreover, despite high death rates associated with *epidemic* infections such as plague, they may have had less effect on the general level of mortality than the *constantly* high death rate from *endemic* infections, such as tuberculosis. Unfortunately, the steady, unchanging impact of endemic infections makes accurate quantitative assessment of their contribution to mortality rates in the past impossible.

The pattern of infectious diseases was not static in pre-industrial Europe: plague appeared suddenly in 1348 and disappeared just as suddenly in 1666. Another example is leprosy, a disease which affects particularly the skin and nerves, and which, without treatment, can destroy nerves, thus leading to gross deformities. Leprosy appears to have been prevalent throughout Europe and the Mediterranean for many centuries, with around 19 000 leprosaria (institutions for sufferers of leprosy) in existence in 1300. However, the arrival of plague in Europe was associated with a massive decline in the number of lepers, an association that so far lacks any widely accepted explanation. Leprosy remains widespread in many parts of Asia, Africa, South America and in middle-Eastern countries such as Afghanistan and Iran.

One important feature of historical research is that, although the events themselves may be long over, information and theories about them are constantly changing. For example, interpretations of historical outbreaks of disease have been up-dated in recent years by a greater understanding of the ability of micro-organisms to change their characteristics (mutate) and hence the pattern of disease that they cause.

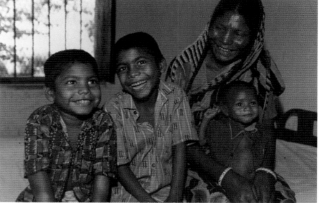

Leprosy is widespread in many developing countries; here a woman with leprosy and her three children (the two oldest are also infected) attend a clinic in India. (Photo Andy Crump/WHO)

A good example of the ability of micro-organisms to adapt to changing circumstances is the causation of three diseases — *yaws*, *pinta* and *syphilis* — by the same bacterium in different circumstances. All three diseases are found in parts of West and Central Africa, Latin America and Asia, and are distinguished by the type and location of ulcerating skin lesions, the extent of damage to internal organs and the route of transmission. Yaws, pinta and so-called endemic syphilis are transferred by any contact with open sores, whereas venereal syphilis is transferred by sexual contact. In warm climates and conditions of overcrowding and poverty, direct skin contact is so common that the bacteria most commonly multiply in the non-sexually transmitted diseases. But it is thought that the bacterium adapted to sexual transmission in the temperate climates of northern Europe and North America, where casual contact with the skin of an infected person is limited by clothing.

Another problem for the medical historian is that historical accounts of some illnesses have proved insufficient to identify them in terms of modern categories of disease. The best example of this is the 'English Sweat' or 'sweating sickness' which first struck in London in 1486, and then spread across England, without ever reaching Wales or Scotland. In 1529 it crossed to the Netherlands, Germany and Switzerland, and by 1551 had disappeared from England completely, its true nature lost in the mysteries of time. From contemporary descriptions it was probably a disease caused by a virus (some historians have suggested it may have been an early form of influenza) that affected the heart and lungs, causing rheumatic pains, fits of shivering and profuse sweating. Victims were often dead within hours of its onset, though in demographic terms it rarely caused more than a doubling of the mortality rate, compared with ten- to twelve-fold increases during plague epidemics. The appearance given by contemporary records that the disease particularly struck the eminent and famous (unlike almost all other infections) probably reflects the chroniclers' interest and concern rather than its true social distribution.

6.2.4 Local patterns of disease

Only a few parish registers survive that are complete enough to indicate the pattern of mortality in a whole community, and we have no way of knowing if these are representative even of the part of the country they came from, much less of the country as a whole. One such example is for the parish of St Botolph without Aldgate in London for the years 1583–99. As the size of the population of the parish for this period is not known (the first census was not taken in England until

1801) it is not even possible to determine the overall mortality *rates* for specific diseases, let alone the age-specific or sex-specific mortality rates. So all we know are the *number* of deaths in the parish between certain dates.

● How could the number of deaths from a particular disease in 1583–99 be meaningfully compared with the number occurring in the present day? (Think back to Chapter 3.)

■ One way in which this has been done is to compare the *percentages* of all deaths that were caused by the particular disease. This is known as the *proportional mortality*.

Note that this measure does not express the *risk* of dying from the disease, only the proportion of all deaths caused by that particular disease. For example, the number of deaths occurring at different ages in the Parish of St Botolph in 1583–99 can be compared with similar data for England and Wales, and South Africa, at present, and this is done in Figure 6.3.

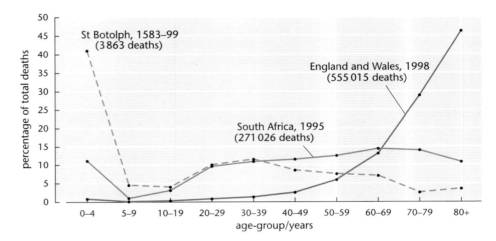

Figure 6.3 *Proportional mortality by age-group; St Botolph without Aldgate 1583–99, England and Wales, 1998 and South Africa, 1998. (Data from St Botolph derived from Forbes, T. R. (1979) By what disease or casualty: the changing face of death in London, in Webster, C. (ed.)* Health, Medicine and Mortality in the Sixteenth Century, *Cambridge University Press, Cambridge, p. 124; England and Wales, 1998, derived from the Office for National Statistics (1999)* Mortality Statistics: Cause 1998, *ONS Series DH2, No. 25, The Stationery Office, London, Table 5; South Africa, 1995, derived from United Nations (1999a)* United Nations Demographic Yearbook 1997, *UN, New York, Table 19)*

● What are the main differences between the mortality experiences in St Botolph at the end of the sixteenth century and England and Wales in 1998?

■ There was a much higher infant and childhood mortality, and a higher mortality in young adulthood during the earlier period. Over 40 per cent of all deaths occurred before the age of 5. In contrast, most deaths (75 per cent) in England and Wales in 1998 occurred in people aged over 70 years — an age that few people reached in the sixteenth century.

● How does the pattern of mortality in St Botolph at the end of the sixteenth century compare with that in modern South Africa?

■ In both cases there is a high proportion of deaths in infancy and childhood: 41 per cent in the sixteenth century, and 12 per cent in modern South Africa. However, a proportionally much greater number of people in South Africa than in the St Botolph records survive middle age and die after the age of 60.

Proportional mortality for the ten most common 'causes' of death in the parish of St Botolph is shown in Table 6.1.

These data once again raise an issue already encountered in this chapter: the problem of interpretation. Plague, for example (which the table indicates to be responsible for a higher proportion of deaths than any other cause), was often used to denote any epidemic disease rather than specifically that caused by plague bacteria (*Yersinia pestis*). Similarly, consumption and convulsions could be confused because records often only state the abbreviation 'con', and finally the meaning of a term such as 'pining' is open to misinterpretation, though it is thought to refer to tuberculosis.

The notion of 'cause' has also altered since the sixteenth century. 'Infancy' was seen as sufficient explanation for dying (though the current use of 'cot death' could be viewed as a modern equivalent, in the sense that the underlying biological cause is unknown).

Although plague only occurred intermittently it was nevertheless responsible for almost a quarter of all deaths. The impact of plague epidemics at the end of the sixteenth century can be seen in the fluctuation in the annual number of burials at that time (Figure 6.4). No other disease caused such fearful loss of life in relatively short periods of time. In contrast, tuberculosis, a chronic endemic infection (recorded as 'consumption' and 'pining') showed no epidemic pattern.

Returning to Table 6.1, the dominance of infectious causes is striking, particularly when it is considered that the apparently non-infectious causes probably conceal an infectious basis. These include 'childbed' (maternal mortality) which led to the death of 23 women per 1 000 deliveries, and 'teeth' which denoted deaths in infancy. Of every 100 babies born in St Botolph's parish, about 30 died before their first birthday, a further 22 died in the next 4 years, and only about 30 survived to the age of 15.

The difficulties of interpreting historical information on diseases are especially well illustrated by one of the few historical records from before 1680 that tell us about non-fatal diseases and disabilities (i.e. morbidity): the diary kept by a country physician named Richard Napier, who lived and worked in the area approximating to modern Milton Keynes. His diary is not only a rich source of data on the

Table 6.1 Proportional mortality (per cent) from the ten most common 'causes' of death, St Botolph's, 1583–99.

plague	23.6
consumption/convulsions	22.2
(not stated)	14.1
pining, decline	13.2
ague, fever	6.1
flux, colic	2.5
smallpox	2.4
childbed	1.5
teeth	1.1

Data from Forbes, T. R. (1979) By what disease or casualty: the changing face of death in London, in Webster, C. (ed.) *Health, Medicine and Mortality in the Sixteenth Century*, Cambridge University Press, Cambridge, Table 2, p. 127.

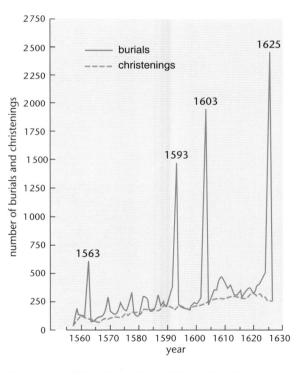

Figure 6.4 *St Botolph without Aldgate, burials and christenings 1558–1626. (Data from Forbes, T. R. (1979) 'By what disease or casualty: the changing face of death in London', in Webster, C. (ed.)* Health, Medicine and Mortality in the Sixteenth Century, *Cambridge University Press, Cambridge, p. 126)*

prevalence of conditions but also on how people described their complaints. Uniquely in such diaries, Napier recorded his patients' own descriptions of their illnesses. Two examples of consultations (from the many thousands he wrote) reveal both the ease and the difficulty of interpreting such data in modern terms. The first example is the case of Alice Billington of Fenny Stratford (see bottom right corner, Figure 6.5), 60-years-old, who was seen by Napier on 10 June 1605 at 6.50 p.m.

> Hath complained of sickness at her hart this week.
> This morning fell into a swoone and now lyes speechless.

This woman had probably suffered a stroke, and was prescribed 'cinamon water an ounce'. Contrast this with the case of Joane Nickson (also Figure 6.5) aged 38, of Wavendon. Seen earlier the same day, she complained of:

> A payne in her hart
> hath had worms of late
> yesterday voided some downwards
> had an Impostume brake upwards 9 yeeres since
> feares the like agayne
> had them last week
> her breath very strong.

The worms were probably roundworms (still common in developing countries today), but the nature of the 'Impostume' she fears (some sort of abscess) is not clear to us. We should of course remember that random scrutiny of the present-day records kept by a general practitioner could be equally puzzling! Unfortunately, few such records of morbidity before 1680 survive (or maybe ever existed).

- ● Before leaving Napier's diary, can you suggest what the strange diagrams in his records might represent? (Remember this was written in 1605 when medicine still contained many traditional beliefs.)

- ■ They are astrological charts. Napier used astrology to augment his clinical methods in deciding on a diagnosis and suitable treatment.

You have seen that, despite the existence of historical data on mortality and population size that are better than for almost any other country, our understanding of the health and disease experience of pre-industrial society in England is still hampered by a lack of knowledge. However, our knowledge has deepened considerably in recent years. This suggests that lack of interest, as much as lack of data, has been a reason for our previous ignorance and doubts about the interaction of population, disease, and food. Peter Laslett, a contemporary historian who has done a great deal to assert the importance of such interactions, has summed up the position as follows:

> Why is it that we know so much about the building of the British Empire, the growth of Parliament, and its practices, the public and private lives of English kings, statesmen, generals, writers, thinkers and yet do not know whether all our ancestors had enough to eat? ... Why has almost nothing been done to discover how long those earlier Englishmen lived and how confident most of them would be of having any posterity at all? Not only do we not know the answers to these questions, until now we never seem to have bothered to ask them. (Laslett, 1971, p. 134)

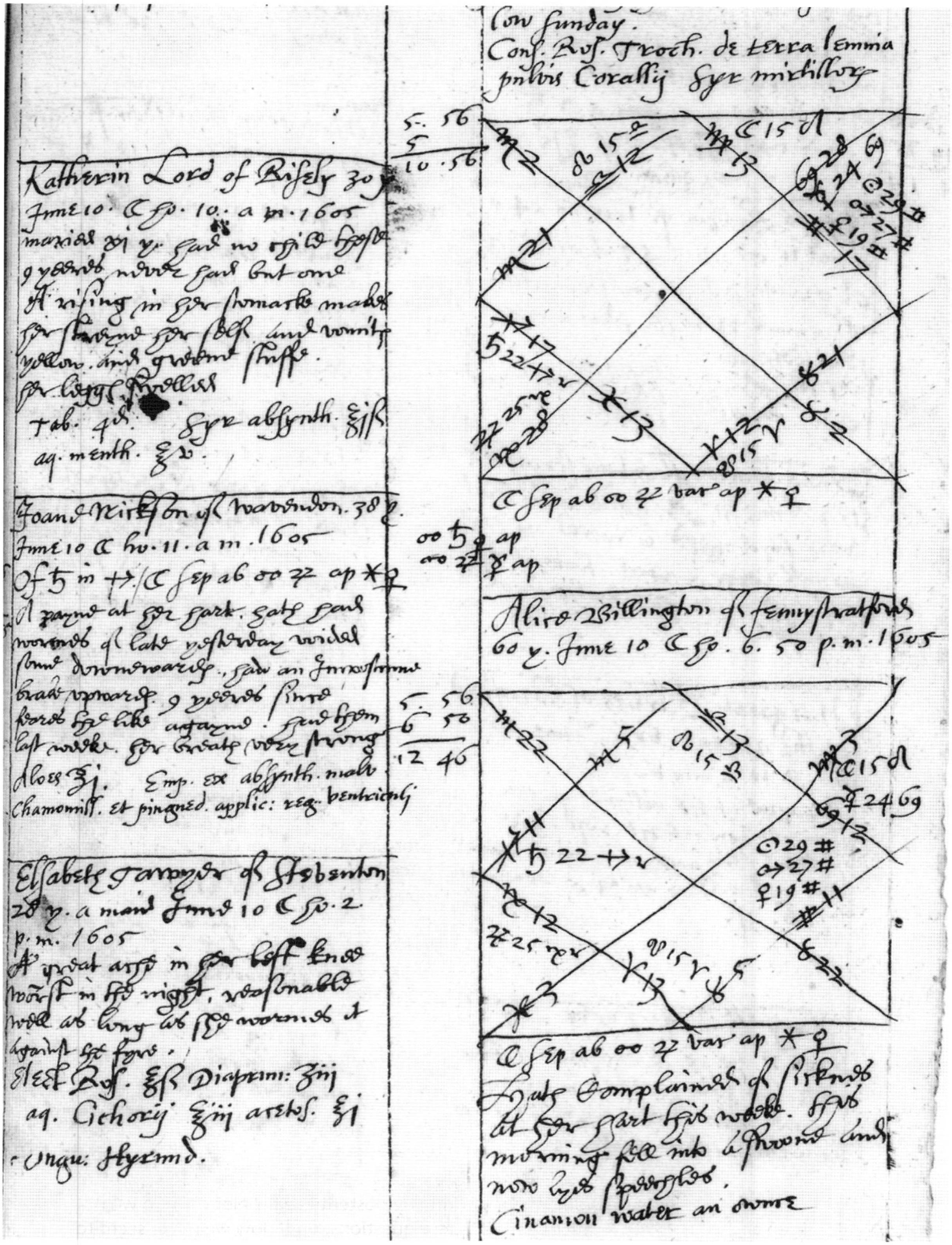

Figure 6.5 *Extracts from the diaries of Richard Napier, seventeenth-century physician (© Bodleian Library, MS Ashmole 216, Folio 116r)*

6.3 Disease and population, 1680–1850

The transition from the disease and mortality patterns of pre-industrial society in which infectious diseases and food shortages were the main causative factors, to the present pattern dominated by chronic non-infectious diseases (such as heart disease and cancers) took place over a period of about 250 years. This was accompanied by an unprecedented increase in the size of the population. As you have seen, the population of England in 1680 was around 5 million (Figure 6.1), and birth and death rates were roughly in balance. Over the following 170 years however, the population is estimated to have trebled to reach almost 17 million by 1851, and in the later part of this period the growth rate is thought to have been the highest in Europe. Whether this surge of growth was the result of a fall in mortality, a rise in fertility, or both, has been the subject of much debate.

6.3.1 Trends in fertility and mortality 1680–1850

Let us now return to Figure 6.2 (p. 108) and pick up the story of fertility and mortality trends in England between 1680 and 1850.

● Describe the main features of Figure 6.2 between about 1680 and 1850.

■ The crude birth rate increased throughout the eighteenth century and reached a peak in the first half of the nineteenth century. The crude death rate moved erratically during most of the eighteenth century, showing no clear sign of a trend, but in the early nineteenth century appeared to begin a long but erratic decline.

Over the same period, the expectation of life at birth also fluctuated erratically, as Figure 6.6 shows, but started to rise at some point towards the end of the eighteenth century to reach almost 40 years by 1851.

● List as many factors as you can think of that could have contributed to the rise in the crude birth rate.

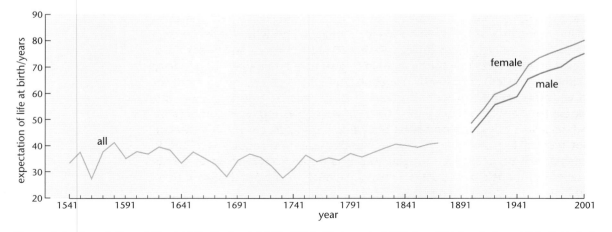

Figure 6.6 *Expectation of life at birth, England, 1541–2001. (Data up to 1871 from Wrigley, E. A. and Schofield, R. S., 1989,* The Population History of England 1541–1871: a Reconstruction, *Cambridge University Press, Cambridge, Table A3.1; from 1871 Registrar General, various years,* Annual Abstracts of Statistics, *HMSO or TSO, London)*

■ Some of the factors are:

An increase in the proportion of women of childbearing age in the population.

Earlier age for marriage, leading to more pregnancies during a woman's reproductive life.

A greater proportion of women marrying and having children, that is, increased nuptiality.

Shorter intervals between successive pregnancies.

Improvements in the health of women, leading to greater fecundity (reproductive capacity), earlier on-set of menstruation (menarche), later menopause, and fewer stillbirths.

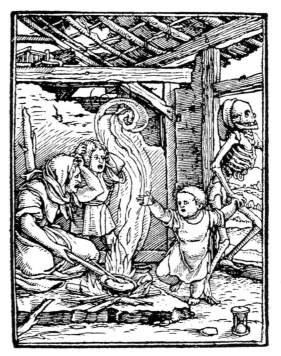

Investigation of parish registers and marriage documents have demonstrated that the rise in the birth rate during the eighteenth century was due primarily to changes in marriage patterns, in particular earlier and more universal marriage. Average age at first marriage in those parishes studied dropped from 26 to 23 years and the proportion of unmarried women fell from 15 to 7 per cent.

It appears, therefore, that the expansion in population between 1680 and 1850 resulted from both a rise in fertility and a decline in mortality. The birth and death rates quoted above are of course *crude* rates that do not take into account the population's age structure, but once this has been done it can be calculated that the rise in the birth rate contributed *two and a half times as much* to the increase in population as did the decline in the death rate.

Death takes a child victim in this engraving, dating from the early eighteenth century. There is little evidence of a sustained decline in English death rates until the early nineteenth century. (Source: Royal Collection)

6.3.2 Explaining fertility and mortality changes, 1680–1850

Although it is now clear that rising fertility was a much more important reason than declining mortality for the increasing population during the period 1680–1850, the latter reason has been debated much more extensively than the former. One reason for this emphasis is that until relatively recently many historians believed that falling mortality was the main reason for population growth. Another reason may be that it is relatively more straightforward to explain rising fertility: the most recent evidence indicates that the changes in nuptiality that underlay rising fertility were fairly strongly and consistently related to changes in real incomes, broadly in accord with the Malthusian model: as real incomes rose, so nuptiality rose. But possible explanations for any decline in mortality are more complex, in part because of a lack of solid information on causes of death, and in part because the decline was not regular, but took place towards the end of a long sequence of erratic movements. It is precisely such irregularities and unpredictable series of events that theoretical models of population change — such as the Malthusian one — tend to be bad at accommodating.

As the main causes of death in the early eighteenth century were infectious diseases, it is fairly certain that the main reason for the decline in mortality towards the end of the period 1680–1850 was a fall in the number of deaths from infectious diseases, though fewer deaths resulting from chronic food shortages may also have contributed. Potential explanations for a decline in deaths from infectious diseases can be grouped into three broad types:

1   Biological — such as a decrease in the virulence of the micro-organisms, or an increase in immunity or resistance in the human hosts.

2   Environmental and social — such as less exposure to infections, for example through improvements in living conditions such as housing and water supplies, in turn related to a rising standard of living.

3   Medical — such as an improvement in the effectiveness of medical intervention in the treatment of infectious diseases.

We shall look at each in turn. First, as you have seen, biological explanations of historical changes in disease patterns are difficult to establish. The best evidence is often simply the failure to substantiate any other explanation. However, it is sometimes possible to provide circumstantial evidence, such as a decrease in the reported *case-fatality rates* (the number of cases of a disease that result in death in a year, expressed as a rate), which may suggest that, for instance, the virulence of a micro-organism had changed. This is thought to have been the case with the decline of scarlet fever, and may also have been true of plague and some other infectious diseases.

Second, changes in the social environment that are claimed to have been responsible for the decline in mortality in this period were improvements in nutrition and in general social conditions. A leading advocate of the importance of nutrition has been Thomas McKeown, a doctor and prominent sceptic about the impact of health care on mortality decline. However, his arguments have been made with particular force in relation to the nineteenth century, and we will return to them below. McKeown has argued that other social improvements had little or no impact until after 1820, but some historians have suggested otherwise. They have pointed to such factors as the drainage of land which led to less malaria (though this was never more than a localised problem in Britain), the replacement of wooden with brick or stone buildings after the urban fires of the seventeenth century, which provided less refuge for vermin and so led to improved domestic hygiene; and the introduction of mechanised cotton cloth manufacture, which may have contributed to reducing the incidence of typhus, a disease spread by body lice, as a result of the greater availability of cotton clothes which could be boiled during washing.

Whatever the balance of evidence on these factors, the evidence that long-term economic trends can explain changes in mortality levels in England during this period is far from clear. Real wages, which were introduced in Chapter 5 as one measure of the standard of living, rose during some periods when mortality was also increasing, and were falling during some periods when mortality was declining — the opposite of what the Malthusian model predicts. One possible explanation for these findings is that, although rising wages may improve the standard of living and reduce mortality if the social and economic environment remains otherwise unchanged, it is likely that rising wages over a period of time will be associated with other changes, such as a growth in urbanisation or in industry, which may initially tend to increase rather than lower mortality. Or there may be long lags between improvements in income and improvements in health; for example, it may take a generation before better social conditions during pregnancy and infancy are reflected in greater longevity.

An alternative hypothesis put forward by some economic historians is that the direction of causality is two-way: economic growth contributed to improved nutrition and health, but these in turn also contributed to economic growth by increasing the productivity of individuals in work and the numbers able to work, and by reducing some of the economic costs of morbidity (which we considered in Chapter 3). For example the American economic historian Robert Fogel has estimated that up to 30 per cent of the growth in income per person in Britain between 1780 and 1979 could be attributed to improvements in health and nutritional status. Using historical data on agricultural output, body size and energy requirements, Fogel estimates that in 1790, even allowing for the generally much smaller stature and weight of the population, at least 20 per cent of the English population were subsisting on such poor diets that they had insufficient energy for more than a few hours of light work per day. As their nutritional status and health improved, so their ability to work productively improved. The issues raised by Fogel's analysis will be examined in more detail in Chapter 11, but they do suggest that the concept of subsistence used by Malthus has limitations:

> Subsistence is not located at the edge of a nutritional cliff, beyond which lies demographic disaster. The evidence ... implies that, rather than one level of subsistence, there are numerous levels at which a population and a food supply can be in equilibrium, in the sense that they can be indefinitely sustained. However, some levels will have smaller people and higher 'normal' (non-crisis) mortality than others. (Fogel, 1994, p. 377)

The third possible explanation of the decline of mortality towards the end of the period 1680–1850 is an improvement in medical intervention. Most commentators have considered the contribution of medicine during the eighteenth century to have been slight or even in some instances harmful. However, the historian Peter Razzell has argued that the introduction from Turkey of smallpox inoculation in 1717, and its widespread use from 1760, helped to reduce mortality from this condition long before the introduction of Edward Jenner's cowpox vaccine from 1796 onwards. The wife of the British Ambassador to Turkey, Lady Mary Wortley Montagu, popularised the practice of deliberately introducing matter from smallpox pustules into the skin or mucous membranes to induce a (hopefully) milder case of the disease. Innoculation was already widespread in Turkey, North Africa, India and the Middle East, and spread among the English elite after 1717. Some researchers have also suggested that hospitals — especially the voluntary general hospitals which increased in number during the eighteenth century — were not as ineffectual or even possibly harmful (by spreading infection or using damaging treatments) as is generally supposed, and may in fact have contributed to the falling death rate. However, hospital populations were probably too small to be of demographic significance in the eighteenth century.

On balance, Wrigley and Schofield (whose work is widely used as the basis for discussion of this period) provide the following assessment of influences on mortality trends during this period in England:

> It is doubtful ... whether the course of real wages was ever the dominant influence on mortality trends. A slowly changing balance between infective parasites and their human host was probably a weightier factor, a balance which tilted to and fro largely outside the consciousness of men and, with few exceptions, quite outside their power to influence. (Wrigley and Schofield, 1989, p. 416)

Finally, it is important to bear in mind that over the period 1680–1850, and especially up to the end of the eighteenth century, there is less of a decline in mortality to be explained than has often been thought.

6.4   Mortality and fertility since 1850

Returning to Figure 6.2 (p. 108), let us complete this account of mortality and fertility changes in England by examining the period from 1850 to the present.

● Describe the main features revealed in Figure 6.2 for the period 1850–2001.

■ Death and birth rates began to fall even more steeply around 1861 and continued to do so until well into the twentieth century. The rate of population growth fell from its peak of approximately 1.5 per cent per annum around the mid-nineteenth century to its present value close to zero.

Referring back to Figure 6.6 (p. 116), you will also see that the expectation of life at birth rose at an accelerating rate: from an average of approximately 40 years in 1850, to 50 years by 1911, 60 by 1931 and by 2001 had reached 80 for women and 75 for men. The difference in life expectancies between males and females has also been calculated in Figure 6.6 from 1871 onwards. Although the expectation of life has increased for both sexes, the increase for males has been slightly less than that for females. The consequence of this has been a widening of the difference between the sexes. Some possible explanations for such sex-differences will be discussed in Chapters 8 and 9.

6.4.1   Changes in the cause of death since 1850

In contrast to the situation pre-1850, more reliable information on cause of death is available from around 1850 onwards as a result of the introduction of death certification in 1838 (although we should always bear in mind possible inaccuracies in death certificates — then and now). In addition, the establishment of a decennial (l0-yearly) census in 1801 provided the means of determining mortality rates not only for the whole population, but for specific age groups, for each sex, and, from 1921, for social classes. However, this only represents a relative improvement in our knowledge of the causes of death, and many problems can still arise unless care is taken in interpreting the evidence:

> Problems arise both from vagueness and inaccuracy of diagnosis and from changes in nomenclature and classification. For example, there must be doubts about the diagnosis of tuberculosis at a time when it was not possible to X-ray the chest or identify the tubercle bacillus. In the Registrar-General's classification scarlet fever was not separated from diphtheria until 1855, nor typhus from typhoid before 1869. Even the less exacting task, so important for the present discussion of distinguishing infectious from non-infectious causes of death, presents difficulties. For example, deaths attributed to diseases of the heart and nervous system included a considerable but unknown number due to infections such as syphilis. (McKeown, 1976, p. 50)

Some of these problems can be avoided by adopting a simple classification based on groups of conditions rather than specific causes. Table 6.2 groups causes of death under four broad headings: infectious disease caused by airborne micro-organisms, water- or food-borne micro-organisms, and other micro-organisms, and all other (that is, non-infectious) diseases.

Table 6.2   Reasons for the reduction in Standardised Death Rates in England and Wales between 1848–54 and 1971.

Cause of death	Per cent contribution to total fall in Standardised Death Rate		
	1848–54 to 1971	1848–54 to 1901	1901 to 1971
airborne micro-organisms			
respiratory tuberculosis	17.5	9.0	8.5
scarlet fever; diphtheria	6.0	4.0	2.0
smallpox	1.5	1.5	0
bronchitis, pneumonia, influenza	7.0	3.0	10.0
other	6.5	1.0	5.5
water/food-borne micro-organisms			
cholera; diarrhoea	11.0	3.5	7.5
typhoid; typhus[1]	6.0	5.0	1.0
other (e.g. dysentery)	4.5	1.0	3.5
other micro-organisms	12.5	4.5	8.0
sub-total all micro-organisms	*74.5*	*27.5*	*47.0*
other conditions: (non-infectious)	25.5	2.5	23.0
total (all causes)	**100.0**	**30.0**	**70.0**

[1]Typhus should be in the 'other micro-organisms' category, but was not distinguished from typhoid before 1869.

(Data from Szreter, S. (1988) The importance of social intervention in Britain's mortality decline, c. 1850–1914: a re-interpretation of the role of public health, *Journal of the Social History of Medicine*, p. 8)

The first data column shows the percentage contribution of each disease to the decline in the death rate between 1848–54 (that is, the average sampled over these 6 years) and 1971, standardised for changes in the age and sex structure of the population between these dates. In the second and third columns, it then sub-divides this period of roughly 120 years into the period 1848–54 to 1901, and the period 1901 to 1971. This allows a comparison of the extent to which a cause of death was declining in the period *before* 1901 and *after* that date. For example, the table shows that the decline in deaths from cholera and diarrhoea accounted for 11 per cent of the total fall in the death rate between 1848–54 and 1971, and that 3.5 per cent of this reduction occurred *before* 1901 and the remaining 7.5 per cent *afterwards*.

⬤   Overall, what was the relative contribution of infectious diseases and non-infectious diseases to the fall in death rates between 1848–54 and 1971?

◼   Between 1848–54 and 1971, three-quarters of the improvement in death rates was due to the decline in infectious diseases, while non-infectious conditions accounted for the remaining quarter.

⬤   For each of these two broad categories of disease, how much of the contribution to falling death rates came (a) before, and (b) after 1901?

◼   For both categories of disease, most of the contribution came *after* 1901. This is especially the case with the non-infectious diseases.

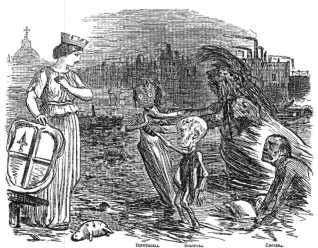

FATHER THAMES INTRODUCING HIS OFFSPRING TO THE FAIR CITY OF LONDON.
(A Design for a Fresco in the New Houses of Parliament.)

A cartoon drawn by Tenniel in 1858 shows a keen awareness of the hazardous state of the River Thames. The 'offspring' are named Diphtheria, Scrofula and Cholera (Punch, 3 July 1858)

Within each of these two general categories of disease there was considerable variation in the pattern of the decline of different diseases. Of the airborne infections, respiratory tuberculosis was the single most important disease to decline, accounting for as much as 17.5 per cent of the fall in overall mortality (from all causes) between 1848–54 and 1971. Whereas deaths from tuberculosis fell throughout this period, there was actually a small increase in deaths from bronchitis, pneumonia and influenza between 1848–54 and 1901, with a decline only occurring during the twentieth century. Before 1901 water-borne infections (such as typhoid) declined more than those that were food-borne (such as dysentery). Though the mortality rate for all infectious diseases and all non-infectious diseases fell between 1848–54 and 1971, this was not true of some non-infectious causes of death. In particular, the death rates for cardiovascular disease and cancers increased substantially.

The overall effect of all these changes in the causes of death can be seen in Figure 6.7. Infections (infectious diseases with tuberculosis shown separately) have undergone a spectacular decline and by 1998 were responsible for less than 2 per cent of all deaths. The decline of diseases of the nervous system was because of changes in diagnosis and classification: in 1851 many people were certified as dying from convulsions, others from insanity and delirium tremens, none of which would be commonly recognised as causes of death today.

These principal causes of mortality have been replaced in recent years by three categories in particular: heart disease, strokes and cancers. Though most of their increase is relative, due to the decline of other causes and the survival of more

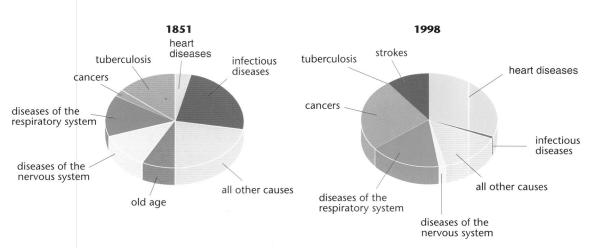

Figure 6.7 *Causes of death in England and Wales, 1851 and 1998. (Data for 1851 from Registrar-General (1855)* England and Wales Report; *for 1998 from Registrar-General (1999)* Annual Abstract of Statistics 1999, The Stationery Office, London, *Table 5.19, p. 55)*

people to ages in which these diseases occur, some of the increase is thought to have resulted from an absolute rise in incidence. The current pattern of causes of death in the United Kingdom will be considered in greater detail in Chapter 9.

A final comment on the historical changes in patterns of disease in England must be made. Most of the discussion has been concerned with *mortality* and changing causes of death. This is unfortunate as it provides only one indication of the health of a population. In particular, it ignores two aspects of ill-health — morbidity and disability — which may also be important indicators of the health of a population. The reason for their omission is simple and no doubt obvious — a lack of historical data. However, they are considered in the discussion of contemporary epidemiology in Chapter 9.

In summary, it seems that the decline in mortality since 1850 has followed a very broad sequence as regards the type of condition causing death: first water-borne and then food-borne infections declined, followed by airborne infections, and finally some non-infectious conditions. Of course, these changes in mortality rates have not been mutually exclusive and, as you have seen, within some categories the incidence of specific diseases has actually increased at times. The timing of these changes should help us to understand how they came about but, as you will see, fierce controversy continues to surround this area.

6.5 Explanations for the modern decline in mortality

As you saw earlier in this chapter, explanations of falling mortality in the period from 1680 up to 1850 did give credence to the possibility of a biological explanation — changing virulence of infectious organisms, for example. However, the influence of biological factors on the *overall* pattern of change has largely been dismissed on the grounds that the virulence of many different micro-organisms would have had to decline more or less simultaneously — an event that is regarded as most unlikely to have happened. The debate on the **explanations of the modern decline in mortality** and, in particular, reasons for the dramatic decline since 1850 in mortality rates attributable to infectious diseases, have had a different emphasis, concentrating on three points:

1   the impact of medical intervention;

2   the establishment of public health administration and legislation;

3   improvements in nutrition and standards of living.

6.5.1 The McKeown hypothesis

For many years, the major contribution to the decline in mortality was considered to have been from medical advances. However, from the 1960s this view was challenged vigorously, largely as a result of the work of Thomas McKeown. In his work, McKeown focused on England and Wales during the period from the mid-nineteenth century to the mid-twentieth century. Rapid industrialisation and population growth was occurring during this period, with the national income per person growing on average by 1 per cent a year. An extract entitled 'The medical contribution' from McKeown's book *The Modern Rise of Populations*, presents his views and appears in *Health and Disease: A Reader (Open University Press, 2nd edn 1994; 3rd edn 2001)*. Open University students should read it now.

● On what grounds does McKeown argue that medical measures made only an insignificant contribution to the overall decline of mortality from infectious diseases since 1850?

■ He does this principally by demonstrating that mortality had declined or was declining *before* the introduction of relevant medical measures (e.g. in the cases of measles and respiratory tuberculosis).

● Despite this, medical measures appear (a) to have made a dramatic contribution to the decline of one infection, and (b) to have accelerated the decline in mortality from two others since the 1940s. Which diseases are these?

■ These are (a) smallpox, in which the decline was mainly due to vaccination, and (b) respiratory tuberculosis, with the introduction of chemotherapy, and diphtheria, with the widespread use of immunisation.

● As an assessment of the contribution that doctors have made to the overall decline in mortality, what are the main limitations of McKeown's thesis?

■ Quite explicitly, McKeown is only concerned with the decline in infectious diseases, ignoring the possible effect doctors may have had on the other types of condition that account for 26 per cent of the overall decline. However, a more important limitation is that he concentrates on the *biomedical* role of medicine and ignores the *preventive* work carried out by doctors, both in the area of individual advice to people and in the establishment of public health measures.

McKeown not only rejected the importance of medical intervention, but attributed the decline in mortality to improvements in nutrition and standard of living, and this became known as the **McKeown hypothesis**.

6.5.2 Critiques of the McKeown hypothesis

The McKeown hypothesis rapidly acquired the status of a new orthodoxy, and it became commonplace to assert that the impact of medical intervention on health improvements was negligible. However, this view has itself come under increasingly critical scrutiny. The historian Winter, for example, has argued that

> … when a doctor advises a change in diet or the removal of unsanitary debris, he may very well improve the survival chances of his patients. Simply because doctors do not require a medical education to make such statements is no reason to conclude that such indirect medical intervention was unimportant in the process of mortality decline. (Winter, 1982, p. 111)

A more sustained critique has been mounted by the historian Simon Szreter, and extracts from his paper 'The importance of social intervention in Britain's mortality decline, *c.* 1850–1914', are also reprinted in *Health and Disease: A Reader* (Open University Press, 2nd edn 1994; 3rd edn 2001). (Open University students should read it now.)

The objective of Szreter's work is not to question McKeown's *negative* conclusion, that modern scientific medicine cannot be awarded much credit for the historical decline of mortality — on this point the two agree. Szreter counters McKeown's *positive* conclusion that nutritional improvements and a rising standard of living were the main causes of declining mortality. Szreter's argument proceeds on a number of fronts. First, he argues that McKeown reached his conclusions about the importance of nutrition and the standard of living on methodologically suspect grounds, by eliminating *other* possible causes so that, by default, only nutrition and rising standards of living could have been responsible for the decline in mortality, through improving the natural defences of individuals to infectious diseases, especially airborne diseases. Szreter also accuses McKeown of subsuming far too much under the term 'standard of living', and as a result implying incorrectly that a whole range of social, cultural and political factors are the automatic corollary of changes in a country's per capita real income. Second, he argues that McKeown misinterpreted the evidence on the contribution of different diseases to declining mortality, and on the chronology of the decline.

● Which particular airborne disease does McKeown's argument heavily rely on, according to Szreter?

■ Respiratory tuberculosis (TB), which in the mid-nineteenth century was the single most important cause of death.[1]

● According to Szreter, what are the flaws in McKeown's reliance on the decline of respiratory TB to substantiate his thesis?

■ First, respiratory TB was only one of a group of important airborne diseases. Two others declined for reasons not related to nutrition: smallpox as a consequence of the spread of inoculation, vaccination and isolation procedures; and scarlet fever probably as a result of immunological changes in the population or in the micro-organism's virulence. Another group of airborne diseases — bronchitis, pneumonia and influenza — actually *increased* substantially during the second half of the nineteenth century. Thus respiratory TB cannot be taken as typical of the airborne diseases. Second, Szreter claims that McKeown places too much faith on unconvincing evidence of the *early* decline of TB. Third, he argues that the prevalence of TB might best be viewed as a *consequence* of other debilitating diseases, and therefore declined as a result of the decline of other diseases. (An interesting modern parallel of this final point is the resurgence of TB as a consequence of the AIDS epidemic.)

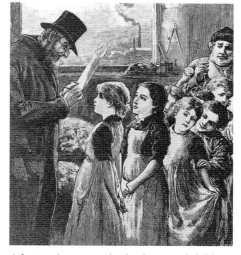

A factory inspector checks the age of children at work. The factory inspectorate was one example of the public health measures introduced in the nineteenth century. After 1833 it was illegal to employ children below the age of nine in factories.

Having moved the focus of attention from the airborne to the water- and food-borne diseases, Szreter argues that these probably rose earlier in the nineteenth century as the population of urban areas expanded rapidly, and experienced conditions such as those described by Engels and discussed in Chapter 5. But these water- and food-borne diseases were finally pushed back towards the end of the century as the result of a whole series of public health measures undertaken primarily by local authorities, and including sanitation and clean water supplies, and the increasing regulation

[1] The history of tuberculosis and factors contributing to its decline are discussed in *Medical Knowledge: Doubt and Certainty* (Open University Press, 2nd edn 1994; colour-enhanced 2nd edn 2001), Chapter 4.

of food and drink. The airborne diseases took longer to decline, perhaps because of the lack of effective public health intervention directed against them until the twentieth century.[2]

Szreter thus concludes that there is no automatic reason to think that nutritional improvements can come about without effective public health intervention, or that a growing economy will be translated into health gains: if economic growth results in rapid urbanisation, poor working conditions and growing pollution it might be harmful to health. The key factors, therefore, are *how* nutritional improvements are brought about and *how* the consequences of economic growth are used. Here Szreter emphasises strongly the role of public health measures in improving food and water supplies and the urban environment, but he also stresses the issue of distribution: unless such measures, and other benefits of economic growth, are distributed widely across the population, the potential health gains will be undermined.

If Szreter's analysis and conclusions are broadly correct, they may be of some wider significance: they suggest that McKeown's thesis, which has been so influential, may mislead countries which are still attempting to lower their population mortality. Social and medical intervention, and especially public health measures, may be central to securing nutritional improvements and ensuring that economic growth results in lower mortality. Moreover, the *distribution* of such interventions to the whole population becomes an important issue of public policy. An improved technology and science of social and medical intervention since the nineteenth century is likely to make the historical lesson drawn by Szreter even more pertinent today. These are issues we will return to in the following two chapters.

[2] The history of the public health movement in the United Kingdom is described in *Caring for Health: History and Diversity* (Open University Press, 2nd edn 1993; 3rd edn 2001).

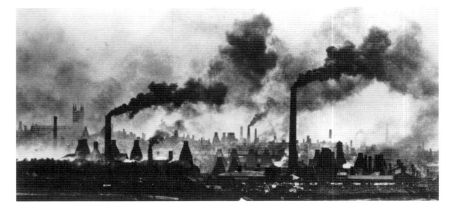

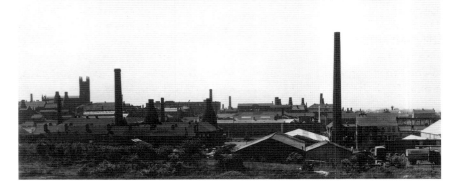

Factory chimneys in Longton, Staffordshire, in 1910 (above), and 1970 (below). Clean air legislation was not effective until the second half of the twentieth century. (Source: Oxford University Press)

6.6 Health transition and demographic transition

6.6.1 Epidemiological or health transition

Finally, does the English case examined here provide a broader insight into links between population change, health, and social and economic development? First, you have seen how the transition from an agricultural society to an industrial society was accompanied by a complete change in disease and mortality patterns, in which infectious diseases and diseases caused by food shortages gave way to the chronic non-infectious diseases such as heart disease and cancers which now predominate. Increasingly this process of change has come to be described as the **epidemiological transition** or the **health transition** (the two terms are used interchangeably in academic discourse). Demographers and epidemiologists argue that the health transition has two main components:

> … the first is the epidemiologic transition strictly speaking, which is defined as the long-term process of change in the health conditions of a society, including changes in the patterns of disease, disability, and death. The second component, which may be called the health care transition, refers to the change in the patterns of organised social response to health conditions. (Frenk *et al.*, 1991, p. 23)

As the case of England demonstrates, this health transition is associated with many different factors: demographic, socio-economic, biological, technological, political and cultural changes were all involved in one way or another. Because of this complexity, it would be misleading to generalise across countries about the health transition. It should also be noted that even within a population, the health transition may be at different stages, with infectious disease still dominant in some groups or locations, while chronic and degenerative diseases predominate in others. Finally, as with all such models, it is all too easy to assume that the health transition inevitably proceeds in just one direction. In fact, it is possible that infectious diseases may undergo resurgences which increase their importance in the pattern of disease and death.

● Can you recall from Chapters 2 and 3, or your wider reading, any examples of changes in disease patterns that run counter to the general direction of the health transition?

■ The global emergence of the viral disease AIDS during the 1980s is a particularly striking example. Even in countries such as the USA, which made the health transition many years ago, this infectious disease has become a leading cause of death. Malaria is an example of an infectious disease that has not declined steadily, but rather has undergone a widespread resurgence. Another infectious disease on the increase is TB, the resurgence of which is partly related to the AIDS epidemic. Some new infectious diseases also gained ground in the 1990s, including Ebola fever, *E. coli* 0157 and Hanta virus pneumonia.

Despite these qualifications, the concept of the health transition is a useful reference point from which to view the experience of individual countries.

6.6.2 Demographic transition

The English case, then, provides evidence relevant to the health transition. But it also throws some light on another link between population change, health, and social and economic development. As the Industrial Revolution progressed in England and spread to other countries, so evidence accumulated that the massive social and economic changes involved were accompanied by changes in birth and death rates that first accelerated and later retarded population growth. In the 1930s and 1940s, attempts were made to construct a more formal theory linking population change to industrialisation — this came to be known as the theory of **demographic transition**. And although this theory was originally intended to fit the demographic experience of industrialised countries such as England, it has been used to try to explain demographic trends in developing countries, and indeed some analysts categorise these countries as 'demographically developing'.

Figure 6.8 depicts the demographic transition for a hypothetical population before and after industrialisation. In this model, the demographic transition has four stages. Stage 1 is characterised by a high death rate and a high birth rate, so any population growth is very slow. This is the pre-industrial stage in the model. In Stage 2, the death rate starts to fall sharply, but the birth rate remains high.

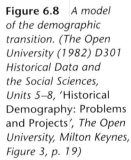

Figure 6.8 *A model of the demographic transition. (The Open University (1982) D301 Historical Data and the Social Sciences, Units 5–8, 'Historical Demography: Problems and Projects', The Open University, Milton Keynes, Figure 3, p. 19)*

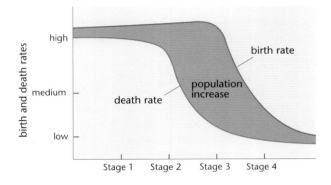

● What hypothesis could you suggest to explain Stage 2?

■ One hypothesis that could be supported from the evidence in the previous chapter is that increases in agricultural productivity have removed the Malthusian 'checks' of famine and disease, allowing the population to expand. Another hypothesis, along the lines advanced by McKeown, is that improved nutrition and rising living standards have resulted in lower mortality. Finally, social and public health interventions may have played a part.

By Stage 3 of the transition, the birth rate also falls sharply, while the fall in the death rate begins to level off. Stage 4 is reached when both the birth rate and the death rate have levelled off at a low level, and the total population size is again fairly stable (but much larger than at the start of the cycle).

This hypothetical model of demographic change can be compared with Figure 6.2 (p. 108), which shows changes in the birth rate and death rate in England between 1541 and 2001. It is clear that the demographic transition model is a considerable simplification of what actually happened. In particular, the sixteenth and seventeenth centuries, when the birth rate was falling and the death rate if anything was rising, do not appear to fit the model very well.

● However, from the early eighteenth century onwards, can you discern periods that correspond approximately to the four stages of the demographic transition model?

■ From 1700 to 1740 the birth and death rates are both high and are quite similar (Stage 1). Then the death rate begins to fall while the birth rate remains high and, in fact, rises to a peak around 1821 (Stage 2). The death rate continues to fall, and around 1861 the birth rate also begins to decline (Stage 3). Finally, from around 1941, both birth and death rates come together again and start stabilising at a much lower level (Stage 4).

This four-stage model of demographic transition has been criticised, as some aspects do not fit the facts of population change in many of the now industrialised countries: for example, in France it appears that the birth rate began falling before there was any significant industrialisation. In this respect the demographic transition model is little different from models in many other science and social science areas, which are often criticised for failing to deal with exceptional cases, erratic and irregular sequences of events, or simply with individual cases: simplification of the real world is simultaneously their strength and their weakness. Critics have also argued that there is no real theoretical basis for the theory of demographic transition, even if it does have some descriptive value. Despite these criticisms, however, and returning to the starting point of this chapter, it can be seen as a valuable descriptive account of the link between social and economic development and population change. The model is a useful starting point from which to consider demographic trends, and experience to date does support it as a generalisation. The following two chapters will take up its relevance for the developing countries of today.

OBJECTIVES FOR CHAPTER 6

When you have studied this chapter, you should be able to:

6.1 Define and use, or recognise definitions and applications of, each of the terms printed in **bold** in the text.

6.2 Explain what is meant by a mortality crisis and describe the features of (a) a mortality crisis caused largely by a shortage of food, and (b) one resulting from an autonomous infectious epidemic.

6.3 Discuss the difficulties of estimating mortality and interpreting the cause of death and illness in historical sources such as parish registers and personal accounts.

6.4 Describe changes in English population size, life expectancy, mortality and fertility, since 1680.

6.5 Describe the main changes in the causes of death since 1850, and summarise and comment on different explanations for the decline in mortality in England during the nineteenth and early twentieth centuries.

6.6 Describe the model of demographic transition, and be able to interpret data on birth and death rates from specific countries with reference to its main stages.

QUESTIONS FOR CHAPTER 6

1   (*Objective 6.2*)

Looking at Figure 6.4, what do you think were the likely causes of the mortality crises in the parish of St Botolph in 1593, 1603 and 1625? What features of these crises determined your answer?

2   (*Objective 6.3*)

Can you suggest three reasons why it is impossible to compare meaningfully the prevalence of a condition such as hysteria in 1550 with its prevalence today?

3   (*Objective 6.4*)

Assess the relative contributions to population expansion of changes in mortality and in fertility in England between 1680 and 1850.

4   (*Objective 6.5*)

In what way does the critique of McKeown mounted by Szreter rely on a distinction between airborne and water-borne diseases as contributors to mortality decline during the nineteenth century?

5   (*Objective 6.6*)

To what extent can the model of demographic transition be fitted to the trends in birth rates and death rates in England between 1541 and the start of the eighteenth century? What conclusion can be drawn concerning the validity of the model?

C H A P T E R   7

Health in a world of wealth and poverty

Study notes for OU students

At the start of Section 7.6 you will be asked to read an extract entitled 'Entitlement and deprivation' by Jean Drèze and Amartya K. Sen, taken from their book, *Hunger and Public Action*. The extract appears in *Health and Disease: A Reader* (Open University Press, second edition 1995; third edition 2001).

If you have not yet watched the video 'South Africa: Health at the Crossroads' you should do so during your study of this chapter.

We extend the discussion (begun here) of the health impacts of European colonial expansion, and influences on the development of health services in Asia and Africa in a later book — *Caring for Health: History and Diversity* (second edn 1993; third edn 2001).

7.1 Introduction

Only a few countries in the world were involved in the first wave of the Industrial Revolution, and the majority of the world's population still lives in countries that are not fully industrialised. As the example of England has shown, health and disease are intimately related to processes of social change and development, and it is clear that the solution to the health problems of developing countries must involve some kind of social and economic development. How this might come about, however, is one of the biggest problems of our time. It raises a series of questions about the origins and present features of the problems besetting low-income countries, and the relationship between social and economic development and health. Let us begin by considering the origins of the current development status of low-income countries.

7.2 The Industrial Revolution and world development

Before the Industrial Revolution, the differences in economic wealth between the major regions of the world were almost certainly much smaller than they are today. If we go back several hundred years, fragments of evidence come to us from the observations of travellers on the condition of the population and the wealth or poverty of the lands they visited. Most famous of all, perhaps, was Marco Polo, who in the late thirteenth century spent 24 years travelling widely throughout the Middle East and Asia taking detailed notes on what he saw. He was a successful merchant and trader (a merchant of Venice) and he had a seasoned eye for the details of commercial life and the clues and signals of economic activity.

In his travels, Marco Polo was

> quick to notice the available sources of food and water along the route, the means of transport, and no less quick to observe the marketable products of every district, whether natural or manufactured, and the channels through which flowed the interlacing streams of export and import. (Latham, in *Introduction to the Travels of Marco Polo*, 1968 edition, p. xix)

Following Marco Polo through his travels, the picture that emerges is quite different from the modern world's low- and middle-income countries, which now includes many countries he passed through: Armenia: 'a land of many villages and towns, amply stocked with the means of life'; Northern Persia: a ride 'through a fine plain and a fine valley and along fine hillsides, where there is a rich herbage, fine pasturage, fruit in plenty, and no lack of anything'; Cathay

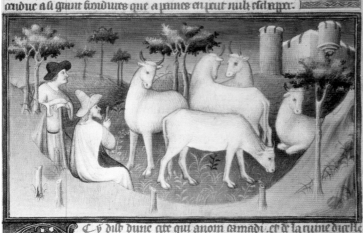

Marco Polo travelling through lands of plenty on his journeys through the Middle East and Asia in the late thirteenth century (from an illuminated manuscript — the Livres de Merveilles *(c. 1407–13) by Boucicaut Master (fl. 1390–1430), in the Bibliothèque Nationale, Paris). (Photo: Bridgeman Art Library)*

(North-East China): 'when harvests are bountiful corn is accumulated in huge granaries, along with wheat, barley, millet and rice to be distributed when crops fail'; Bengal: 'the people live on meat, milk and rice. They have cotton in plenty. They are great traders, exporting spikenard, galingale, ginger, sugar and many other precious spices'; and Northern India: 'They live by trade and industry. They have rice and wheat in profusion. The staple foods are rice, meat and milk. Merchants come here in great numbers by sea and by land with a variety of merchandise and export the products of the kingdom'. Venice may have been a 'jewel on the shores of the Adriatic', about to take its place in the forefront of the Renaissance, but Marco Polo at least gives no indication that it was unimaginably more advanced than many other places he passed through.

Even between 1750 and 1800, as the Industrial Revolution was getting well under way in Britain, the economic historian Paul Bairoch has calculated that the average levels of production and wealth in what are now developing countries were not so very different from those in the countries that are now industrialised: in China they may even have been higher.

7.2.1 Expansion of European colonial territory

As the Industrial Revolution gathered pace in a small number of countries, it gave them a tremendous advantage over the rest of the world in economic, technological and military power, and a gap rapidly opened and widened. Propelled by an immense increase in trade and exchange between different parts of the world, there began a great wave of **colonisation**, empire-building, and annexation of territories. As every British schoolchild used to be taught, by the late nineteenth century 'the sun never set' on the many countries of the world that were part of the British Empire, and there were very few areas of the world in which control or influence was not exercised or fiercely contested by the newly industrialised countries, including France, Germany, Italy, Belgium, Holland, Spain and Portugal.

Overseas expansion was not of course a phenomenon new to the period of industrialisation. We have only to think of the Romans, whose influence and power in Europe and much of Asia is witnessed even today, not only by the many relics of buildings, but by the location of towns, the routes taken by roads, the language, laws, currencies and measurements that still mould our lives. We must also note that other examples of European conquest, which have already been mentioned (for example the conquest of the Americas by the Spaniards) occurred from the sixteenth century onwards, well before the Industrial Revolution reached full speed.

However, the expansion that occurred in the wake of the Industrial Revolution was unprecedented in scope and scale. Between 1846 and 1930 over 50 million Europeans migrated to other parts of the world in a great wave of humanity, settling in the Americas and Australasia, and temporarily taking control of most of Africa and much of Asia. Pushed by the rapidly growing population of Europe and pulled by the prospect of open lands and escape from hunger and poverty, they helped to diffuse the Industrial Revolution and to transform the world. The population of Europe was growing at more than double the rate of the rest of the world, but the rate of growth of the settler populations in these newly colonised lands was almost unchecked, with relatively low death rates coupled to some of the highest fertility rates ever recorded.

One consequence of this expansion was that the 'white' or 'Caucasian' population of the world surged from around one-fifth of the global total in 1800 to over one-third by 1930. Although this share of population was not long held, however, the

Contemporary engraving depicting ill-treatment of native Americans by the Spanish colonialists in the sixteenth century.

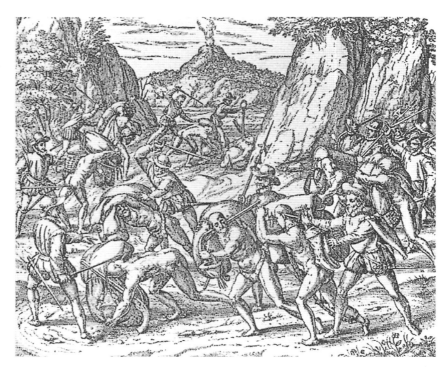

surge in their population did give the Europeans a more permanent advantage: the settlement of territories comprising almost one-quarter of the world's land surface. Furthermore, these newly settled territories, including the United States of America, Canada, Argentina, Uruguay, New Zealand and Australia, turned out to be vastly productive agricultural lands, able to feed not only their own burgeoning settler populations, but also to produce huge surpluses for anyone able to purchase them.

Of course the lands settled by European emigrants were not empty of other inhabitants, and these native populations were dispossessed and often suffered demographic collapse as a result of the devastating impact on them of infectious diseases imported with the European settlers.[1] In New Zealand, for example, the native population of Maori was estimated to be around 150 000–180 000 at the beginning of the nineteenth century. However, numbers had collapsed to barely 40 000 by the end of that century as a result of infectious diseases such as measles and sexually transmitted diseases introduced by the Europeans, and also as a result of social and economic collapse manifesting itself in alcoholism, infanticide, malnutrition and sheer despair.

7.2.2 Impact of colonisation

As Europe's rush of colonial acquisition proceeded, key aspects of the political, social and economic systems prevailing in these territories were greatly altered in a way that was essentially geared to the needs of the colonialists rather than the local populations. In the Americas and the Caribbean, the first major change introduced was the establishment of plantations to provide cotton, and later coffee and tobacco,

---

[1] Reciprocal influences on the health of settlers and indigenous peoples in European colonial territories are discussed in *Human Biology and Health: An Evolutionary Approach* (Open University Press, 2nd edn 1994; 3rd edn 2001), Chapter 5. The impact on health care in the colonies is a theme in several chapters of *Caring for Health: History and Diversity* (Open University Press, 2nd edn 1993; 3rd edn 2001).

for Europe. In the first instance, this required the importation of labour on a massive scale, in large part to compensate for the collapse of the native population through the epidemics. These were the origins of the slave trade, which not only dislocated the social and economic system of much of Africa, but again set off new waves of infectious disease.

The other important aspect of this process was that the entire pattern of agriculture and farming in colonised territories was changed beyond recognition, with the most fertile land being devoted to the production of **cash crops** that were grown for export rather than to meet the needs of local populations. As the economic, technological and political predomin-

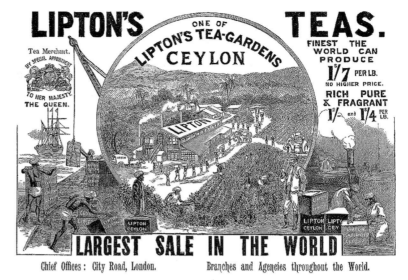

An advertisement for Lipton's Teas depicts Ceylon (Sri Lanka) as the 'tea garden' for the British consumer. (Illustrated London News, 21 November 1896)

ance of the industrialised countries grew, many parts of the world were transformed into satellite economies producing the raw materials and foodstuffs required by the industrial countries: tea from India and Ceylon (Sri Lanka), coffee from Brazil and Kenya, rice from Burma and Thailand, rubber from Malaya, guano fertiliser from Peru, and so on. For these countries, whether formally administered as colonies or informally administered by European commercial enterprises, the needs of distant industrial economies were placed foremost, and the needs of the local populations and of indigenous development were very much secondary considerations.

This dependence on the export of raw materials has continued to the present day: in 1998 only 20 per cent of the total exports of the high-income countries were comprised of raw materials and foods, compared with 45 per cent in the low-income countries, and no less than 85 per cent in the Sub-Saharan countries. In India, 52 per cent of all exports in 1996 were low-technology manufactured goods, and a further 31 per cent were unfinished raw materials, leaving just 17 per cent of all exports in the medium- and high-technology categories.

The industrialised countries have thus exerted a powerful influence over agriculture and industrialisation around the world. But, in addition to their role as producers of foodstuffs and raw materials, the colonised or partly colonised countries of the world were affected in other ways as a world economy developed around the industrialised countries. In particular, they became markets for the industrial goods being manufactured in Britain and elsewhere. The frequent result of this need for new markets, and of the technological superiority of the industrial countries, was that traditional manufacturing industries in the colonised countries were destroyed. India's textile industry, for example, was devastated as cotton fabric imports from Britain soared from one million yards in 1814 to 51 million yards by 1830.

In an attempt to calculate the effects of this process on what are now categorised as developing countries, the economic historian Paul Bairoch has assessed changes in total world manufacturing production from 1750 onwards, and some results are shown in Table 7.1 overleaf.

The figures in Table 7.1 are expressed in terms of an index in which the volume of production in the UK in 1900 is taken as equal to an index number of 100. Thus, in 1880, manufacturing production in the USA had an index number of 47, which means that it was approximately equal to 47 per cent of UK production in 1900.

Table 7.1 The development of world manufacturing production, 1750–1980 (relative to production in the United Kingdom in 1900, which is given an index number of 100).

Year	Industrialised countries			Developing countries
	UK	USA	All	All
1750	2	–	34	93
1800	6	1	47	99
1830	16	5	73	112
1850	45	16	143	83
1880	73	47	253	67
1900	100	128	481	60
1913	127	298	863	70
1928	135	533	1258	98
1938	181	528	1 562	122
1953	262	1 373	2 870	200
1963	334	1 804	4 699	439
1973	471	3 089	8 432	927
1980	454	3 475	9 718	1 323

Data from Bairoch, P. (1982) International industrialization levels from 1750 to 1980, *Journal of European Economic History*, **11** (2), pp. 269–333, Table 2.

● What happens in the developing countries from 1750 onwards?

■ From 1750 to 1830 the developing country index rose from 93 to 112 (i.e. by 1830 it exceeded by 12 per cent the production of the United Kingdom in 1900). From 1830 onwards, however, as the process of colonisation we have described gathered pace, manufacturing production in these countries started to fall, and by 1900 it was barely half the level it had been at the beginning of the nineteenth century. Not until 1938 did manufacturing production in developing countries regain its earlier level, but after 1938 it grew more rapidly.

● Now compare the relative positions of the UK, USA and developing countries in 1980.

■ In 1980 the UK's manufacturing production is still equivalent to more than one-third of the manufacturing production of all the developing countries combined, while the USA's manufacturing production is more than two and a half times that of the entire developing world.

It seems clear, therefore, that social and economic changes in the developing countries have been influenced powerfully by the Industrial Revolution, and in particular by the countries that are now industrialised. In order to explore the implications of this for health and disease patterns, let us now take stock of the differences in social and economic development in the world today.

7.3 Measuring social and economic development

One way of looking at the world, already encountered in this book, is to draw up a list of countries and then order them into a league table according to some indicator such as life expectancy or infant mortality. International agencies such as the World Health Organisation present data in this way, and so also do organisations such as the World Bank, which publishes data on social and economic development. Such league tables are therefore a convenient starting point, although they have limitations, which we will discuss later.

7.3.1 Gross National Product

One of the most commonly used indicators of social and economic development is **Gross National Product (GNP)** per capita (per head). The GNP is a measure of the total output of a national economy expressed in money terms. It includes wealth produced abroad but brought into a country, and excludes wealth produced in a country but taken abroad. For example, millions of people — migrant workers — go abroad to earn money and send remittances back to relatives in the country they left. Their remittances are included in the GNP of the country the remittances are sent to, and excluded from the GNP of the country the remittances were earned in. Profits which companies earn in one country and move to another are included in the GNP of the country that receives them. The GNP is thus an attempt to place a figure on the total wealth that accrues to the residents of a particular country, and GNP per capita is simply the total GNP divided by the number of residents in the country.

The GNP and other measures of economic activity — known collectively as the **national accounts** — have been described as one of the most significant social inventions of the twentieth century, and their influence is pervasive. They are used to divide and describe the countries of the world; politicians use the GNP as a measure of national potency, of their successes and their opponents' failures; small changes in GNP can trigger policy changes and influence public mood by determining whether a country is in or out of recession, growing steadily or 'overheating'.

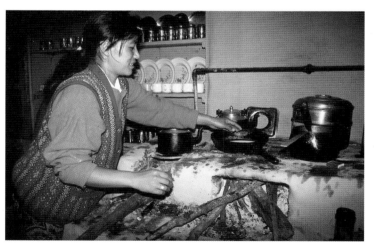

The economic value of housework is the largest item excluded from calculations of national wealth; if all domestic labour such as the cooking, cleaning and washing done by this Nepalese woman were included, her country's GNP would rise significantly. (Photo: Hartmut Schwarzbach/ Still Pictures)

Despite the tremendous influence of national accounts, they have defects and weaknesses. For example, one of the limitations of using GNP to measure wealth is that it only includes goods or services exchanged by a financial transaction in a market, and excludes goods and services that contribute to wealth but are not bought or sold.

- What common examples of goods and services can you think of that contribute to wealth but would be excluded from the GNP?

- In all countries of the world, a great deal of cleaning, washing, cooking and other domestic work is done in households, mainly by women. Because no formal payment is made for this work it is not included in the GNP.

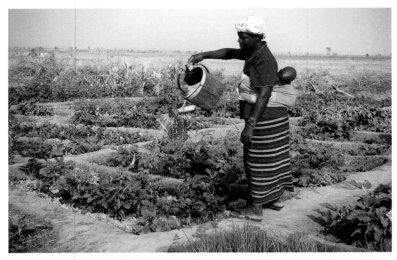

GNP calculations exclude the value of food produced for consumption within the family from subsistence farming, back-yard vegetable plots as here in Mali or as breast-milk. (Photo: Giacomo Pirozzi/Panos Pictures)

Housework is probably the largest single item excluded from GNP, and it has been estimated that including this sort of work might increase measured GNP by anything up to 30 per cent. This kind of measurement problem can be found in all countries, but is particularly acute in developing countries: subsistence farming, for instance, is by definition an activity in which food is consumed by the people who produce it. As they do not sell it in a market, it is not included in the GNP. Similarly, a breast-fed baby does not contribute to GNP but a baby fed on formula milk does, as the milk has to be manufactured and purchased and therefore enters the national accounts.

Another criticism sometimes levelled at the GNP as a measure of economic progress is that it does not reflect the depletion or despoliation of natural resources. For example, if a country's main source of wealth was its forests, and it felled them and sold them while making no attempt to replace them or use them in a sustainable way, its GNP would for a while increase. However, it would in fact be destroying the basis of its future prosperity, rather like a factory owner tearing up the floorboards to feed the boilers. Thus the GNP would give a very misleading impression of economic progress. A variety of ways of dealing with this problem have been proposed, but so far none has been adopted.

For these reasons, GNP measurements should not be accepted uncritically as a measure of wealth: like measures of health such as mortality they have the advantage of being relatively easy to arrive at, but they present only one part of the story.

7.3.2 Comparing GNP between countries

Figures for GNP per capita and various other social and economic measurements are published by the World Bank for most countries in the world. (The main countries for which no information on GNP was available in 1998 are Cuba, Iraq, the People's Democratic Republic of Korea (North Korea), Sudan and Somalia.) The reported countries are grouped by the World Bank into five categories, as shown in Table 7.2.

The 'low-income' countries are those with an annual GNP per head of up to US$760 in 1998; they include China and India, which are shown separately from the others. The 'middle-income' countries had an annual GNP per head greater than $760 but less than $9 360, and are shown split into a 'lower' ($761–$3 030) and an 'upper' ($3 031–$9 360) category. The lower-middle-income group of countries includes, for example, Sri Lanka, Romania, Egypt, South Africa and the Russian Federation. Examples of countries in the upper-middle-income group include Brazil, the Republic of Korea (South Korea), Poland and Malaysia. The high-income countries all had an annual GNP per head of $9 360 or above; they include the United Kingdom, USA, Japan and Canada.

● What proportion of the world's population live in countries with low-income or lower-middle-income economies?

Table 7.2 World[1] shares of population and GNP, 1998.

Country group	GNP per head /US dollars	Percentage of world population	Percentage of world GNP	Percentage of world GNP using purchasing power parities
low-income economies (less than $760)				
China	750	21.0	3.2	10.9
India	430	16.6	1.5	4.5
other low-income	380	22.0	1.7	5.0
middle-income economies ($760–$9 360)				
lower-middle-income	1 710	15.4	5.4	10.1
upper-middle-income	4 860	10.0	9.9	12.6
high-income economies (more than $9 360)				
all high-income	25 510	15.0	78.3	56.8

[1] 'World' excludes Cuba, Iraq, People's Democratic Republic of Korea, Sudan, Somalia. Also excluded are a number of countries with populations less than 1.5 million.

Data derived from World Bank (2000) *Entering the 21st Century: World Development Report 1999/2000,* Oxford University Press, Oxford and New York, Table 1.

■ About 75 per cent of the world's population lives in these countries (mainly in the low-income countries).

Perhaps the most striking thing about Table 7.2, however, is the column showing the share of total world GNP taken by each group of countries.

● What proportion of world GNP is taken by the countries with upper-middle-income and high-income economies (broadly the industrialised countries), and how does this compare with the share taken by the low-income countries?

■ The 25 per cent of the world's population living in the upper-middle-income and high-income economies take almost 90 per cent of the world's GNP, whereas the 60 per cent of the world's population in low-income countries take only a tiny 6 per cent of the world's GNP.

The final column of Table 7.2 shows a somewhat different version of the distribution of world GNP, calculated on the basis of **purchasing power parities**. Exchange rates, which were used in the previous column to calculate each country's GNP in the common denominator of US dollars, can fluctuate for many reasons and are not always a good guide to relative prices within countries. Purchasing power parities attempt to get round this problem by calculating an exchange rate based on equivalent purchasing power: for example, if a bundle of goods and services such as a taxi fare, a haircut, a snack lunch and a pair of socks cost $35 in Washington and £45 in London, then the purchasing power parity exchange rate is $1.28:£1 (45/30), irrespective of the market exchange rate. On this basis, the distribution of world GNP is not quite so starkly disproportional to population, although the poorest 60 per cent of the world's population still take only 21 per cent of the world's GNP.

7.3.3 Development indicators

Many measures other than GNP per head are often used to illustrate differences in social and economic development, and Table 7.3 shows a number of these **development indicators**, using the same income groupings used in Table 7.2.

● In one sentence each, summarise the main conclusions from the data in Table 7.3 on (a) adult literacy and education; (b) daily calorie supply; and (c) urbanisation.

■ (a) The table reveals that although adult literacy and secondary education are the norm in the high-income countries, they are only common to between one-half and two-thirds of the population in low-income countries. (b) The average daily supply of calories per person in the high-income countries is over half as much again as in the low-income countries. (c) Over three-quarters of the population in the high-income countries live in towns and cities, compared to less than one-third in most low-income countries.

● What evidence does Table 7.3 contain of a gender gap?

■ In terms of literacy, women do much worse than men in the low-income countries, but the gap narrows or disappears as we move up the national income scale.

Looking across all the development indicators listed in Table 7.3, the general pattern is that each indicator is better when national income is higher. This suggests that the World Bank's approach of classifying countries strictly on the basis of GNP per head does give a fair guide to many features of development, and Table 7.4 bears this out by showing a wider variety of development indicators by income level.

Table 7.3 Selected development indicators, 1998.

Country group	Percentage of adults who are illiterate (1997)		Average daily calorie (kcal) supply per person (1998)	Percentage of relevant age group reaching 5 years of education (1996)		Percentage of population living in large towns and cities (1997)
	males	females		males	females	
low-income economies						28
China	9	25	2 844	93	94	32
India	33	61	2 415	59	n/a	27
other low-income	30	47	2 145	64	n/a	26
middle-income economies						
lower-middle-income	11	18	2 695	74	n/a	42
upper-middle-income	9	13	2 815	79	n/a	74
high-income economies						
all high-income	<1	<1	3 347	>99	n/a	76

Data derived from World Bank (2000) *Entering the 21st Century: World Development Report 1999/2000*, Oxford University Press, Oxford and New York, Tables 1, 28, 29, 31 and 32; and United Nations Development Programme (1999) *Human Development Report 1999*, Oxford University Press, Oxford and New York, Tables 10 and 20. (n/a = not available)

Table 7.4 Development indicators by income group, 1998 or nearest date.

Indicator	Low income	Middle income	High income
total population in millions, 1998	3 515	1 496	885
(and as a percentage of world population)	(60)	(25)	(15)
life expectancy at birth: males	62	66	74
females	64	72	81
infant mortality rate per 1 000 live births	69	33	6
electricity consumption per capita (kilowatt hours)	433	1 902	8 121
per cent of roads paved 19	51	92	
radio sets (per 1 000 people)	147	383	1 300
daily newspapers (per 1 000 people)	13	75	286
personal computers (per 1 000 people)	4.4	32.4	269.4
internet access points (per 10 000 people)	0.17	10	470

Data derived from World Bank (2000) *Entering the 21st Century: World Development Report 1999/2000,* Oxford University Press, Oxford and New York, various tables.

7.3.4 The Human Development Index

Before leaving this survey of measures of social and economic development, let us look at an attempt to construct a more general 'Human Development Index'. In 1990, the United Nations (UN) published the first in a series of reports, which argued that development was essentially the process of increasing people's options:

> … the most critical choices that people should have include the options to lead a long and healthy life, to be knowledgeable and to find access to the assets, employment and income needed for a decent standard of living. (United Nations Development Programme, 1991 p. 88)

Taking this view, development cannot be measured by income alone, and so the new **Human Development Index** (**HDI**) proposed by the UN was based on three separate components: life expectancy, educational attainment, and a measure of income which gives a progressively lower weight to income above the poverty level. (The thinking behind this last component is that, above a certain level, the additional contribution of an extra unit of income to human development has progressively less impact.)

● Consider the main components of the HDI. Can you think of any important items that are omitted?

■ One important omission is that the index does not embrace any measure of human freedom: freedom of speech or assembly, enfranchisement, freedom from arbitrary rule or illegal arrest or torture, and so on.

Despite this and other limitations, the HDI has proved a useful innovation. In all, the United Nations applied the index to 174 countries in its 1998 report. When they are ranked from best (= 1) to worst (= 174) using the index, it is perhaps not surprising to find that the overall ranking is broadly similar to that which would be obtained if the same countries were to be ranked simply on the basis of GNP per head. However,

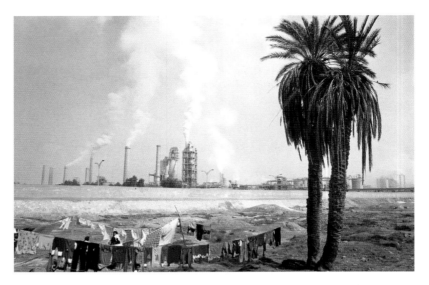

Women from a makeshift squatter camp hang washing alongside a Tawa cement factory on the outskirts of Cairo, Egypt. The uneven progress of development, which creates such contrasts, is typical of many developing countries. (Photo: Jorgen Schytte/Still Pictures)

some interesting differences do emerge: some countries have a human development ranking well *below* their GNP ranking, while others do much *better* on the HDI than might have been predicted on the basis of their GNP per head.

Figure 7.1 attempts to illustrate these discrepancies for a small sample of countries. If GNP rank and human development rank are the same, the country will be on the diagonal line. Below the line, countries are doing worse in terms of human development than their GNP per head would indicate, suggesting that they have the resources to improve their performance in life expectancy and educational provision. Above the line, human development is higher than would be predicted on the basis of GNP, suggesting that health and education have been higher priorities for spending in these countries, or that resources have been used more effectively.

Figure 7.1

Scattergram showing relationship between GNP rank and Human Development Index (HDI) rank, 1998. Rank ordering: best = 1. (Data derived from United Nations Development Programme (1999) Human Development Report 1999, *Oxford University Press, Oxford and New York, and World Bank (2000)* Entering the 21st Century: World Development Report 1999/2000, *Oxford University Press, Oxford and New York)*

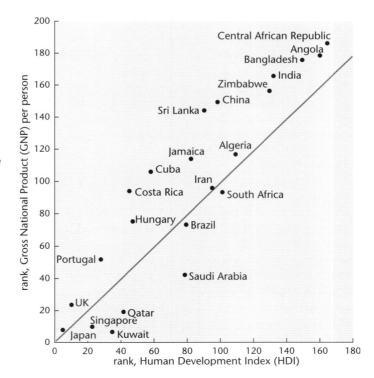

● Looking at Figure 7.1, how would you describe the broad association between GNP and human development?

■ The association is strongly positive for most countries in the sample. Countries with a high ranking on GNP per head (e.g. Japan, the UK) also tend to have a high ranking on the HDI, and those with a low ranking on one index also tend to rank low on the other (e.g. Central African Republic, Angola, Bangladesh).

● Which countries appear to diverge most markedly from this pattern?

■ Sri Lanka and China, for example, are ranked in terms of GNP per head at a point similar to Zimbabwe, but their rank on the HDI is much better. Cuba has a rank of GNP per head not very different to that of Algeria, but does significantly better on the HDI. And Saudi Arabia, Kuwait and Qatar have high GNP per head ranks, but do much less well in human development terms.

Those countries that do diverge from the more general pattern of health and development give some interesting clues as to the limitations of the 'league-table' approach. In the first place, it can be grossly misleading to talk about national averages. South Africa, for example, had a per capita GNP of US$2 880 in 1998, putting it among the 'lower-middle-income' group of countries. But within South Africa the legacy of apartheid is that, on average, 4.5 million whites have health and income levels comparable with those of Western Europe, whereas the 38 million black and 'coloured' (mainly Asian) peoples have average health and income levels more similar to the pattern in low-income countries.[2] Figure 7.2 shows infant mortality rates for the main racial groups in South Africa between 1984 and 1994.

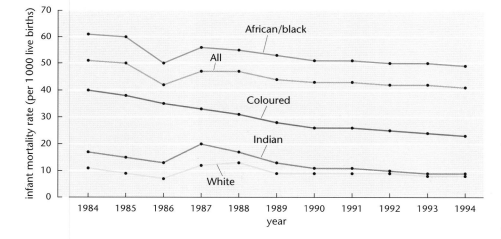

Figure 7.2 *Infant mortality rates by ethnic group in South Africa, 1984–1994. (Data from South African Institute of Race Relations (2000) South African Survey, 1999/2000, Johannesburg)*

● In one sentence, make a comparison between the infant mortality rates shown in Figure 7.2 and the data on infant mortality shown earlier in Table 2.4 (p. 29).

■ The infant mortality rates for whites and Indians in South Africa are similar to the average rate for the developed countries, while the infant mortality rate amongst the African/black population in South Africa is similar to the average rate for the developing countries.

---

[2] The video 'South Africa: Health at the Crossroads', produced for Open University students, is relevant here.

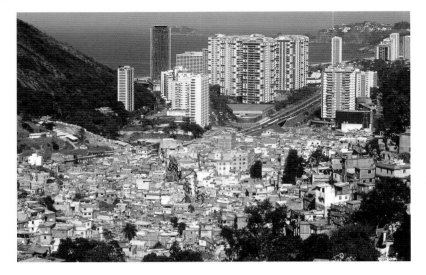

The divisions of income and opportunity in Brazil are strikingly revealed in this view of Rio de Janeiro; the shanty district (or 'favella') is crammed onto the slopes, while the luxury apartment blocks and business skyscrapers are spread out along the sea shore. (Photo: Mark Edwards/Still Pictures)

In Brazil, over the period from 1960 to 1995, the share of national income taken by the poorest 50 per cent of the population fell from 17 per cent to around 13 per cent, while the share of the wealthiest 1 per cent rose from 12 per cent to 19 per cent. Thus, although the average per capita GNP of Brazil grew, the distribution of income within the country became even more unequal. In turn, the average values of Brazil's health indicators conceal very wide variations between a wealthy elite and a great mass of rural poor and urban shanty dwellers.

By contrast, one of the reasons for Sri Lanka's relatively good health indicators is that, although GNP per capita is not high, attempts have been made to pursue a more equitable distribution. In particular, the Sri Lankan government has long operated a food-distribution programme, issuing ration books or coupons for essential commodities, running a state system of food subsidies to the low-income sections of the population, and providing special protein-enriched food supplements to school children. In Chapter 8 we will look in a little more detail at the policies for improving health that low-income countries such as Sri Lanka have pursued.

Distribution, therefore, is as important as any average figure or total amount of wealth or health. This is particularly so of poor countries, where there are often major concerns about **equity**: that is, the fairness or justice with which health, wealth, income or other aspects of society are distributed. Note that equity does not necessarily mean **equality**: equity may or may not require an equal distribution, depending on society's views about fairness and justice. Equity is also an important issue in industrial countries, as you will see when you study the United Kingdom in Chapters 9 and 10 of this book.

7.3.5 Health and development in the former socialist economies

Another facet of the relationship between health and development can be seen in the experiences of the countries of central and Eastern Europe, including the former USSR. During the years when these countries formed a prominent political and economic bloc, they constituted what became known as the *Second World,* in relation to the West's *First World* and the developing countries' *Third World.* However, since the late 1980s when communist rule in these countries collapsed and the bloc began to fragment, they have sometimes come to be categorised more prosaically as the **former socialist economies** of Europe, or **FSEs**.

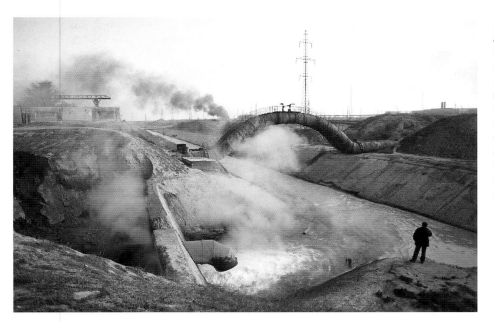

Petrochemical plant in Azerbaijan. Rapid and uncontrolled industrialisation in the former socialist economies of Eastern Europe wreaked widespread environmental damage and contributed to the declining health status of the population. (Photo: Caroline Penn/ Panos Pictures)

During the decades when these countries were run as 'command' economies, planners in government offices attempted to direct the economy by issuing directives and decrees which laid down wages, prices and levels of production. This system seemed for a time to produce rapid rates of economic growth and industrialisation, but at tremendous human and environmental cost, resulting in severe and widespread social malaise, which eventually contributed to the collapse of the old regimes. These problems in turn seem to have had a significant impact on the health of populations in these countries (although detailed documentary evidence on this only began to be made available after the collapse of communist rule).

Figure 7.3 shows some data from the USSR on trends in average life expectancy. The figure shows that average life expectancy in the USSR seems to have improved steadily until the mid-1950s. However, this trend appears to have gone into reverse during the late 1970s and early 1980s, and during the early 1990s, life expectancy

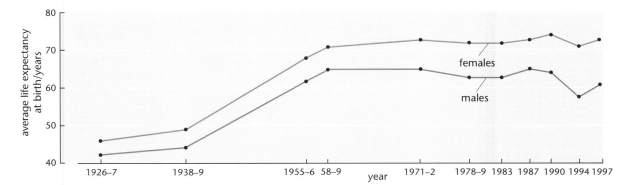

Figure 7.3 *Average life expectancy (in years) of men and women in the USSR (to 1990), and Russian Federation (from 1990), trends from 1926/27 to 1997. (Data to 1987 from Rockney, B. P. (1991) Soviet Statistics since 1950, Dartmouth, Aldershot, Table 38, p. 81. Data for 1990 and 1994 from Notzon F. C. et al. (1998) Causes of declining life expectancy in Russia, Journal of the American Medical Association, **279**, pp. 793–800. Data for 1997 from United Nations Development Programme (1999) Human Development Report 1999, Oxford University Press, Oxford and New York)*

actually fell spectacularly — by around 6 years for men and 3 years for women to a degree unmatched in the peacetime experience of any other industrialised country. At best, average life expectancy in the Russian Federation at the beginning of the twenty-first century is now little better than it was 20 or even 40 years previously.

● Drawing on the evidence presented so far in this book on factors influencing health and disease, suggest reasons for this rapid decline in health?

■ First, there may have been changes in the level or distribution of income or wealth. Second, there may have been changes in nutrition. Third, there may have been changes in risk factors such as smoking and drinking. Fourth, the health care system may have deteriorated. Finally, it is possible that the apparent increase in mortality is mainly a result of poor quality data collection.

One way of exploring this issue is to look in more detail at causes of death. Table 7.5 provides some evidence on death rates per 100 000 by cause in Russia in 1994, the percentage change in these death rates between 1990 and 1994, and the Russian death rates as a ratio of the American death rates in 1990 and 1994.

● Was the increase in mortality in Russia between 1990 and 1994 evenly spread across all causes of death?

■ No. The overall increase in mortality was 33 per cent, but it was much higher in some areas, such as pneumonia and influenza (135 per cent increase) and other alcohol-related causes (266 per cent), while in some areas such as malignant neoplasms (cancers) there was very little change.

Table 7.5 Age-standardised death rates for selected causes of death in Russia and the United States, 1990 and 1994 (males and females).

Cause of death	Deaths per 100 000 in Russia in 1994	Percentage change in death rate between 1990 and 1994	Death rate in Russia as ratio of death rate in USA in: 1990	1994
all causes	1 582	33	1.5	2
infectious diseases	21	65	0.6	0.8
diseases of the heart	478	40	1.3	2
cerebrovascular disease	297	21	4.8	6.1
malignant neoplasms (cancers)	205	4	1	1
pneumonia and influenza	18	135	0.3	0.7
chronic obstructive pulmonary disease	41	15	1.1	1.2
chronic liver disease and cirrhosis	24	68	1.3	2.3
other alcohol-related causes	44	266	4.3	6.1
motor vehicle crashes	23	−5	1.3	1.5
suicide	42	54	2.2	3.5
homicide and legal intervention	31	123	1.5	3.4
other injuries	117	83	3.5	6.3

Data from Notzon, F. C., Komarov, Y. M., Ermakov, S. P., Sempos, C. T., Marks, J. S. and Sempos, E. V. (1998) Causes of declining life expectancy in Russia, *Journal of the American Medical Association*, **279**, pp. 793–800.

● How did death rates in Russia compare with those in the USA in 1990 and 1994?

■ For almost every cause of death, the death rate in Russia was significantly higher than in the USA, a major exception being malignant neoplasms, where death rates were similar. But the table shows clearly that death rates in Russia were already higher than in the USA in 1990 — that is, even before the sharp deterioration in Russian health occurred, which is apparent by 1994.

Using these and other data, researchers have concluded that the increase in mortality in Russia cannot be explained by inaccuracies in the statistics. More than half of the decline in life expectancy can be attributed to cardiovascular diseases and to injuries. The underlying reasons for these changes are still being researched, but almost certainly include a combination of factors such as economic and social instability, which has caused unemployment, poverty and stress; a rapid increase in alcohol consumption; and a poor health-care system in which many drugs considered essential in the West are barely available. It follows that reversing this situation will require far-reaching changes to the Russian economy, society and health-care system. Finally, the experience of Russia in the 1990s illustrates that the tremendous improvements in life expectancy achieved in the industrialised countries during the twentieth century rely on a functioning economy, social order and health-care system, and cannot be assumed to be permanent.

7.4 Closing the gap?

So far, you have seen that it is not always easy to define or measure the link between national wealth and measures of human development such as education and health. This is crucially important when considering policies to improve health, as you will see in the following chapter. However, another major issue is that GNP league tables suggest a ladder of progress, with different countries on different rungs but all heading in the same direction (upwards), and separated only by the time they set off. How true is this?

Clearly there are very wide differences in both wealth and health between developed and developing countries. It could be argued, however, that this is the inevitable short-term consequence of some countries industrialising before others, that where there are pioneers there must also be late-comers, but in time the late-comers will catch up. We can begin to explore the validity of this catching-up concept by looking at the relative rates of growth of GNP in different countries. The first column of Table 7.6 shows the average annual rate of growth of total GNP for each of the three main groups of countries over the period from 1975 to 1995.

● Do the data in the first data column of Table 7.6 support the idea that the developing countries of the world are catching up with the industrialised countries?

Table 7.6 World rates of economic growth, 1975–95.

	Average annual growth rate (%) in	
	total GNP 1975–95	GNP per person 1975–95
least developed countries	2.3	−0.2
all developing countries	4.4	2.3
of which: China	9.1	7.7
of which: India	5.0	2.8
industrialised countries	2.6	1.9

Data derived from United Nations Development Programme (1999) *Human Development Report 1999*, Oxford University Press, Oxford and New York, Table 11.

■ The average annual growth rate of total GNP was substantially higher in the developing countries than in the group of industrialised countries, suggesting that there was some narrowing of the gap. However, in the least developed group of countries, GNP was growing more slowly than in the industrialised countries.

● Now look at the second data column of Table 7.6, which shows the average annual rate of growth of GNP *per person* over the same period. What is the reason for the difference between the first and second columns?

■ The GNP per person is calculated by dividing the total GNP by the population number. The differences between the two ways of representing a nation's resources are explained by differences in population growth rates.

If the population of a country is increasing, the GNP per person will not grow as quickly as total GNP. The bigger the difference between the two columns the higher the increase in population must be. For the industrialised countries the difference between GNP growth and GNP per person growth is less than 1 percentage point, but for the other groups of countries it is much wider: between 2.1 and 2.5 percentage points. As a result, although the total GNP in the developing countries grew substantially more rapidly than in the industrialised group, the gap between them in GNP per person hardly closed. And for the least developed countries — which (as you saw in Chapter 2) contain almost 570 million people — per capita GNP actually *fell* over this period.

It is important to remember that by bundling a lot of countries into just three groups, many differences will be lost among average figures. Looking more closely at Table 7.6, for example, you can see that the growth in GNP per person in the developing countries has been strongly influenced by the above average performance of China; for many of the other developing countries the gap dividing them from the rest of the world appears to have been growing.

One last step in this exploration is taken in Figure 7.4. It shows that, for most of this period of over 30 years, the high-income countries of the world generally experienced a higher rate of growth in GNP per person than any of the other

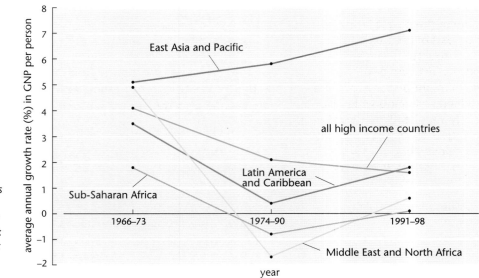

Figure 7.4 *World rates of economic growth, by region, 1966–98. (Data derived from World Bank (1999) Global Economic Indicators Database, Appendix 2)*

regions or categories of country, with the exception of East Asia and Pacific, which includes China, Korea and India. And from the mid-1970s onwards, some groups of low-income countries — notably in the Middle East, North Africa and Sub-Saharan Africa — began falling behind, not only relatively but in absolute terms. There, around 500 million of the poorest people in the world have been getting poorer, with everything that implies for their health, welfare and prospects for survival. There is no single reason for the experience of these latter countries; in some, wars or revolutions have caused economic and social dislocation, others have been affected by droughts or other ecological changes to which they have been unable to respond unaided. However, an underlying problem has been that any growth in *total* GNP was outstripped by their population growth rate.

Once again, therefore, we can see that population change is inseparable from social and economic development, which in turn is linked to health and disease patterns, although, in the developing countries — as in the case of England — these links are not straightforward. Many of the same issues arise when we consider one aspect of economic activity that is fundamentally important to health: food production.

7.5 Food production

7.5.1 The global distribution of food production

In order to make comparisons of food production around the world, we must be able to measure a country's food production accurately, but this raises many of the same difficulties encountered in measuring GNP. The normal procedure for **food production measurement** is to estimate the amount of food that comes onto the market in a country by first calculating, for each type of food crop, the total area planted multiplied by the yield per unit of area. Then all types of food crops and all the producers in a country are added together to obtain a total. Imported food is added, and exports and any food grains fed to animals are subtracted. A correction is then made for losses in storage and during milling and processing and the remainder is converted into equivalent amounts of nutrients (protein, fat, etc.) and energy, using average figures for the chemical composition of each foodstuff. Finally, the result is divided by the current estimate of the total population of the country to give an estimate of food supplies per person.

Some of the pitfalls in this method are obvious. In developing countries, where a large part of production is in the hands of small family farms, many of these stages are a source of systematic under-reporting: farmers all over the world are conservative and pessimistic about their prospects and wary of giving information which might be used to assess land and production taxes. Their estimates of food retained for their own families tend to be minimal. Many countries have long and poorly regulated borders and, if price differences across these borders provide incentives to import or export illegally, there may be large volumes of unreported food movement. And when times are bad, because of drought or recession, large numbers of small farmers may simply withdraw from the market, return to a subsistence pattern of life and wait for better times.

In industrialised countries, the basic statistics of land use, yields, imports and exports are probably much more accurate and the numbers of producers very much smaller. The problems are more in the distribution system. Somewhere in between primary production and the purchase of food by households, around 20–30 per cent of food measured by its energy value goes astray. The more highly industrialised the food processing and retailing system, the greater the losses. Probably a good deal of this is not actual waste, but represents a diversion of some by-products of the food industry into other non-food processes. These systematic errors in the recording of food production create a tendency to underestimate available food in predominantly agricultural populations and to overestimate it in industrial countries.

With these problems in mind, what is the current pattern of food production in the world? Table 7.7 shows the way in which world production of a variety of foods is split between developed and developing countries.

Table 7.7 Total food production of the world, developed and developing countries, 1999.

Food type	Total annual production/million metric tonnes					
	All world	(%)	Developed	(%)	Developing	(%)
cereal (wheat, rice, coarse grain)	1 970	100	832	42	1 138	58
marine fish catch	91	100	32	35	59	65
meat	225	100	104	46	121	54
milk	561	100	340	61	221	39
sugar	1 521	100	303	20	1 225	80
Population/millions	**5 930**	**100**	**1 181**	**20**	**4 748**	**80**

Data from Food and Agriculture Organisation (2000a) *FAOSTAT database*.

● What strikes you about the distribution of food production in 1999 shown in Table 7.7, compared with the distribution of the world's population?

■ The developed world, with only 20 per cent of the world's population, produces over one-third of the world's marine fish catch, over 40 per cent of the world's most important foodstuffs (cereals), almost half of the world's meat, and over 60 per cent of the world's milk.

This dominance of the developed world as a whole in global food production is paralleled in the world trade in foodstuffs. The developed countries have a dominance of the international food trade greater than the Middle East has ever attained in the oil trade: for example, during the 1990s they accounted for almost three-quarters of wheat exports.

7.5.2 Trends in food production

Although the developed world dominates global food production and trade, there was a large increase in food production in the developing countries as a whole during the 1980s and 1990s. However, these average figures disguise many variations in different regions and countries of the world and, as with GNP growth, they have to be adjusted to take into account population growth. Figure 7.5 shows an index of food production per person for major regions of the world, taking the level of production in each region in 1961 as an index number of 100, and covering the period to 1999.

● Summarise the main features of Figure 7.5.

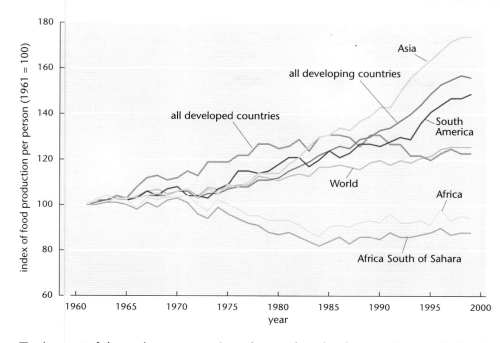

Figure 7.5 *Index of food production per person in major world regions, 1961–1999 (relative to their production in 1961 = index number of 100). (Data from Food and Agriculture Organisation (2000a) FAOSTAT database, 2000)*

■ In most of the regions or groupings shown, there has been an increase in food production per person since 1961. However, in Africa as a whole and particularly in Sub-Saharan Africa there has been a long-term decline in food production per person, going back to the early 1970s.

The difficulties of accurately measuring a country's food production were noted earlier, and these should be borne in mind when considering the data in Figure 7.5. First, there may be questions concerning the equitable distribution of food production within countries, even where overall food production per person has been increasing. In addition, there is an argument that food production in Sub-Saharan Africa has deteriorated *less* than the official figures indicate, and that a substantial amount of food production, exchange and consumption goes unrecorded. If the official figures were telling the whole story, continues this argument, then one would *not* expect to observe life expectancy continuing to rise and infant mortality rates continuing to fall in the region. And yet these indicators have steadily improved, as Chapter 2 indicated.

Despite these qualifications, it does seem that Sub-Saharan Africa faces uniquely difficult problems: as you saw earlier in this chapter, GNP per person also declined during the 1980s, and many other indicators of health and development are the worst of all the world's major regions. As with the GNP decline, there are also many possible reasons why it might be difficult for food production to keep pace with population growth.

One factor is the physical environment, which is very poor for farming: a large portion of the continent is desert or too sandy to farm, much of the land is almost unusable because it is infested with tsetse flies, which transmit to humans and cattle the parasites (*Trypanosoma* species) that cause sleeping sickness (trypanosomiasis) — a slowly progressive infestation of the nervous system resulting eventually in abnormal behavioural patterns, coma and death. Rainfall is low and droughts are normal. Historically, farmers in Africa have adapted their farming methods to these conditions, for example by leaving land fallow sufficiently long for it to recover from cropping. However, these sustainable farming methods have been jeopardised by growing population pressures, so that, for example, land is given insufficient time to recover from cropping, or vegetation is removed for fuel-wood, which is the major source of energy in this region. Another factor has been damaging policies, such as price controls on foods, which give farmers little incentive to increase production. Or there may have been too much investment in urban areas at the expense of rural roads and towns.

Finally, a substantial number of countries in this region have been afflicted since the 1970s by political instability and at worst by civil or international wars: the list includes Angola, Chad, Eritrea, Ethiopia, Mozambique, Nigeria, Somalia, Sudan, Uganda, Sierra Leone and Rwanda. These wars have disrupted food production, created large numbers of refugees, hindered aid efforts, and diverted scarce resources into military expenditure.

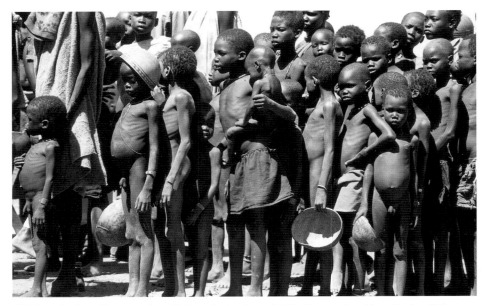

Children displaced by armed conflicts wait at a food distribution centre, Akon, Sudan. War disrupted food production in many African countries throughout the 1980s and 1990s. (Photo: Hartmut Schwarzbach/Still Pictures)

However, the countries of Sub-Saharan Africa affected by this gap between population growth and food production would not necessarily be headed for crisis if they were able to purchase food from other countries. After all, many countries of the world — the United Kingdom is a good example — no longer grow enough food to feed themselves, but do not have any problem feeding their populations because they are able to export other commodities in exchange for food imports. It could be argued, therefore, that the fundamental problem in the Sub-Saharan region is not so much that food production in this part of the world has failed to keep pace with population growth, as that the region is not earning enough from its exports to afford enough imported food to meet its requirements.

This raises a general issue: if we are interested in the ability of a nation to feed itself, it is misleading to focus on national food production without taking into account the ability of that nation to obtain its food requirements from elsewhere. And what is true at the national or regional level is also true of individuals: obtaining food does depend in part on what is produced, but it also depends on such crucial issues as distribution, access and 'entitlement'. As you will see below, this important point is dramatically illustrated by famines.

7.6 Entitlement, food and famine

One image of developing countries that is all too familiar is probably that of a black child with arms and legs of skin and bones and a swollen belly, caught in the middle of drought, famine or simply pervasive and chronic malnutrition and poverty. Insufficient food is a major contributory cause of much death and disease, and seems to be another defining characteristic of developing countries. In a tragic and acute way, **famines** raise the need to take into account the social and economic circumstances in which they occur. They have been the subject of a great deal of research, and one theory which helps to explain their occurrence and the persistence of other forms of **food insecurity** has been developed by the economist Amartya Sen. An extract called 'Entitlement and deprivation' from a book by Sen and Jean Drèze, *Hunger and Public Action,* is included in *Health and Disease: A Reader* (Open University Press, 2nd edn 1994; 3rd edn 2001).

- Write down as briefly as possible your own view of why famines occur. (Open University students should then read the extract and compare your view with Sen and Drèze's comments on how famines occur.) Are there any differences between your view and theirs?

- Of course, we can't claim to know what your earlier views were. But most probably you would have held to the common assumption that famines occur because of a shortage of food. However, Sen and Drèze argue that it is quite misleading to focus only on food supply; what is much more important, they argue, is entitlement, the ability of people to procure food.

The system of **entitlement relations**, which govern whether or not people can get hold of or (in economists' language) *command* food, is of central importance to Sen and Drèze.

- Why do Sen and Drèze claim that it is misleading to focus only on the *supply* of food?

- Even if there is no overall shortage of food, famines can occur because some groups have no 'entitlement' to what is available.

© Gerald Scarfe, 1970.

7.6.1 The 1974 famine in Bangladesh

To illustrate their argument, Sen and Drèze examine a famine that occurred in Bangladesh towards the end of 1974. You have already seen that it is often extremely difficult to obtain reliable health statistics in developing countries, and not surprisingly there is no agreement over how many people may have lost their lives as a consequence of this famine: the absolute minimum is approximately 26 000 deaths, but the estimates range up to 1.5 million deaths. Between June and August in 1974, severe flooding occurred in northern Bangladesh as the Brahmaputra river burst its banks (you may wish to look back at the map in Figure 4.2). This event seemed to point to the common-sense conclusion that the food supply had

Table 7.8 Availability of food-grains in Bangladesh, 1967–76, compared with availability in 1967 (given an index value = 100).

Year	Grain availability per day/ounces per person	Index (1967 = 100)
1967	15.0	100
1968	15.7	105
1969	16.6	111
1970	17.1	114
1971	14.9	99
1972	15.3	102
1973	15.3	102
1974	15.9	106
1975	14.9	99
1976	14.8	99

Data from Drèze, J. and Sen, A. (1989) *Hunger and Public Action*, Clarendon Press, Oxford, Table 2.1, p. 27.

been badly hit and people went hungry in consequence. Once again, however, a careful look at the data reveals a much more complex picture.

● Table 7.8 shows the average availability per capita of all food-grains in Bangladesh for the years 1967–76, measured in ounces per day. What do you notice about 1974, the year the famine occurred?

■ The availability of food-grain in this year was actually higher than in the surrounding years.

Not only was 1974 the least likely year for a famine to have occurred if we look at total food supply, but the districts of Bangladesh most seriously affected by famine tended to be those which, if anything, had *increased* their food supply in 1974 by more than the average for the country as a whole. In fact the Bangladesh famine of 1974 is a good illustration of the way in which an initial event can trigger a series of changes which may compound and magnify the consequences, further destabilising the situation instead of returning it to equilibrium.

In the language of systems technology, we might think of **positive and negative feedback loops**: a thermostat which responds to an increase in an oven's temperature by reducing power to the oven and so maintaining equilibrium is an example of negative feedback, whereas a thermostat which responds to a rise in the oven's temperature by further increasing the supply of power to the oven and thus accentuates the disequilibrium is an example of positive feedback. Complex models of biological systems such as the human body have now been devised, with many coexisting positive and negative feedback loops.[3] But some simpler models fail to acknowledge that positive feedback may occur. For example, the Malthusian model of population change outlined in Chapter 6 suggests a world of negative feedback loops that automatically restore equilibrium.

In the Bangladesh famine of 1974, those most seriously affected by the famine were the wage labourers, because their employment opportunities, and therefore income, were severely reduced by the flooding. At the same time, the price of food

[3] These models are discussed in *Human Biology and Health: An Evolutionary Approach* (Open University Press, 2nd edn 1994, 3rd edn 2001).

rose very sharply in response to an expectation of a damaged harvest in 1975, and also perhaps because of panic buying or hoarding. These price rises compounded the reduction in the entitlement to food of these wage labourers and their families, leading to destitution, famine and, for many, death.

7.6.2 The 1845–49 Irish famine

One of the best-known famines occurred in the nineteenth century: the 1845–49 potato famine in Ireland. During this period, it seems likely that the population of Ireland fell by almost one-third, from roughly 9 million to 6.5 million. Of this 'lost' 2.5 million, nearly one million people emigrated, and the rest died of hunger, disease and fever. A conventional view of this event would be that the potato crop, a staple in the diet of most of the Irish population at the time, had been ruined several years in a row by a blight or disease, leading to a straightforward food shortage.

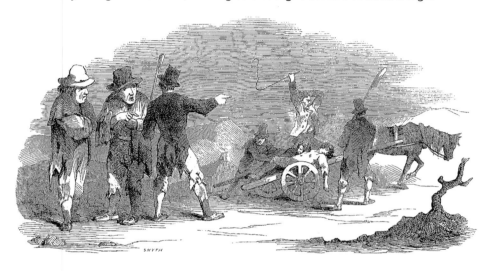

*The famine in Ireland — a funeral at Skibbereen, from a sketch by Mr H. Smith, Cork. (*Illustrated London News, *30 January 1847)*

The closer we look at this event, however, the more the facts seem to fit the 'entitlement' approach. In the first place, large quantities of cattle, corn and other foodstuffs were being produced normally throughout the famine years and exported to England in quantities that would have been sufficient to avert the famine had the Irish population had the means to obtain them. Second, although the English Parliament cheapened the price of grain in 1846 by repealing the Corn Laws in a proclaimed attempt to make grain more accessible to the Irish, the reality of the situation was that the Irish tenant farmers grew grain to pay rent to the landowners, and the falling price of grain increased their rent and thus their poverty, and made them liable to eviction through an inability to meet the landowners' demands. Again, the social and economic organisation of Ireland, and its colonial relations with England, were of more importance than the absolute quantity of food being produced in Ireland at the time. Hence the Irish saying 'God sent the blight; but the English landlords sent the Famine!'

7.6.3 Aspects of entitlement

Famine, of course, is only the most spectacular instance of a breakdown in the system of entitlements to food, and these systems can vary widely from one country to another with correspondingly different consequences. In India, for example, periodic famine no longer occurs, but substantial sections of the population suffer from chronically inadequate access to food. In China, by contrast, the normal lot of the population is much better, and entitlement to food is comprehensive. But it now seems clear that occasional large-scale famines have occurred. In 1959–61, for example, it has been estimated that up to 15 million people may have died in China, because of famine conditions that emerged during a period of economic and political turmoil. (The impact of this event on the subsequent demographic structure of the Chinese population was noted in Chapter 2.)

Amartya Sen has suggested that the difference between India and China may be due to the political processes which affect and influence the system of entitlements. In India, relatively independent media and competing political parties act to ensure that sudden famine is at least newsworthy and considered a political liability to be avoided, but chronic long-term hunger among the poorest sections of society is neither newsworthy nor politically intolerable to the main parties. In China, the state is committed to and can ensure regular access and a more equal entitlement to food. But because its political system is centralised, Sen argues, it can pursue policies which may have consequences that are completely unintended and (for a time) unknown to the rest of the world. Indeed not until 1983, over 20 years after the 1959–61 famine, was its occurrence officially acknowledged by the Chinese Government, following publication of a detailed account by a Chinese economist in the *New York Review of Books*.

One other aspect of entitlement that requires greater emphasis relates to gender. Chapter 3 discussed the phenomenon of 'missing' women, and noted that it occurs mainly in areas of the world (especially in the Indian sub-continent and China) where, in comparison with men, women have restricted access to paid employment, fewer land rights, and less freedom of movement. They thus have fewer opportunities to secure entitlement to goods and services, and there is a good deal of evidence that they receive less parental attention and that their entitlement to health care is less than that of males.

7.7 Conclusion

In conclusion, therefore, the concept of entitlement seems to be a valuable aid to understanding the relationship between health and disease patterns and social and economic development. Sen's work in this area was acknowledged in 1998 when he was awarded the Nobel Prize for Economics for his contributions to the theory of social choice, definitions of welfare and poverty and studies of famine. Equipped with the concept of entitlement, it no longer seems so paradoxical, for example, that many of the countries in the world which had inadequate food supplies for their own populations were also net food-exporters.

The entitlement approach also opens a new perspective on the contribution of Malthus (Chapter 6) to the debate on the relationship between population and food. By rejecting Malthusian pessimism on the grounds that food production at the global level is keeping ahead of population growth, we may run the risk of falling into an equally unwarranted trap of Malthusian optimism: that as long as food production is keeping ahead of population growth there is nothing to worry about. The point is that food production is just one of a range of factors determining entitlements, and to focus on some ratio of food to population, as Malthus and many others have done, is to see only one element of a much more complex picture.

Similarly, as you saw earlier in this chapter, it cannot be assumed that the level or rate of growth of GNP per person can be equated with levels of health or human development: again, there is some connection, but it is much less direct than is sometimes thought.

Finally, it should be clear from the evidence in this chapter that population growth remains a crucial factor in understanding trends in GNP and in food production in different regions of the world. So the next chapter begins by examining these population trends.

OBJECTIVES FOR CHAPTER 7

When you have studied this chapter you should be able to:

7.1 Define and use, or recognise definitions and applications of, each of the terms printed in **bold** in the text.

7.2 Discuss some of the main consequences of the Industrial Revolution for the countries that are now classified as 'developing', particularly in agriculture and industry.

7.3 Explain what Gross National Product (GNP) and the Human Development Index (HDI) measure and what their main limitations are.

7.4 Evaluate the evidence on whether the gap in income per capita between rich and poor in the world is narrowing or widening.

7.5 Outline recent trends in food production in different areas of the world, and some of the problems in interpreting these data.

7.6 Describe and illustrate the entitlement approach to famine.

QUESTIONS FOR CHAPTER 7

1   (*Objective 7.2*)

During the Industrial Revolution, the United Kingdom was often described as 'the workshop of the world'. From Table 7.1, how true was this?

2   (*Objectives 7.3*)

The United Nations Development Programme has argued that the Human Development Index (HDI) broadens the development dialogue from a discussion of mere means (GNP growth) to a discussion of the ultimate ends. To what extent do you think the HDI does succeed in doing this?

3   (*Objective 7.4*)

'The developing countries may be a lot poorer, but by sheer weight of numbers they must account for a big share of total world economic activity. After all, India is one of the top ten world industrial producers.' How valid is this line of reasoning?

4   (*Objective 7.5*)

In what ways do the measurement of food production per capita and the measurement of GNP per capita face common difficulties?

5   (*Objective 7.6*)

The entitlement approach argues that food availability is an inadequate and misleading way of viewing famine. Does this mean that food availability and entitlement are not linked?

CHAPTER 8

Population and development prospects

Study notes for OU students

This chapter builds on material in Chapters 6 and 7 to consider the relationship between economic development and the demographic transition. You may wish to look back at Figure 7.1 and the 'in-text questions' which relate to it, before starting Chapter 8. There is no additional set reading for this chapter.

8.1   Introduction

In Chapter 7 you saw that there is no simple link between national wealth and levels of health or human development. Some countries have lower mortality and longer life expectancy than might be predicted on the basis of their GNP per person, others do less well. This chapter begins by placing such findings in a broader context: it looks in more detail at population change in developing countries, then considers the evidence of a link between economic development and the demographic transition described in Chapter 6. It then looks at some of the ways in which countries have attempted to promote the demographic transition, not simply by relying on economic development, but by pursuing policies explicitly aimed at lowering their birth rates and their mortality rates. The chapter concludes with a brief survey of some of the major obstacles to development facing developing countries.

8.2   Population change in developing countries

8.2.1   Global trends

As Chapter 7 illustrated, rates of **population growth** are a crucial factor in understanding trends in GNP and in food production in different regions of the world. They also represent one of the main differences between the industrialised and the developing countries. Figure 8.1 shows some features of the rate of population growth in the more developed and less developed countries, based on United Nations estimates; (the dashed lines from 2000 onwards signify projected rates).

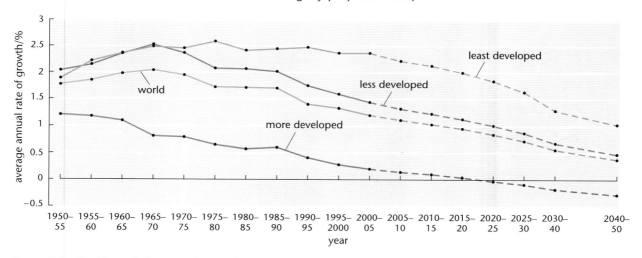

Figure 8.1   *World population growth rates, 1950–2050. (Data from United Nations, 1999d,* World Population Prospects 1998, *Volume 1 (ST/ESA/SER.A/177), UN, New York, Table 1)*

● First look at the data for the world as a whole from 1950 to 2000, what patterns do you detect, and what effects would these trends have on population size?

■ From 1950 to approximately 1970, the rate of annual growth was actually increasing, so the pace of population growth accelerated quickly. Growth rates then started to fall, seemed to reach a plateau during the 1980s, and then continued a downward path. So although the world population was still growing in 2000 (by about 1.3 per cent a year) the *rate* of increase had begun to slow down.

●   Now compare the population growth rates of the more, less and least developed countries in Figure 8.1. How have they changed from 1950 to 2000?

■   The growth rate in the less developed countries is substantially higher than in the more developed countries. For example, in the years 1995–2000, it averaged 1.6 per cent per year in the less developed countries, and 0.3 per cent in the developed countries. However, growth rates in the less developed countries seem to have continued a downward trend at around the same time as in the more developed countries — around 1985–90. Amongst the least developed countries, population growth rates are higher than in any other group and remained around 2.5 per cent per annum between 1965 and 1995.

8.2.2 Projections

The United Nations makes regular projections of the world's population, covering every country and territory from Pitcairn with a population of 46 to China with 1.2 billion inhabitants. Figure 8.1 also shows the projections (made in 1998) of annual rates of population growth up to the year 2050. These indicate that the downward trends in growth rates will continue, with the least developed countries also showing slower rates of growth from around 2000 onwards. By the year 2020 the UN anticipates that the population of the developed countries as a whole will no longer be growing, and by 2045–50, it is likely that at least 56 countries will be experiencing negative growth (that is, falling population size).

How do these growth rates translate into actual numbers? Figure 8.2 shows that the *central estimate* (that is, in the middle of a range of high and low estimates) of projected world population predicts an increase of 50 per cent from 6 billion in 2000 (in fact 12 October 1999 was designated by the United Nations as the 'Day of 6 Billion') to almost 9 billion by 2050. And because growth rates are falling, the number of additional people per year in the world has also begun to fall. This annual increment peaked during the period 1985–90 when an additional 85 million people were being added each year to the world's population. By 1995–2000 this had fallen to 78 million more per year, and by 2045–50 is projected to have fallen to an additional 30 million each year. This is still a lot of extra people — equivalent to a new Canada every 12 months — but the trend is clearly set downwards.

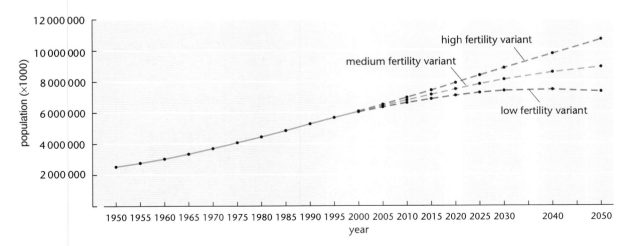

Figure 8.2 *The projected population of the world, 1990–2050. (Data from United Nations, 1999d,* World Population Prospects 1998, *Volume 1 (ST/ESA/SER.A/177), UN, New York, Table 1.)*

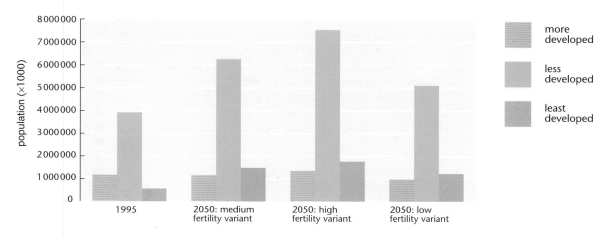

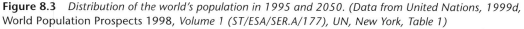

Figure 8.3   *Distribution of the world's population in 1995 and 2050. (Data from United Nations, 1999d, World Population Prospects 1998, Volume 1 (ST/ESA/SER.A/177), UN, New York, Table 1)*

Figure 8.3 shows how the projected population increase to the year 2050 is distributed between developed, developing and least developed countries, and also how this is influenced by different assumptions about future fertility rates.

● According to Figure 8.3, where is most of the population growth likely to occur?

■ Almost all the increase is occurring in the developing countries (in fact 97 per cent of the projected increase in population between 2000 and 2050 will be in the 'less' and the 'least' developed regions).

● What is projected to happen in the 'more' developed regions?

■ On all projections apart from the high fertility model, population size is expected to *fall*.

● How do different assumptions about fertility rates affect the projected total population?

■ They have a very large effect: even over a 50-year period the projected total world population varies from 7 billion to 11 billion depending on which fertility assumptions are used.

The United Nations Population Division also produces much longer term world population projections, stretching into the middle of the twenty-second century. In 1998 it estimated that world population would rise to 10.4 billion by 2100 and 10.8 billion by 2150, eventually stabilising around 2200 at just under 11 billion. However, these long-term projections are even more subject to uncertainty, with the projected population in 2150 varying from a low estimate of 3.6 billion (barely half *current* world population) to a high estimate of 27 billion (which far exceeds most current estimates of the world's *carrying capacity*, as you will see in Chapter 11). This wide range is mainly dependent on future fertility rates. The importance of these rates is illustrated by the fact that the high and low fertility scenarios differ by only *one child* per male/female pair. We will look at fertility in more detail shortly.

Such long-term projections are highly speculative, and the passage of a fairly short time can lead demographers to change their assumptions and forecasts quite substantially. In 1982 the UN projected a peak world population of under 11 billion, then in 1992 increased this by about 10 per cent, mainly because the downward trend of birth rates — which was apparent during the 1960s and 1970s — slowed during the 1980s. The estimate made in 1998 has come down by around 0.7 billion, mainly due to larger than expected declines in fertility in many countries.

Nevertheless, as you will recall from the discussion of population pyramids in Chapter 2, a population structure has a tremendous amount of in-built momentum: for example, the cohorts of individuals who will be childbearing adults in 10 or 20 years are already alive. In consequence, even quite rapid changes in birth rates or death rates take time to feed through into changes in growth rates and age structure. To illustrate, even if all couples in the world had begun to bear children only at the replacement level of just over 2 per couple in 1995, the growth momentum of the world's age structure would still ensure that the population rose by two-thirds to 9.5 billion by 2150. Consequently, although forecasts beyond the middle of the twenty-first century are uncertain, it *is* certain, barring calamities, that by 2050 the world's human population will be several billion more than in 2000.

8.2.3 The potential impact of AIDS

One such possible calamity, the impact of which is still hard to predict, is the AIDS epidemic, which gained ground throughout the 1980s and 1990s. In 1999 the United Nations Population Division published an assessment of the impact of HIV/AIDS in the 34 countries most affected by the epidemic — that is the countries with an adult HIV prevalence of 2 per cent or more, plus Brazil and India with adult HIV prevalence of around 1 per cent but because of their large populations having many affected individuals. 29 of these countries were in Africa, 3 in Asia, and 2 in Latin America. Table 8.1 summarises the likely impact of AIDS on the population size of these countries up to the year 2015, and the impact on life expectancy.

- According to Table 8.1, what impact will AIDS have on projected population growth between 1985 and 2015 in the 34 countries most affected by the epidemic?

- The population will be around 3.5 per cent lower by 2015 than it would have been in the absence of HIV/AIDS.

This may sound a relatively low figure, but as Table 8.1 shows, the absolute difference in numbers is almost 80 million people, a horrifyingly large total. In the 9 countries with the highest prevalence of HIV/AIDS, population size by 2015 is projected to be reduced by 15 per cent as a result of the epidemic.

- Now look at the second part of Table 8.1, which shows the predicted impact of HIV/AIDS on life expectancy in these countries. How would you summarise these data?

- Across the 34 countries most affected, life expectancy will continue to rise, but by much less than would otherwise be the case: average life expectancy at birth would probably have reached 65 years by 2015 without AIDS, but the epidemic is predicted to reduce this to less than 61 years. Furthermore, in the 9 most affected countries, the consequence of the epidemic is expected to *reduce* average life expectancy over the period 1985 to 2015, thus reversing many decades of progress.

Table 8.1 Potential impact of AIDS on population growth and life expectancy in the 34 countries most affected by the epidemic.

	Population size/millions in:			
	1985	**1995**	**2005**	**2015**
all 34 countries:				
with AIDS	1 308	1 616	1 916	2 204
without AIDS	1 308	1 622	1 953	2 283
absolute difference	0.2	6	37	79
percentage difference	0	0.4	1.9	3.5
9 countries with more than 10% HIV prevalence[†]				
with AIDS	94	119	143	163
without AIDS	94	120	155	191
absolute difference	0	1	12	28
percentage difference	0	1.1	7.8	14.6

	Life expectancy/years in:			
	1985–90	**1995–2000**	**2005–10**	**2010–15**
all 34 countries:				
with AIDS	55.4	57.0	58.7	60.7
without AIDS	55.8	59.7	63.4	65.1
absolute difference	0.4	2.8	4.7	4.4
percentage difference	0.7	4.6	7.5	6.7
9 countries with more than 10% HIV prevalence				
with AIDS	53.4	47.6	43.8	47.1
without AIDS	54.2	58.0	61.8	63.4
absolute difference	0.9	10.4	18.0	16.3
percentage difference	1.6	17.9	29.1	25.6

[†] The nine countries with more than 10% HIV prevalence in 1997 were Botswana (22%), Kenya (10%), Malawi (13%), Mozambique (12%), Namibia (16%), Rwanda (11%), South Africa (12%), Zambia (17%) and Zimbabwe (21%).

Data from United Nations (1999b) *The Demographic Impact of HIV/AIDS*, ESA/P/WP.152, New York.

Such projections are of course subject to many uncertainties, but they do indicate that HIV/AIDS is having a serious impact in many countries, sufficient to erode or even reverse some of the modest development gains achieved in areas such as life expectancy. Indeed, it is drastic enough to reverse population growth in some countries. The AIDS epidemic will impose a very heavy burden on the economies and health services of some of the poorest countries in the world.[1]

[1] The impact of HIV/AIDS on developing countries is further discussed in *Caring for Health: History and Diversity* (Open University Press, 2nd edn 1993; 3rd edn 2001), Chapter 8, and *Experiencing and Explaining Disease* (Open University Press, 2nd edn 1996; colour-enhanced 2nd edn 2001), Chapter 4.

8.2.4 Mortality and fertility trends

What factors have most influenced the population changes that have occurred in recent decades in the developing world? Arithmetically, population growth occurs when the crude birth rate exceeds the crude death rate. As Figure 8.4 shows, the birth rate has been falling around the world for many years and is projected to continue falling, but the crude death rate has also been falling at around the same rate, so the population has continued growing. In the more developed regions, however, most of the major reductions in mortality have already occurred, so the falling birth rate has greatly slowed the rate of population growth. In the less developed regions, a similar flattening off in mortality decline is projected to occur from around 2015 onwards, in time slowing the rate of population increase.

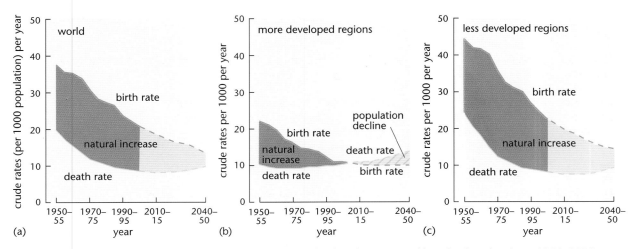

Figure 8.4   *Crude birth and death rates for the world, more developed regions and less developed regions, 1950–2050. (Data from United Nations, 1999d,* World Population Prospects 1998, *Vol 1 (ST/ESA/SER.A/177), UN, New York, Table 1)*

Turning to birth rates, we encounter a familiar measurement problem, namely that the crude birth rate cannot be considered in isolation from information on the age structure of the population, as with the crude death rate. To overcome this, a good measure of the underlying trend in the birth rate is the **total period fertility rate (TPFR)** — the average number of children a woman would give birth to if she experienced the prevailing age-specific birth rates as she passed through the childbearing ages. When a population has a low overall mortality rate, it will replace itself if each woman has 2.1 babies on average. If overall mortality is high, as it is for example in most of the least developed countries, the replacement rate would be around 2.7 babies per woman. Figure 8.5 shows this fertility rate and how it is changing.

● How would you summarise the data in Figure 8.5?

■ The TPFR is much higher in the less developed than in the more developed countries (which fell below their replacement level of 2.1 in the 1970s, although this takes time to feed through to actual population decline). TPFR is highest of all in the least developed group, where the rate is well above the replacement rate of 2.7 and in consequence produces strong population growth. The TPFR has been falling in all groups of countries, including the less and least developed groups as a whole, and this is projected to continue. In all areas of the world the TPFR is currently projected to have fallen below replacement level by around 2040.

However, this does not mean that the world's population will start falling at the same time, again because of the momentum of the existing population structure:

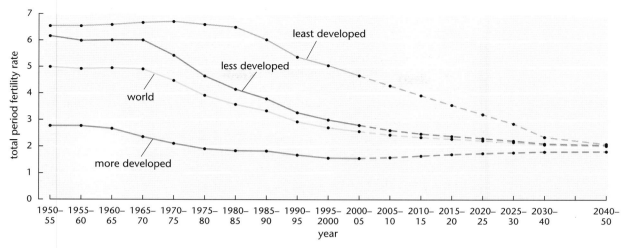

Figure 8.5 *Total period fertility rate estimates, 1950–55 to 2040–50. (Data from United Nations, 1999d,* World Population Prospects 1998, *Volume 1 (ST/ESA/SER.A/177), UN, New York, Table 1)*

as the data above show, the TPFR in the developed countries fell below replacement level in the 1970s, but the total population in the developed countries is not predicted to start falling until around 2020, some 50 years later.

8.2.5 Demographic transition?

How do changes in birth rates and death rates in the developing countries compare with the pattern of change laid out in the model of demographic transition? Figure 8.6 shows available data on birth and death rates for the developed and developing countries from 1775 onwards. (It should be emphasised that the estimates for earlier periods, especially those for the developing countries, are fairly speculative.) Using the model of demographic transition shown in Chapter 6 (Figure 6.8), it is possible to try to fit the four different stages of transition onto Figure 8.6. For the developed countries, it looks as if Stage 1 is at the left-hand edge of the figure, that is, up to the late eighteenth century. By 1800 the death rate has begun falling while the birth rate remains high: this approximates to Stage 2. By around 1880 the birth

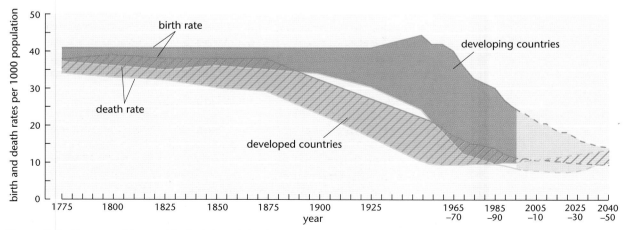

Figure 8.6 *Demographic transition? Birth and death rates in current developing and developed countries, from 1775 to 1995 and projected to 2050. (Data from World Bank, 1982,* World Development Report 1982, *Oxford University Press, Oxford and New York, Figure 3.4, and United Nations, 1999d,* World Population Prospects 1998, *Volume 1 (ST/ESA/ SER.A/177), UN, New York, Table 1)*

rate has also started falling, while the decline in the death rate continues to accelerate: this is the broad pattern of Stage 3. By 1960 the death rate and the birth rate are beginning to stabilise at a much lower level — Stage 4 of the transition.

Among the developing countries, it seems that high birth rates and death rates (Stage 1) existed until around 1900. Then the death rate began to fall, but the birth rate remained high (Stage 2) until about 1960, when it too started to fall in a number of countries (Stage 3).

Although there are some apparent similarities between the past experience of the industrialised countries and present trends in the developing countries, a number of differences should also be noted. First, the rate of population growth in developing countries since World War II has been unprecedented. Even at its peak, the average annual rate of growth of England's population did not go above 1.7 per cent, and for most of the Industrial Revolution was well below this, as Figure 6.2 showed. In some developing countries, the annual rate of population growth has gone as high as 4 per cent. Birth rates were never as high in England as they have reached in many developing countries. Mortality decline in England and other industrialised countries took place over a long period of time, whereas in the developing countries it has been happening quite rapidly. Furthermore, the industrialising countries of the nineteenth century were able to export a large portion of their population growth in the form of international migration.

Cumulatively, these differences help to explain why rapid population growth has sometimes been seen as an obstacle to development in developing countries, in a way that was generally not the case in the history of the industrialised countries.

8.2.6 Problems of population growth

Despite almost two centuries of research and debate, opinion on the relation between population change and economic development is still divided much as it was in the age of Malthus and Godwin. Pessimists, such as the biologist Paul Ehrlich, argue that if population continues to grow it will inevitably collide with finite resources at some not-too-distant point, and the result will be a return on a grand scale of the old Malthusian checks of epidemics and famines (Ehrlich *et al.*, 1970). Optimists, of whom an outspoken example was the American economist Julian Simon, argue that resource limits are not fixed, but depend on technology, which is constantly advancing. From this perspective, human beings are the 'ultimate resource', and population growth could actually augment economic growth in developing countries (Simon, 1981). So far, any evidence on the impact of population growth on economic development has been much less strong than are the opinions of these different protagonists. However, most surveys have concluded that, on balance:

> … economic growth in many developing countries would have been more rapid in an environment of slower population growth.
> (Kelly, 1988, p. 1 715)

Examples of the negative consequences of rapid population growth are not hard to find: overgrazing and other land pressures have led in many areas to land degradation, erosion, deforestation (also caused by the search for fuel) and sometimes the creation of desert. Unemployment and underemployment lead to migration to the cities and the break-up of families. Apart from the human costs, high birth rates in countries where child mortality remains high have economic consequences. For example, a substantial portion of agricultural output may be consumed by people who die before reaching an age when they can contribute their labour.

8.3   Development prospects and problems

In addition to the population pressures discussed above, the development prospects of many developing countries are uncertain. You saw in Chapter 7 that rates of economic growth vary widely across the developing countries, with some of the lowest rates of growth — and indeed some absolute declines in GNP per person — among the world's poorest countries. Looking to the future, it seems likely that this pattern will persist. In 2000 the World Bank conceded that the

> … broad picture of development outcomes is worrisome … Rich countries have been growing faster than poor countries since the Industrial revolution in the mid-nineteenth century … Such findings are of great concern because they show how difficult it is for poor countries to close the gap with their wealthier counterparts. (World Bank, 2000, *World Development Report*, p. 14)

8.3.1   Indebtedness

One major unsolved problem many developing countries face is **indebtedness** to the industrialised countries. For most of the post-war period there was a net flow of resources from private banks and government agencies in the industrialised countries to the low-income countries. This grew rapidly during the 1970s, but much of the money was poorly invested or was simply used to buy consumer goods, while world interest rates rose, so that it became very difficult for many countries to repay these loans. They began sliding further and further into debt, until by 1999 total developing country debt had reached 2.2 trillion (thousand billion) dollars. In consequence, the less developed countries by 1999 were making a net transfer of approximately US$60 billion per year to the richest countries of the world. Particularly badly hit have been the **41 heavily indebted poor countries**, or **'HIPCs'**. Only 2 of these countries have achieved per capita growth rates greater than 2 per cent per annum since 1980; in 1998, 29 of these countries were spending more on debt service repayments than on health care. Numerous proposals have been made to deal with this debt problem, and some progress on debt cancellation was made to mark the millennium in 2000. Even so, the problems of heavy indebtedness and its legacy will not be speedily resolved.

8.3.2   Resource depletion

One final problem faced by developing countries (and another difference compared with the historical experience of the industrialised countries) is that these countries have to find their place in a world whose natural resources have already been depleted and whose environment has already been degraded by the first waves of

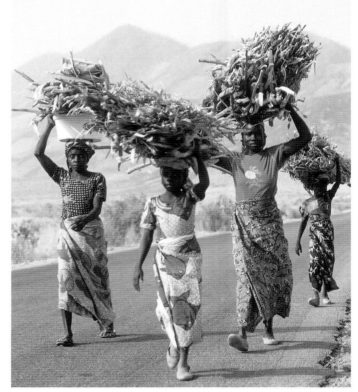

Women collecting firewood in Cameroon. Deforestation is increasingly recognised as a major problem in many areas of the world. (Photo: Mark Edwards/Still Pictures)

industrialisation. In 1996, for example, energy consumption per person in the high-income countries of the world was 5 350 kilograms of oil equivalent per person, or 8 times higher than in the low-income countries. As a result, the 15 per cent of the world's population in these countries were responsible for almost one half of global emissions of carbon dioxide, one of the principle **greenhouse gases** implicated in global warming (World Bank, 1999, Table 10).

Looked at another way, many global environmental problems — such as global warming, deforestation, over-fishing, resource depletion, soil degradation and desertification — are still primarily the responsibility of the industrialised countries, even though most of the world's population and population growth are located in poor countries. If consumption of raw materials and energy use per person were to rise in developing countries to the levels currently prevailing in the industrialised world, an aspiration that cannot be criticised from the perspective of the current high-income countries, it is hard to see how the colossal growth in environmental threats to health and well-being could be contained without massive world-wide changes in social and economic organisation. This tension between the desire of four-fifths of the world's population to participate fully in industrialisation, and the many pressing environmental problems already confronting the world, has been presciently and succinctly stated by the economic historian Carlo Cipolla:

> In order to improve their miserable standards of living, the underdeveloped and developing countries must undergo the Industrial Revolution. If they fail, they are condemned to abject misery. If they succeed, they will add greatly to the problems of pollution and depletion plaguing our planet today. (Cipolla, 1974, p. 120)

These are some of the most complex and possibly intractable problems that humanity has had to face so far: all that can be said with any certainty is that present trends cannot continue indefinitely. But, if they are to be stopped by the

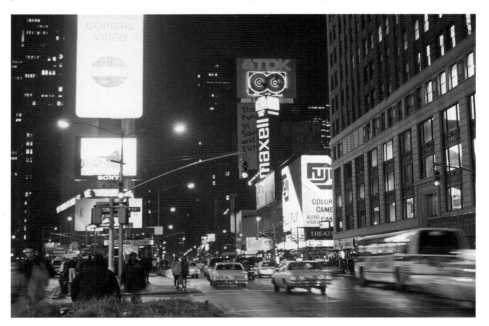

The high-income countries contain 15 per cent of the world's population, but produce almost 50 per cent of the greenhouse gases responsible for global warming; Time Square, New York, USA. (Photo: Richard T. Nowitz/Corbis Images)

adoption of some more stable and sustainable relationship between humans and their natural environment, many observers believe that it will be necessary actively to promote policies to accelerate the decline in fertility rates in developing countries. And, given the uncertain development prospects facing some major regions of the world, and the many obstacles to development that have to be overcome, it will also be necessary to look for ways of trying to improve health and further reduce mortality. In short, economic development cannot be relied upon alone to propel the demographic transition. Let us look first at policies to reduce fertility rates.

8.4   Promoting the decline of fertility rates

8.4.1   Influences on fertility

As you saw in Chapters 5 and 6, there are a number of influences on fertility, including marriage patterns, breast-feeding customs (breast-feeding suppresses ovulation and makes a woman significantly less likely to become pregnant), and the availability and reliability of contraception. The factors that might be related to fertility decline have been extensively studied in recent decades, and three broad areas have been identified: general socio-economic development, the cultural setting including prevailing religious beliefs, and government population policy.

Although these studies confirm that progress in economic development has the strongest influence in reducing fertility rates, they also show that some aspects of development are more important than others. In particular, higher levels of education (especially for women) and better child survival seem to be especially powerful influences, and these — together with the presence of well-organised family planning programmes — explain most of the variation between countries in fertility rates. Other measures of development, such as economic indicators of production or income, appear to add very little. The powerful contribution of improved child survival to reducing fertility rates has been quantified by some studies, which have indicated that this factor has an impact on fertility decline up to three times stronger than that of family planning programmes.

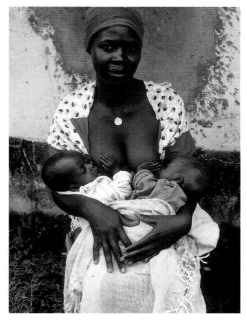

● Why might child survival rates be such an important influence on fertility rates?

■ When child survival rates are low, parents are likely to adopt an 'insurance' strategy, having more children than they actually want in case some die. As child survival improves, parents are more likely to have additional children only if existing ones die. In addition, lower infant mortality is likely to mean lengthened periods of breast-feeding, and this in turn increases the intervals between pregnancies. (You may recall the discussion in Chapter 3 about the two-way association between birth spacing and infant mortality.)

However, as Chapter 4 described, the birth rate began falling in Bangladesh even before infant mortality began to decline, suggesting that under certain circumstances the provision of accessible contraception may be a *more* important influence on fertility rates.

A Kenyan woman breast-feeding twins. Breast-feeding has major advantages for child health and for birth spacing. (Photo: Paul Harrison/ Still Pictures)

Table 8.2 World use of contraceptives, 1998 or nearest date.

Country group	Contraceptive prevalence rate[1] (1998)	TPFR 1997	Annual population growth rate (1975–97)
all less developed countries	55	2.9	2
Africa	19	4.9	2.8
Asia	60	3.4	1.5
Latin America	66	2.7	2
all more developed countries	70	1.7	0.6
world	**58**	**2.7**	**1.8**

[1] The percentage of married women of childbearing age who are using, or whose husbands are using, any form of contraception: that is, modern or traditional methods.

Data from United Nations (1999c) *Levels and Trends of Contraceptive Use as Assessed in 1998*, United Nations, New York, and World Bank (2000) *World Development Report 1999/2000*, Table 7.

Table 8.2 summarises data on the current prevalence of contraceptive use in the world. The table indicates that there is a substantial gap in contraceptive prevalence between the more developed countries, where approximately 70 per cent of married women of childbearing age or their partners practise contraception, and the developing countries, where the comparable proportion is barely one-half. The contrast with particular regions such as Africa is especially marked: there, fewer than one in five women of childbearing age or their partners currently use contraception. And since the most available form of contraception is the condom, which also offers some protection against sexually transmitted diseases, Table 8.2 also sheds light on the spread of HIV/AIDS.

Contraceptive prevalence rates for a number of individual countries are shown in Figure 8.7, which also indicates each country's GNP per capita.

● What is the relationship between contraceptive prevalence and GNP per capita?

■ There seems to be a broadly positive relationship, but it is quite weak, and no direction of causality can be assigned.

On the evidence of these data, it seems that there is a relationship between contraceptive prevalence and broad level of development, but that there is a great deal of variation between countries that are at similar levels of economic development. All these indicators suggest that there is substantial scope for expanding contraceptive prevalence and thus reducing fertility rates and population growth. In fact significant growth of contraceptive prevalence has occurred in almost all developing countries, and in almost 70 per cent of countries with trend data, contraceptive prevalence increased by at least 1 percentage point per year during the 1990s. However, contraceptive prevalence at the global level will need to increase substantially (to at least 75 per cent in the more developed regions and 67 per cent in the less developed regions) if the United Nations medium-variant projections of fertility decline that we examined earlier are to be attained. This is particularly the case in Africa, where the projections depend on a doubling of the contraceptive prevalence rate between 1993 and 2005, with further increases thereafter.

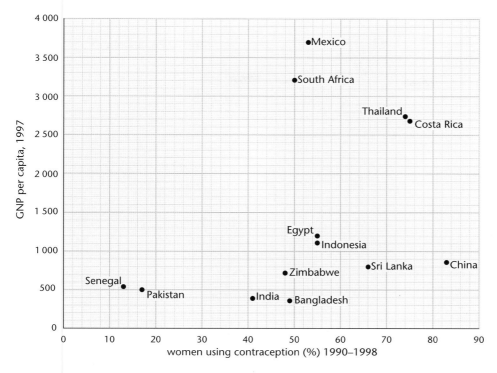

Figure 8.7 *Percentage of women of childbearing age using contraception in 1998 (or nearest dates) in various countries, compared with the GNP per capita in those countries. (Data from* Human Development Report 1999, *Tables 11 and 16)*

8.4.2 Population planning

Among the countries that have achieved greatly improved access to education and increased child survival, and that have also ensured a wide availability of family planning programmes, are China, Costa Rica, Thailand and Sri Lanka (see Figure 8.7). These countries have all attained rapid declines in fertility rates. Conversely, countries with poor child survival, low levels of education and poor family planning services, such as Afghanistan and many countries in the Middle East and North and Sub-Saharan Africa, have experienced much slower fertility declines.

Such data suggest that a range of measures to accelerate falling fertility rates can be a highly effective means to slow the growth in world population, and that effective methods of birth control are an essential component of any such strategy. Of course, there are many cultures in which a large family size may bring greater social or political prestige in a community, and increase the likelihood of favourable settlement of disputes over land or water rights, legal disputes, or straightforward feuds. Economically, children may be highly valued from a very early age as agricultural and domestic workers. It must also be borne in mind that in many developing countries social security provision against unemployment, old age, or sickness is either negligible or non-existent. Children may therefore be valued for the financial support they could eventually provide. In other words, large family size is a positive choice in many areas of the world, and not an accident or mistake. This view is supported by attitude surveys in many countries.

There may also be legal or religious obstacles to the use of contraception. This is especially so in areas of the world where a substantial amount of political power is exercised by the religious hierarchies of Islam or Roman Catholicism: as in Central

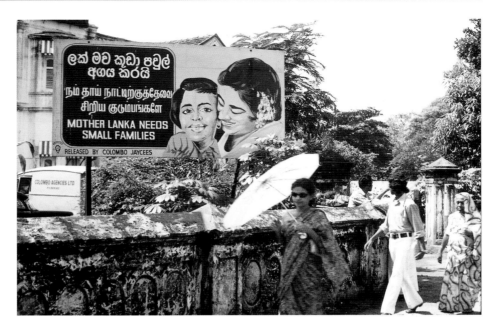

Despite its relatively low GNP per person (see Figure 8.7), Sri Lanka has above average contraceptive prevalence rates for a developing country, due to investment in education, health care and family planning. (Photo: Paul Harrison/Still Pictures)

and Southern America, parts of North Africa and the Middle East, Pakistan, Bangladesh and the Philippines. However, such problems are not insuperable. A well-organised government population programme in Bangladesh has helped to produce a large fall in the TPFR, from 6.3 in 1971–75 to 5.1 in 1983, 4 in 1991 and 3.3 by 1996–97, giving tremendous hope that such changes can occur even in very poor countries that are not experiencing particularly rapid economic development.

Notwithstanding these qualifications, there is often a gap between fertility preferences and contraceptive practice, and this is sometimes used as a measure of the 'unmet need for contraception'. This unmet need is highest in Sub-Saharan African countries, where an average of 27 per cent of women in family union in the 1990s had fertility preferences either for family size limitation or for the spacing of births that were not matched by contraceptive practice.

Family planning programmes have often been treated with suspicion when a ruling elite has used compulsion or removal of individual rights and liberties to reduce the fertility of the general population. The compulsory sterilisation campaign mounted in parts of India during the Emergency of 1975–77 did have a dramatic effect on fertility, but the policy could not survive the return to democracy and the reductions in fertility were not sustained. However, if everyone who wished to control their family size by the most effective means possible were enabled to do so, thus eradicating unmet need, there is little doubt that the world-wide decline in fertility rates and in population growth would be significantly reinforced. The high toll of morbidity and mortality surrounding childbirth that you saw in Chapter 3 would also be reduced.

It is estimated that, in 1999, around US$9.5 billion was devoted to population planning activities in the developing countries, of which almost 80 per cent was provided by the developing countries themselves. The UN Population Fund has also estimated that US$17 billion would be the minimum annual cost of providing worldwide access to modern reproductive health care and family planning services. This is equivalent to one day's worth of personal consumption of goods and services in the USA, and seems a fairly modest cost to attain such an important goal. Even so, international assistance for family planning programmes fell in real terms during the 1980s and 1990s.

8.5   Routes to low mortality?

As you have seen at various points in this book, mortality decline — like fertility decline — is related in a broad way to economic development, but there are many countries performing better or worse than might be predicted on the basis of their national income per person. Let us now look at these countries and try to discover why their mortality is exceptional.

8.5.1   Inferior and superior health achievers

We have identified groups of countries that are furthest above or below average by ranking each country in terms of GNP per person in 1998 and in terms of life expectancy at birth in 1998. The bigger the difference between the two rankings, the more exceptional the country's mortality in relation to its income level. The countries with the highest life expectancy in relation to income level form one group (referred to hereafter as **superior health achievers**), and those with the lowest life expectancy relative to income form another (the **inferior health achievers**). Very small countries, and countries for which very limited information is available are not included. Table 8.3 shows the results of this exercise.

Table 8.3   Countries with high and low mortality relative to level of income, 1998.

	Low mortality relative to income level[1]	High mortality relative to income level[2]
average GNP per person, 1998/US$	2 672	3 801
average life expectancy at birth, 1998/years	69.3	54.5
average infant mortality rate, 1997/1 000 live births	34	68
average female literacy rate, 1997/100 women	80	72

[1] China, Sri Lanka, Vietnam, Cuba, Madagascar, India, Jamaica, Honduras, Armenia, Costa Rica

[2] South Africa, Angola, Libya, Namibia, Brazil, Uganda, Congo, Gabon, Zimbabwe, Botswana

Data derived from United Nations Development Programme (1999) *Human Development Report 1999*, Oxford University Press, Oxford and New York, Tables 8, 11 and 25.

● Summarise the health indicators relative to income in the two groups of countries shown in Table 8.3.

■ The superior health achievers have an average GNP per person which is US$529 per person lower than the inferior health achievers, but despite their poverty, the superior health achievers have longer life expectancy, lower infant mortality rates and higher female literacy rates than the inferior health achievers.

How have this group of superior health achievers been able to transcend their low income levels and achieve their success, and can they teach other developing countries some lessons? This question has been asked repeatedly and over many years, for some of the countries in this group have been superior achievers for several decades and consequently have been studied extensively. During the 1980s, a report commissioned by the Rockefeller Foundation (Halstead *et al.*, 1985) reported in detail on the way in which mortality was reduced in four populations: China, Sri Lanka and Costa Rica (which were all still in the list of superior achievers in 2000) and Kerala, which is a state of India. The report identified the following ways in which these countries seemed to have achieved 'good health at low cost':

1   political and social will;

2   education for all with emphasis on primary and secondary schooling;

3   equitable distribution throughout the urban and rural populations of public-health measures and primary health care;

4   assurance of adequate calorific intake for all (Halstead *et al.*, 1985, p. 246)

Not all of these elements have been present in equal measure in the countries that have reduced their mortality, despite low income levels. But combinations of them can be found in all the superior health achievers listed in Table 8.3. First, a number of the countries have had long histories of political radicalism and grass-roots activism, or have experienced revolutionary governments dedicated to various forms of egalitarianism and welfare in the post-war period.

Second, women generally hold more equal social positions in the countries which have been superior health achievers, reflected in higher rates of female access to employment, health care and education. Kerala State has achieved a much higher female literacy rate than is the norm in the rest of India; this may be one reason why there are no 'missing' females in Kerala State, unlike the situation in the remainder of India.

Third, the essential feature of public-health measures and health-care provision among the superior health achievers has not on the whole been a higher level of spending (although this has also been true of some of the group), but greater *equity*. Services in these countries are more equally distributed between the rural and urban areas than is often the case in developing countries, and they give more equal access to females, and therefore are more efficient at producing health improvement for a given level of resources.

And, finally, most of the superior health achievers have government supported nutrition programmes. These embrace a variety of mechanisms: for example, free school meal systems; food supplements distributed to expectant and nursing mothers and other social groups; public distribution systems and voucher schemes; food subsidies; and schemes of social insurance and assistance and of public sector employment to maintain income and hence entitlement. In reference to these common elements in the experience of the superior health achievers, the demographer John Caldwell has stressed the striking parallels between Sri Lanka, Kerala and Costa Rica:

> These parallels include a substantial degree of female autonomy, a dedication to education, an open political system, a largely civilian society without a rigid class structure, a history of egalitarianism and radicalism and of national consensus arising from political contest with marked elements of populism. (Caldwell, 1986, p. 182)

However, these similarities are so striking and so rooted in historical experience that, as Caldwell goes on to observe, '... they give pause to any belief that low mortality will be achieved easily in most other countries' (Caldwell, 1986, p. 182). In other words, the characteristics of the countries that have succeeded in lowering mortality despite their low incomes may be so strikingly different to those pertaining in the group of inferior health achievers that the idea of drawing lessons and transferring them from one group to the other is far too simplistic.

This view tends to gain support when the characteristics of the inferior health achievers are also examined. Of the ten such countries listed in Table 8.3, several have particularly high and long-standing degrees of income inequality (such as Brazil), or have deep-seated ethnic or other divisions that have resulted in long-running civil wars and political instability. If we were to widen the list of underachievers we would also find a number of countries that are either predominantly Muslim (such as Saudi Arabia, Iraq, Iran, Algeria, Sudan) or have substantial Muslim minorities (Cameroon, Côte D'Ivoire). In contrast, none of the superior health achievers have anything other than small Muslim minorities.

Why might these differences of religion be related to mortality? Just as you have seen that a country's mortality is not determined by its level of income, so it would be wrong to think that it is determined by its religion. However, one of the most important features of Islamic societies concerns the position of women. Relatively good female access to education and health care is a feature of the countries that have managed to reduce their mortality despite their low incomes. These same factors seemed also to be a crucial factor in reducing fertility rates, as you saw above. Furthermore, as Chapter 3 showed, female education is strongly related to childhood mortality, while the position of women and their ability to obtain employment and hence entitlement is an important factor in explaining differences in female:male population ratios in different areas of the world. In many Islamic countries, women tend to have quite restricted autonomy in a number of spheres, and in particular the secular education of females historically has not been encouraged. This is certainly not the only explanation for the over-representation of Islamic countries among the inferior health achievers, but it is of undoubted importance.

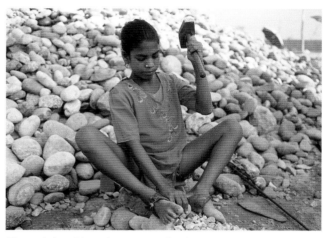

The social position of women and girls tends to be lower than that of males in countries where life expectancy is lower than predicted, given the level of national income. This 11-year-old Bangladeshi girl earns money after school by breaking rocks for road building. (Photo: Shehzad Noorani/Still Pictures)

8.5.2 Aid

One obvious way to promote the human development policies outlined above, with their emphasis on basic education, primary health care, family planning and nutrition programmes, is by means of **Official Development Assistance (ODA)**, that is, donations of money from the industrialised countries to the developing world. ODA amounted to US$48 billion in 1997, or 0.22 per cent of the combined GNP of the donor countries. This is well below the level of 0.7 per cent of GNP set by the UN and agreed by most donor countries as an aid target, and in fact the amount donated has fallen from 0.33 per cent of GNP in 1990.

The total amount of aid to the developing countries is about the same as the net debt repayments from the developing countries to the industrialised countries. For example, in 1997 a total of $13 billion in official development assistance was given to the least developed countries, but most of these countries are also the most heavily indebted poor countries, who have debts of $245 billion and in 1996 paid back $11 billion in debt servicing. Official development assistance is also less than the estimated lost export earnings of developing countries due to trade barriers on their agricultural and other goods.

The distribution of official aid is not related in any obvious way to the poverty of the individuals in the recipient countries. In fact the United Nations Development Programme has estimated that the richest 40 per cent of the population in developing countries receives more than twice as much aid per person as the poorest 40 per cent (UNDP, 1992, pp. 45–6). Even then, only a very small share of official aid is directed into the basic human priority areas identified in this book as being most relevant to health. During the 1990s basic education, primary health care, safe drinking water, family planning and nutrition programmes together were allocated less than 8 per cent of all aid, the great bulk of which was directed to industrial projects, agriculture and infrastructure. International agencies such as the World Bank have begun to accept that support for health and education are not *alternatives* to economic development but important *components* of development, but so far the impact of this on the distribution of development assistance has been small.

8.6   Summary

In summary, the social, cultural and historical differences between the superior and inferior health achievers are often profound, and challenge the idea that there are easy routes to low mortality by simply transferring a few policies from one setting to another. But the steps taken by countries such as China, Sri Lanka or Kerala State to lower mortality and lower population growth rates have been documented in detail, and do demonstrate that low mortality with low birth rates is potentially within the reach of most countries, relatively few of which are poorer than these high achievers. Perhaps above all, the lesson is that these outcomes are unlikely to be attained simply as a side-effect of rising income levels. Because a country is poor it does not follow that the only way health can be improved is to become richer. As the economists Amartya Sen and Jean Drèze noted, in a summing-up of the performance of the superior health achievers:

> At the risk of oversimplifying the problem, it can be argued that a high level of GNP per head provides an *opportunity* for improving nutrition and other basic capabilities, but that opportunity may or may not be seized. In the process of transforming this opportunity into a tangible achievement, public support in various forms … often plays a crucial role. (Drèze and Sen, 1989, p. 181)

In those developing countries facing falling or stagnant incomes per person, the degree to which improvements in mortality can be separated from levels of income may be put to a severe test during the opening decades of the twenty-first century.

In the final chapter of this book we shall look in more detail at nutrition, which has been a recurring theme in our explorations of health in the contemporary developing countries and of health changes in the past of the industrialised countries. Before that, the next two chapters complete our account of world health and disease patterns with a detailed look at contemporary health and disease in an industrialised country: the United Kingdom.

OBJECTIVES FOR CHAPTER 8

When you have studied this chapter you should be able to:

8.1 Define and use, or recognise definitions and applications of, each of the terms printed in **bold** in the text.

8.2 Outline the main features of the recent past and the projected future population of the developing and developed countries of the world.

8.3 Assess the evidence in present trends for a demographic transition in developing countries.

8.4 Discuss the determinants of fertility decline, and describe the role of family planning and other population control policies in influencing fertility rates.

8.5 Give examples of countries that seem to have exceptional (high or low) mortality in relation to their income levels, and discuss some of the characteristics of these countries.

QUESTIONS FOR CHAPTER 8

1 (*Objective 8.2*)

'There are so many uncertainties concerning human population growth that making projections of the future world population is a futile exercise.' Discuss.

2 (*Objective 8.3*)

To what extent does the past experience of demographic transition in the industrialised countries fit present trends in the developing countries?

3 (*Objective 8.4*)

According to most research evidence, what are the main factors that influence fertility decline, and how would you rank them in terms of importance?

4 (*Objective 8.5*)

'Some poor countries may have achieved exceptionally low mortality in relation to their income levels, but this is irrelevant when the objective of most developing countries is not low *relative* mortality, but low mortality in *absolute* terms.' How true is this statement?

C H A P T E R   9

Contemporary patterns of disease in the United Kingdom

Study notes for OU students

This chapter contains a considerable amount of data, presented in several different ways: tables, graphs, pie diagrams, histograms and maps. They have been included partly for illustrative purposes and partly as a useful source of reference, and it is important to realise that you are not expected to memorise the details. This is the second longest chapter in the book, so allow adequate time for it. You may find it helpful to refer to *Studying Health and Disease* (Open University Press, second edition 1994; colour-enhanced second edition 2001*)*, Chapters 6–8, to refresh your memory of epidemiological methods of data-collection and interpretation, and also the calculation of Standardised Mortality Ratios (SMRs). A video called 'Status and wealth – the ultimate panacea?' is associated with this chapter (and with Chapter 10). It looks at the impact of the living and working environment on health inequalities in the UK and examines the interaction of social factors such as poverty with cultural, biological and 'lifestyle' factors in producing social gradients in disease and in expectation of life. Details can be found in the *Audiovisual Media Guide*, which you should read before watching the video. The audiotape on 'Smoking: A global health problem' (associated with Chapter 3 of this book) is also relevant here, and you could usefully listen to it again if you have time.

9.1   Introduction

So far in this book we have examined differences in the patterns of health and disease between industrialised and developing countries, and looked at how these are related to the social and economic environment. In Chapter 6 we have also traced the historical changes in the health of the people of England, from a pattern that in some ways resembled that of a present-day developing country, to that of a modern industrialised state. This chapter now considers in more detail the patterns of health and disease experienced by different social groups in the UK today.

The chapter begins by describing the overall patterns of mortality, morbidity and disability. It then discusses both the nature of the epidemiological approach to understanding how such patterns arise, and some limitations of this approach that should be borne in mind when examining the data it generates. In the remaining six sections we consider the main biological and social determinants of health and disease under six broad headings: gender; age; marital status; ethnicity; geography; and occupation and social class.

9.1.1   Sources of data

This chapter is particularly reliant on many different health measures. It has been suggested (Jette, 1980) that four main criteria should be used in choosing such measures:

(1) *the purpose* — for example, whether the intention is to measure the health of an entire population or to assess the effect of a disease or treatment on individuals or specific groups;

(2) *the conceptual focus* — for example, whether the intention is to look at symptoms, or disease pathology, or changes in health status;

(3) *the properties of the measurement instruments* — for example, whether they are reliable, well validated and sensitive;

(4) *the source of data* — for example, whether they come from voluntary surveys or routinely recorded information.

Here we are particularly concerned with patterns of mortality, morbidity and disability in the population as a whole, so much of the data used in this chapter are drawn from routine statistics compiled by the Office for National Statistics (ONS) in annual publications or major reviews.[1] However, it is important to be aware that these data can be affected by the way they are defined and collected. For example, the *International Statistical Classification of Diseases* (ICD) system, which is used to categorise deaths and diseases, was revised ten times during the twentieth century, and each revision had a potential effect on the apparent trends in disease.[2] When AIDS was identified in the late 1970s, for instance, it was classified by the ICD system in a category containing all the endocrine, nutritional and metabolic diseases and immunity disorders. But in 1993 it was decided to transfer it to the category of infectious diseases. The result was to create an apparent drop in one category and a sudden jump in the other, neither of which accurately reflected the true picture. Many similar instances could be cited, but the point is not to throw doubt on all

[1] For example, *The Health of Adult Britain 1841–1994* (edited by John Charlton and Mike Murphy, 1997, ONS, Series DS No. 12, The Stationery Office, London.

[2] The ICD coding system is discussed in *Studying Health and Disease* (Open University Press, 2nd edn 1994; colour-enhanced 2nd edn 2001), Chapter 7.

routine statistics, but rather to be prepared to consider whether apparent findings in the data are *artefacts* of the way in which the data were collected. (We return to the problems of artefacts in epidemiological data in Chapter 10 of this book.)

9.2 The main causes of mortality, morbidity and disability

9.2.1 An ageing population

In Chapters 2 and 3 you saw how epidemiology and demography interact in developing countries. In the UK and other industrialised countries, changes in the pattern of many diseases have gone hand in hand with alterations in the age structure of the population. And, as Figure 9.1 shows, these changes in the age structure of the population are expected to continue into the foreseeable future. The figure shows population changes by age-group, in the form of an *index* in which the size of each group has been set equal to 100 in 1991. Changes in the size of each group are then calculated in relation to this initial index number, so that, for example, an increase in the size of the total population (all ages) of 10 per cent between 1991 and 2021 is shown as a change in the index from 100 in 1991 to 110 in the year 2021.

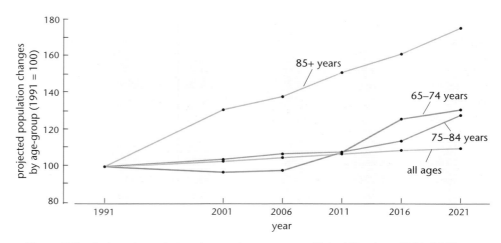

Figure 9.1 *Projected population changes by age-groups, United Kingdom, 1991–2021 (1991 = 100). (Data from Office for National Statistics, 1999,* Annual Abstract of Statistics, *The Stationery Office, London, Table 5.3)*

● What is the percentage increase in size of the three age-groups shown by the year 2021? (Read the approximate value from Figure 9.1.)

■ Compared with 1991, there will be 31 per cent more people aged 65–74, 28 per cent more people aged 75–84, and the numbers of those aged 85 and over will have increased by 75 per cent.

These trends reflect the probability of surviving to any given age, but they also reflect the actual numbers of people born in the past. For example, the fall in the number of people in the age-group 65–74 during the 1990s resulted from a fall in the birth rate during and after World War I.

9.2.2 Mortality

In Chapter 6 you saw how life expectancy in the UK has increased rapidly from the late nineteenth century onwards. By the year 2000, males born in the UK could expect to live for about 75 years, and females for 80 years. One consequence of this improvement in survival has been that **degenerative diseases** (due to cumulative damage and the wearing out of tissues) have become the leading causes of death, as Figure 9.2 indicates.

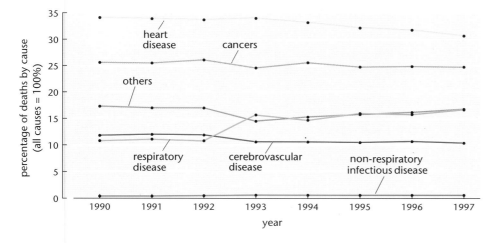

Figure 9.2 *Causes of death in England and Wales, 1990–1997 (percentages of total for all males and females aged 28 days and over). (Data derived from Office for National Statistics, 1999,* Annual Abstract of Statistics, *The Stationery Office, London, Table 5.19, p. 55)*

Figure 9.2 shows the **proportional mortality**, i.e. the percentages of all deaths in England and Wales, attributable to the leading causes of death between 1990 and 1997. (In 1997 the total number of deaths in England and Wales from all causes was 555 281). Two groups of chronic disease associated with degeneration of the arteries together accounted for about 41 per cent of all deaths in 1997: they are *heart disease* caused by deterioration of the arteries supplying the heart muscle (coronary arteries), and *cerebrovascular disease*, in which a similar process of deterioration causes part of the brain to be damaged or destroyed by losing its blood supply, known as a stroke. The proportion of deaths caused by both groups of disease has been declining in recent years, more noticeably in the case of heart disease. (Note that the information in Figure 9.2 is for males and females combined; when they are considered separately a number of differences are evident, as you will see later in the chapter.)

The next two largest categories identified in Figure 9.2 (apart from 'others' to which we return later) are those of cancers and respiratory disease, which in 1997 accounted for 25 per cent and 17 per cent of all deaths respectively. The proportion of deaths caused by cancers remained fairly constant during the 1990s. You will notice an increase in the proportion of deaths from respiratory disease (conditions affecting the lungs) in the middle of the decade. The main cause of death from non-malignant (i.e. not cancer-related) respiratory disease is pneumonia, and these deaths mostly occur in frail, elderly people who are already suffering from chronic lung conditions. Another cause of death in this respiratory group is influenza: deaths from influenza vary between a few hundred and 10 000 a year, reflecting the epidemic nature of this infection. So the sudden increase in the proportion of deaths attributable to respiratory disease was partly a result of a change in the incidence of these diseases, but was also to some extent an artefact of the kind of changes in the classification of diseases in the official statistics that were discussed earlier. In particular, bronchopneumonia appeared to decline during the 1980s because the Office of Population Censuses and Surveys (OPCS, the predecessor to the Office for National Statistics, ONS) changed the rules about selecting a cause of death, giving more emphasis to *underlying* causes of death, and less emphasis to the *immediate* or direct cause of death, which often was bronchopneumonia. However, in 1993 this decision was reversed, and the number of deaths attributable to bronchopneumonia jumped as a consequence.

Infectious diseases other than those affecting the lungs were responsible for just over half of one per cent of deaths in 1997, a fact that graphically illustrates the degree to which the health transition discussed in Chapter 6 has been accomplished in the UK. As Figure 9.2 shows, deaths from all infectious diseases combined rose by almost 40 per cent during this period, but again the picture is complicated by changes in the way the data were collected: as noted earlier, deaths from HIV/AIDS were reclassified from immunity disorders to infectious diseases in 1992, causing a sharp increase in the following year under the infectious disease heading.

The 'cancers' category in Figure 9.2 includes a large number of cancers of different types that arise in different organs. Figure 9.3 shows the age-standardised death rates for the commonest cancers among men and women. In men in 1998 the most common cancer was of the lung, followed by the prostate, colon and stomach. The lung cancer rate has been falling steadily among men since the mid-1970s, and the stomach cancer rate has been falling for even longer; cancers of the prostate show a long-term increase, although this may not have continued through the

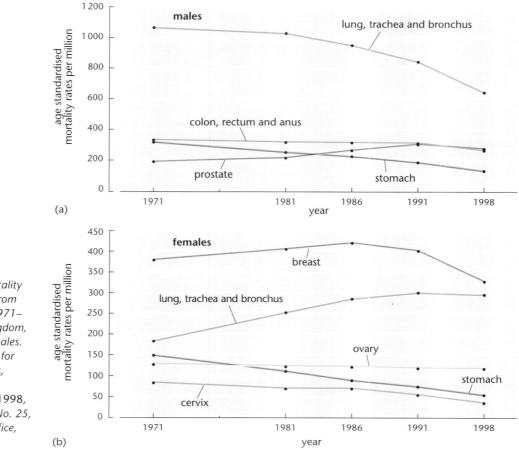

Figure 9.3 *Age-standardised mortality rates per million from cancers by site, 1971–1998, United Kingdom, (a) males, (b) females. (Data from Office for National Statistics, 1999a,* Mortality Statistics: Cause 1998, *ONS Series DH2 No. 25, The Stationery Office, London, Table 5)*

1990s. Notice that the vertical scale on Figure 9.3 for male cancer deaths is much larger than for females. In women the commonest cancer is of the breast, followed by lung cancer. The death rate from breast cancer rose during the 1980s among women in the UK, although this trend may have come to an end. There has been a sharp increase in lung cancer deaths, reflecting the post-war increase in smoking prevalence amongst women, but the death rates from stomach cancer and cervical cancer have been falling among women.[3] Across the population as a whole the top three cancers — of the lung, the female breast, and the stomach — account for around 40 per cent of all deaths from cancer.

Look back at Figure 9.2 and the category labelled 'others', which includes numerous causes of death. The actual number of deaths caused by some of these 'other' causes are shown in Figure 9.4. In 1997 they ranged from 35 deaths of women in labour or childbirth to 3 885 deaths from accidental falls.

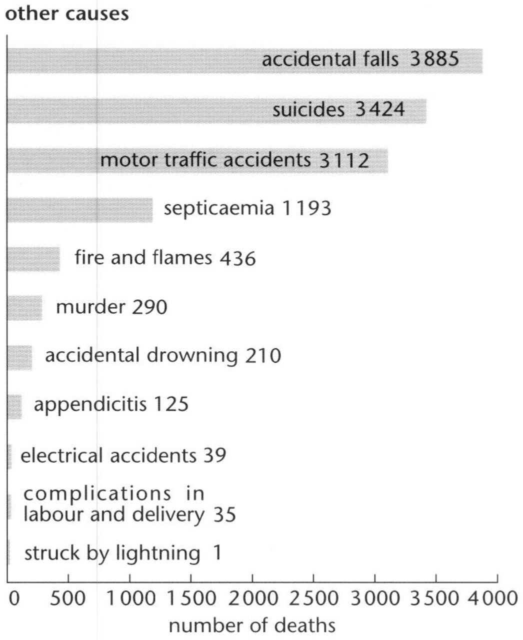

other causes

Figure 9.4   *Some examples of deaths from 'other causes' in England and Wales, 1997. (Data derived from Office for National Statistics, 1998, Mortality Statistics: Cause 1997, ONS Series DH2 No. 24, The Stationery Office, London, Table 2)*

- Consider the following pairs of causes of death. In each pair, which cause is responsible for more deaths, and how much more common is it?

   (1) suicide and murder;

   (2) electrical accidents and burns (fire and flames);

   (3) septicaemia and deaths from falls.

- From Figure 9.4:

   (1) suicide is almost 12 times as common as murder (3 424 ÷ 290 is approximately equal to 12);

   (2) burns cause 11 times as many deaths as electrical accidents;

   (3) falls kill almost 3 times as many people as does septicaemia.

[3] Trends in smoking for males and females in the UK in the twentieth century, and the health consequences, are explored in an audiotape for OU students, called 'Smoking: a global health problem'.

Figure 9.4 also raises a more general issue, concerning perceptions of the risk of dying from various causes.

● Before continuing, note down your estimate of the chance of dying in any one year from (1) smoking 10 cigarettes a day; (2) a road accident; (3) being murdered, and (4) cancer. Then compare your notes with the data in Table 9.1, which shows the chances of dying from a variety of specified causes, during a year of exposure, averaged over the whole population of England and Wales, regardless of sex or age. (You can also think of the chances reported in the table as the number of years a person would have to live and be exposed to that risk, in order to be almost certain to die of it.)

Table 9.1   Risk of a person dying in any one year from various causes, England and Wales, 1998.

Cause of death	Chances of dying
smoking 10 cigarettes a day	1 in 200
circulatory disease (CHD, stroke etc)	1 in 220
cancer	1 in 290
influenza	1 in 5 000
road accident	1 in 8 000
accident playing soccer	1 in 25 000
murdered	1 in 100 000
all forms of food poisoning	1 in 100 000
railway accident	1 in 500 000
salmonella poisoning	1 in 1 000 000
struck by lightning	1 in 10 000 000

Data derived from Office for National Statistics (1998b) *Mortality Statistics: Cause 1997*, ONS Series DH2 No. 24, The Stationery Office, London, and British Medical Association, 1987, *Living with Risk*, BMA, London, p. 23.

■ Table 9.1 shows that the chance of dying in any one year from:
  (1) smoking 10 cigarettes a day is 1 in 200;
  (2) a road accident is 1 in 8 000;
  (3) being murdered is 1 in 100 000;
  (4) cancer is 1 in 290.

We often seem to perceive some risks to be very much greater than the figures in the table suggest is actually the case, while other risks are consistently underestimated. For example, the chances of dying from eating unsafe food are very low, yet as you will see in Chapter 11, this issue can generate enormous controversy and concern compared with other more potent threats to health.

In summary, mortality in the UK population is dominated by a number of chronic and degenerative diseases, which have become the leading cause of death as the average expectation of life has increased. The largest groups are heart disease, cancers and cerebrovascular disease, which together account for around two-thirds of all deaths.

9.2.3 Morbidity

So far we have only considered mortality, but further information on the pattern of diseases can be obtained from studying morbidity. There are four commonly used methods of measuring morbidity.

● Can you suggest what they are?

■ 1 Measuring the *use of health services* (such as the number of people admitted to hospital with a particular disease);

2 *Screening*, in which the whole population or a sample are investigated in some way in order to identify those individuals who might benefit from treatment for a particular disease;

3 *Registers*, in which, for example, all new cases of cancer are recorded, providing valuable data on the incidence of cancers;

4 *Population surveys* or *self-assessment surveys* in which people are examined or asked about their own state of health, but with no prior intention to treat whatever conditions are found.

However, some sources of information fall between these categories: for example, the law requires that certain infectious diseases must be reported to a central agency when they are detected, and the central agency (in England the Centre for Disease Surveillance and Control) is therefore an important source of information on these 'notifiable' diseases.

Most of the routinely published information on morbidity is based on the use of health services. However, information derived in this way reflects not only the presence of ill-health and disease, but also such factors as the availability and accessibility of services, and knowledge, beliefs and attitudes about illness and health care among patients and professionals. The influence of such factors on health service use will vary with the type of condition suffered: almost everyone with a fractured leg will attend a hospital, whereas only some people with low back-pain or influenza will see their doctor.

Another feature of morbidity measures that are based on health service use is that different patterns of morbidity will emerge depending on which part of the service is studied. This can be seen in Figure 9.5 (overleaf), which shows the top groups of conditions as measured by (a) the proportion of hospital beds occupied by patients with each condition; (b) hospital consultant episodes (that is, in-patient spells in the care of a hospital consultant, sometimes called 'finished consultant episodes' or FCEs in official statistics); and (c) general practitioner (GP) consultations. You should note that mental handicap and pregnancy are not included in the figure, despite the fact that a great deal of health care is provided for both conditions, as they are not normally considered illnesses.

● By comparing Figures 9.2 and 9.5, what can you conclude about the contribution of cancers to mortality and to morbidity rates?

■ In spite of being responsible for 25 per cent of all deaths, cancers account for only about 6 per cent of occupied hospital beds, 9 per cent of hospital consultant episodes and do not figure as a major reason for GP consultations. This suggests that cancers are a disease category of high mortality, but of intermediate or low morbidity.

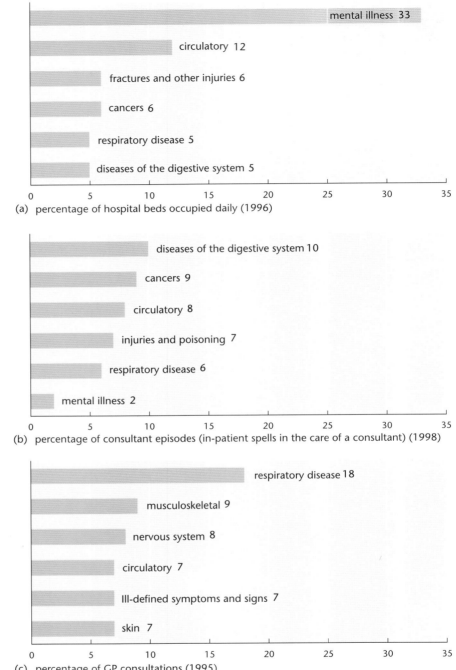

Figure 9.5 *Morbidity patterns for the commonest groups of disorders/diseases in each category in England and Wales. (Data derived from: (a)* Health and Personal Social Services Statistics for England, 1998, *The Stationery Office, London, Table B12; (b) Department of Health, 1996,* Hospital Episode Statistics, *Volume 1, Department of Health, London, Table 1; (c) Royal College of General Practitioners/OPCS/DHSS, 1995,* Morbidity Statistics from General Practice: Fourth National Study, *OPCS Series MB5 No. 3, HMSO, London, Table 23)*

The conclusion for cancers contrasts with a category such as musculoskeletal disorders (for example, arthritis and rheumatism) which are rarely fatal or requiring a period in hospital, but are responsible for almost one tenth of all GP consultations.

⬤ Now compare mental illness with diseases of the digestive system in terms of hospital beds occupied and admissions to hospital in the care of a consultant (Figure 9.4a and b). What differences exist and how might you explain them?

▨ The percentage of hospital beds occupied by people with a mental illness is much higher than the percentage of hospital admissions attributable to mental illness, whereas diseases of the digestive system are responsible for a much higher proportion of admissions than occupied beds. This suggests that patients with a mental illness tend to be in hospital for long periods, whereas patients with diseases of the digestive system have a fairly short length of stay in hospital.

These differences demonstrate the importance of examining a variety of measures of the impact of a disease or group of diseases when assessing its importance on the health of a population. Consider, for example, skin conditions, which, like rheumatism, cause few deaths or admissions to hospital, yet are a common source of distress and discomfort. Table 9.2 indicates how frequently these and other common conditions are encountered in one year in a general practice of fairly average size.

Table 9.2   Annual prevalence of illness and other events in a primary care practice in England in the 1980s, in a population of 2 500.

Condition	No. of sufferers	Condition	No. of sufferers
minor illness		asthma	30
upper respiratory infections	600	diabetes	30
skin disorders	350	varicose veins	30
psycho-emotional problems	250	peptic ulcers	25
gastro-intestinal disorders	200	strokes	20
chronic diseases		*major acute diseases*	
high blood pressure	250	acute bronchitis	100
chronic rheumatism	100	pneumonia	20
chronic psychiatric disorders	100	severe depression	10
ischaemic heart disease	50	acute myocardial infarction (heart attack)	10
obesity	50	acute strokes	5
anaemia	30	new cancers	5
cancers under care	30	acute appendicitis	5

Data derived from Fry, I. (1983) *Common Diseases*, MTP Press, 3rd edn, pp. 22–4, Table 1.4.

⬤ Which were the five most prevalent conditions seen in this general practice?

▨ They are:

(1) upper respiratory infections (600): these include conditions such as tonsillitis and ear infections;

(2) skin disorders (350), such as eczema and warts;

(3) psycho-emotional problems (250);

(4) high blood pressure (250);

(5) gastro-intestinal disorders (200), such as food poisoning, diarrhoea and vomiting.

These data reflect the everyday sorts of health problems which affect nearly all of us at some time or another: a general practitioner would only expect to see one new case of breast cancer and ten heart attacks (acute myocardial infarction in the table) in a year, compared with hundreds of people with emotional problems, skin disorders and chronic conditions.

However, as you have seen above, even data such as these from general practice may fail to reveal a considerable amount of ill-health and disability, such as foot-problems in the elderly which cause difficulty with walking and even complete immobility. Information on the prevalence of such 'minor' conditions has to be obtained from special surveys. One such survey that has been conducted on a number of occasions has focused on the dental health of adults, and some results are shown in Figure 9.6.

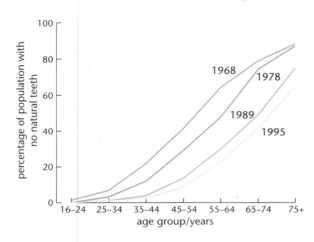

Figure 9.6 *Total tooth loss for different age-groups, Great Britain, 1968–95. (Data for 1968 and 1978 come from OPCS (various years)* Adult Dental Health Surveys, *HMSO, London; 1989 data from OPCS, 1991,* General Household Survey 1989, *OPCS Series GHS No. 20, HMSO, London, Table 4.41; 1995 data from Office for National Statistics, 1997,* Living in Britain: Results from the 1995 General Household Survey, *The Stationery Office, London, Table 9.2.)*

● At what age had 50 per cent of the population lost all their natural teeth in 1968, 1978, 1989 and 1995, and what does this indicate about general standards of dental health?

■ By the age of 45–64 half the population in 1968 had lost all their natural teeth. By 1978 this age had risen to 55–64, and by 1989 it was 65–74. By 1995 it was only in the age group 75 and over that a majority of the population had no natural teeth. This suggests a substantial improvement in dental health, and also changes in dental practice that make dentists more likely to try to conserve teeth.

In summary, different measurement methods suggest quite different patterns of morbidity. For example, data based on use of hospital beds show mental illness to predominate, whereas GP consultations also reflect distress and discomfort caused by upper respiratory infections and 'minor' conditions affecting the skin, muscles and joints.

9.2.4 Disability

Surveys of the prevalence of morbidity in the population sometimes attempt to define illness in terms of its impact on an individual's life. Thus a **physical impairment** may be said to exist if some bodily function is limited, such as having difficulty with breathing, as occurs with chronic bronchitis. If this impairment is sufficient to restrict the person's general physical functioning — for example if chronic bronchitis makes it very difficult or impossible to walk to the shops or climb the stairs — it can be said to constitute a **disability**. Finally, it is sometimes argued that a **handicap** exists if the environment fails to accommodate a person's disability, with the effect that their social functioning is limited. The term 'environment' refers not only to physical structures, such as a lack of wheelchair access to a public building, but also society's attitude to disability which may either be welcoming and accommodating, or hostile and inflexible. For example, severe facial disfigurement may cause physical pain and discomfort, but may also engender social hostility.[4] In other words, disabled people may be handicapped by the able-bodied.

Some indication of the prevalence of disability among older adults in England and Wales is shown in Figure 9.7, using information from a survey performed between 1989 and 1994. The figure shows that fairly severe problems of hearing and sight increase markedly in the older age groups, as does the proportion of people who are housebound, where women over 75 are particularly affected.

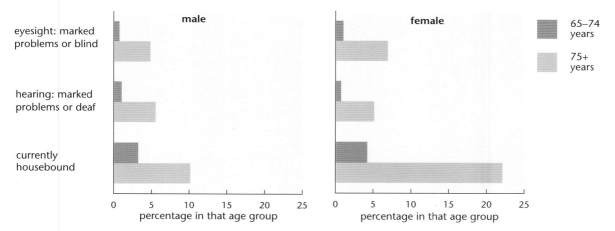

Figure 9.7   *The prevalence of disability among elderly people in England and Wales, 1989–1994. (Data from Parker, C.J., Morgan, K. and Dewey M.E. (1997) Physical illness and disability among elderly people in England and Wales: the Medical Research Council cognitive function and ageing study*, Journal of Epidemiology and Community Health, *51, Table 5, p. 497.)*

In general, deafness and other ear complaints, and eye disorders are the most prevalent disabilities amongst older adults living at home, alongside musculoskeletal diseases such as arthritis, which can severely restrict mobility. In institutions, mental disorders are the most prevalent, followed by musculoskeletal disorders and then disorders affecting the nervous system such as stroke. It is also worth noting that there is no consistent relationship between the disability and the mortality caused by specific disease categories. Cancers, for example, cause a quarter of all deaths

[4] A television programme for OU students, called 'More than meets the eye', explores stigmatisation and facial disfigurement; it is associated with the final book in this series, *Experiencing and Explaining Disease*, (Open University Press, 2nd edn 1996, colour-enhanced 2nd edn 2001).

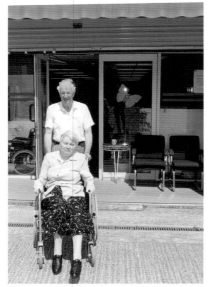

Multiple sclerosis is a progressive degenerative disorder of the nervous system, which interferes with muscular movements and causes disability that typically 'waxes and wanes' episodically over many years. (Photo: Mike Levers)

but are not a prevalent cause of disability. Circulatory disease results in both high mortality and high disability, whereas musculoskeletal diseases cause much disability but low mortality.

Figure 9.7 showed the proportion of older people with a marked problem relating to hearing or eyesight. But a much larger proportion of people — approximately 60 per cent of adult men and nearly 70 per cent of adult women in Britain — wear glasses for at least some activities. In addition some of those who do not wear glasses are thought to suffer from some visual difficulty. So although we tend to think of disabled people as a minority group, in reality there are few fully able-bodied adults.

To give some impression of how the prevalence of disability (and morbidity) may be changing over time, Figure 9.8 shows some data from the General Household Survey, an annual survey of self-reported illness in a sample of the British population which includes a number of questions concerning health. The figure shows the percentage of respondents who reported a long-standing illness, and of these, whether the illness limited their activities in any way. Data are shown separately for men and women.

It is clear that there has been a fairly substantial increase since the early 1970s (when this survey first began) in the proportion of men and women reporting some long-standing illness, and that this proportion now stands at around one-third of the population. There has been a similar increase in the proportion reporting that their activity is in some way restricted by a long-standing illness: around one fifth of the population claim to be restricted by illness.

● What explanations can you think of for the increase over time in the proportion of people who report a long-standing illness?

■ One explanation may be that people's expectations, attitudes and assessments of their health have been changing: remember that these data are self-reported. Another possibility is that the increase simply reflects a changing population

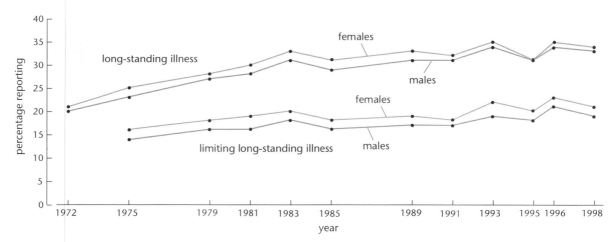

Figure 9.8 *Trends in self-reported long-standing illness by sex, 1972–98, Great Britain. (Data from Office for National Statistics, 2000a,* Living in Britain: Results from the General Household Survey 1998, *The Stationery Office, London, Table 7.1.)*

age structure: with more older people than in the past, there is likely to be more chronic illness. A third possibility is that the increase is associated with rising life expectancy: people may be living longer, but these extra years of life may not be very healthy.

It is very likely that people's attitudes and expectations have changed over time, but there is no easy way to assess whether this has affected rates of self-reported illness: it might also be noted that such changes could have reduced or increased these rates. The second potential explanation, which concerns changes in the age structure of the population, can easily be checked by age-standardising the data, but this does not in fact account for all of the rise in long-standing illness.

9.2.5 The compression of morbidity

The debates sketched above leave open the question of whether rising life expectancy has been accompanied by parallel improvements in health. One view, expressed for example by the American epidemiologist James Fries, is that as life expectancy increases so chronic illness will be restricted to the last few years of life. As a result the *healthy* lifespan will also increase: Fries has described this essentially optimistic outlook as being characterised by the **compression of morbidity**. However, another more pessimistic view is that increases in life expectancy will not be free of illness, and will increase the proportion of life spent sick or disabled.

Figure 9.9 shows one attempt to address these questions. It shows how life expectancy changed for males and females aged 65 from 1976–92 in England and Wales. Figure 9.9 also shows the **healthy life expectancy**, or expectation of life

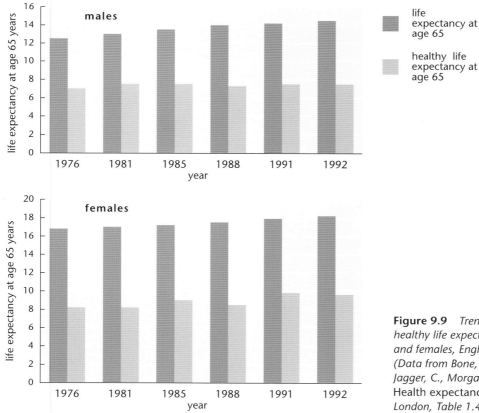

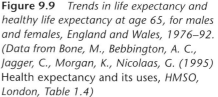

Figure 9.9 *Trends in life expectancy and healthy life expectancy at age 65, for males and females, England and Wales, 1976–92. (Data from Bone, M., Bebbington, A. C., Jagger, C., Morgan, K., Nicolaas, G. (1995) Health expectancy and its uses, HMSO, London, Table 1.4)*

without disability (calculated from the General Household Survey's self-reported data). The figure tends to bear out the view of the pessimists: overall the number of remaining years of life expectancy at age 65 rose significantly for both sexes during this period. But *healthy* life expectancy for 65-year-old men remained almost constant at around 7 more years; for women it may have risen slightly, but not as much as the increase in life expectancy. These results are broadly in line with similar calculations done in Denmark, Finland and elsewhere. However, some American research has produced more encouraging evidence, indicating that chronic disability in the elderly population is declining (Singer and Manton, 1998).

This discussion prompts one final thought concerning the likely future trend in life expectancy. Although many of the initial gains in average life expectancy in countries such as the UK occurred because far more individuals survived infancy, in fact the expectation of life has been rising not just at birth but at every age: for example, a 60-year-old woman in the UK could expect to live for another 14.6 years in 1901, but by 1996 this had increased to over 22 years. This trend is continuing for the present, but for how long? The demographer Bernard Benjamin has constructed various projections based on different assumptions, some of which show life expectancy at birth of 88 years among men and 95 years among women. On these projections 10 per cent of males would survive to the age of 95 and 10 per cent of females would celebrate their 99th birthday. The underlying assumptions may seem far-fetched but, as Benjamin remarks:

> ... It seems at least plausible that there is no predetermined limit to the attainable lifespan. The only statistic we can depend upon is the longest life ever lived and every day the record grows longer. The fault lies not in our stars, but in ourselves that we are mortal. (Benjamin, 1989, p. 227)

Rising life expectancy has resulted in many more older people in Britain, but it is not clear that life expectancy free of illness or disability has increased. (Photo: Homer Sykes/ Network)

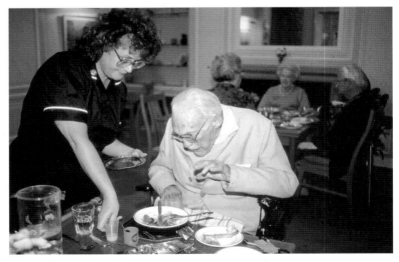

9.2.6 Summary

To summarise: survival to middle and old age has led to a rise in the medical and social importance of chronic degenerative diseases (especially those affecting the cardiovascular and respiratory systems) and cancers. These conditions dominate the causes of mortality. Patterns of morbidity are dependent on how the measurements are made: for example, measuring the use of hospital services does not reflect the everyday experiences of distress and discomfort caused by upper respiratory infections, mental ill-health and emotional problems, and 'minor' conditions affecting the skin, muscles and joints. The causes of disability are primarily musculoskeletal disorders and diseases of the sense organs. The proportion of the population reporting some form of disabling condition appears to be rising, prompting questions about the proportion of life expectancy that is free of disability.

9.3 Studying distributions of health and disease

A widely accepted definition of epidemiology is that it is concerned to interpret the health experience of human communities. More specifically, epidemiology addresses at least three types of questions:

(1) Who gets ill? (2) Why do they get ill? and (3) What should the response be?[5]

● How might these three questions be answered, using the methods of epidemiology?

■ (1) Can be answered by describing the distribution of health and disease in the population and how it changes over time.

(2) Can be addressed by generating hypotheses about the aetiology (or cause) of disease, or establishing associations with other factors such as environment, life history, etc.

(3) Can be answered by evaluating the effectiveness of different treatments and other interventions such as prevention campaigns.

This chapter is primarily concerned with (1) the distribution of health and disease. By describing how particular conditions are distributed in the population, it is possible to generate hypotheses that might explain such patterns.

9.3.1 Methodological problems

Epidemiology is an eclectic science, which has borrowed many of its investigative methods from other areas. Consequently, the kinds of methodological problems that often arise, and which you will encounter at various points in this chapter, are not unique to epidemiology.

The first such problem is that the diseases or health conditions that are most feasible to study are, in general, those that have medical labels, definitions and classifications attached to them. **Classification of diseases** has led to many advances in understanding illness, but it can also limit the scope of epidemiology, by encouraging epidemiologists to study those states of ill-health that are most easily identified and measured, and to neglect those that are not easily verified by a doctor or do not readily fit into the description of a specific disease. For example, feeling 'under the weather' is a common condition, but it is not usually given a specific disease-label and does not attract much serious research effort. Too rigid an adherence to the current classification of diseases may also limit advances in knowledge. For instance, it is possible that our understanding of the causes of coronary heart disease is being impeded because the current disease definition actually comprises several different diseases, each with its own cause (or causes). In practice one of the roles of epidemiology should be to challenge such definitions and help to redefine diseases in more useful ways.

[5] Epidemiological methods are discussed in *Studying Health and Disease* (Open University Press, 2nd edn 1994; colour-enhanced 2nd edn 2001), Chapters 7 and 8.

A second set of problems concerns the factors that may contribute to disease patterns. Studying these often requires **population stratification**: that is, sections of the population are grouped in accordance with the characteristic of interest. This is fairly straightforward for factors such as age and sex, but it may present considerable difficulties with factors such as social class, which cannot be measured directly. (Sociologists refer to complex factors such as social class, which are hard to measure because it is difficult to construct a definition on which everyone would agree, as *contested concepts*.[6]) One solution is to develop 'proxy' or indirect measures, for example, by using country of origin as a measure of ethnic background, or occupation as a measure of social class.

Going beyond these practical difficulties, there is the question of selecting which factors or types of factor to study. For instance, most studies of gastroenteritis (diarrhoea and vomiting) in infants have been concerned with biological factors such as whether or not the mother breast-fed her infant, rather than with social variables such as housing conditions and income. If the conclusion is that gastroenteritis is caused by mothers failing to breast-feed their infants, the recommended change might be to encourage mothers to breast-feed. But an investigation embracing social factors may draw attention to circumstances that discourage some mothers from breast-feeding, such as insufficient advice and support, and so recommend that more breast-feeding counsellors be trained. Policy implications are, therefore, very much dependent on the factors chosen to be studied, and that choice is influenced not only by practical considerations, but also the interests and values of the investigator or the funding body behind the research.

A third problem concerns **interaction between different factors**. A study of the effectiveness of a drug may attempt to simplify the issues by looking separately at two factors: age and sex. It may then show that the drug's effectiveness declines in older age groups and that it is less effective among men than women. But for biological or other reasons the effect of age and sex may not be independent: effectiveness may decline more rapidly in older men than older women, so that the *combined* influence of age and sex is not the same as the separate influence of each factor: there is an interaction between them. Although sophisticated statistical methods exist to cope with the interaction of factors, many epidemiological studies (especially much of the routine descriptive data) make no such attempt.

Finally, it is often very difficult to establish whether an association between, for example, a disease and a factor such as age, is causal, or whether some other possible explanation exists. There are many **levels of causality**: explanations of the cause of a disease may be offered in terms of chemicals and cells at one extreme, and in terms of politics and economics at the other. In theory, a causal relationship can only be assumed after an exhaustive analysis has considered and rejected all other possible explanations — causal and non-causal — of the association. For instance, in our infant feeding/gastroenteritis example, we cannot be certain that the colour of the mother's hair, her astrological sign or her relationship with the infant's father are *not* relevant *unless* these are also studied. In practice, epidemiologists have to decide which factors to study on the basis of a wide range of criteria including clinical, biological, demographic or social plausibility. But they may have a prior inclination to emphasise one group of factors, for example biomedical or clinical factors, and neglect others such as social factors.

---

[6] The use of proxy measures to 'operationalise' other contested concepts including 'health' and 'safety' are discussed in *Studying Health and Disease* (Open University Press, 2nd edn 1994; colour-enhanced 2nd edn 2001), Chapters 5 and 6.

These methodological difficulties which, as noted earlier, are not unique to epidemiology, can be and often are overcome in collaboration with other disciplines. The result of such multidisciplinary approaches has been a major contribution to the study of health and disease. (A recent example of such a collaboration has been the development of *genetic epidemiology*, in which geneticists and epidemiologists have collaborated to explore the distribution of specific genetic characteristics in populations and their relation to diseases.) The rest of this chapter is devoted to describing the contribution of multidisciplinary approaches to the study of health, disease and disability in the UK, and discussing some of the explanations epidemiological work has suggested. Each of the six main demographic characteristics (sex and gender, age, marital status, ethnicity, geographical location and social class as defined by occupation) is discussed below in terms of the following:

- the distribution of mortality
- the distribution of morbidity (and disability where appropriate); and
- possible explanations for such patterns, considering biological and social aspects (and cultural factors where appropriate) and the influence of personal life-histories.

9.4   Sex and gender

9.4.1 Mortality and morbidity

Figure 9.9 showed a feature of the average expectation of life that should now be familiar to you: female lives in the UK are on average around 6 years longer than male lives. As Figure 9.10 shows, this advantage is present throughout life.

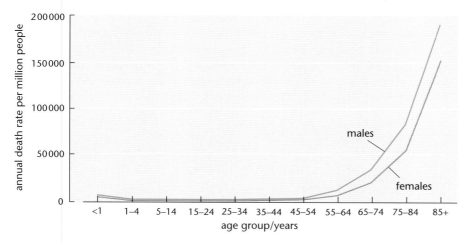

Figure 9.10   *Annual death rates per million people within each age-group for 1997, males and females, England and Wales. (Data derived from Office for National Statistics, 1998b,* Mortality Statistics: Cause 1997, *ONS Series DH2 No. 24, The Stationery Office, London, Table 4)*

● Is there an age-group in which male mortality is lower than that for females?

■ No. In England and Wales the male mortality rate is higher at all ages.

● Can you recall from previous chapters any exceptions to this in other places?

■ This pattern is found is most countries. However, in Table 2.3 you saw that female and male life expectancies are virtually identical at all ages in Bangladesh.

However, the consistently higher overall death rates for males in the UK are not reflected in higher overall *morbidity* rates. Although the morbidity rates for many major chronic diseases *are* higher in males (e.g. coronary heart disease), for other conditions there either does not appear to be any substantial difference, or the female rate is higher. Studies have shown that the incidence of acute conditions, days of restricted activity because of illness, and visits to GPs tend to be higher in women than men. In Figure 9.8 you saw that the proportion reporting long-standing illnesses was consistently higher among women than men. One disease that illustrates this difference in morbidity is rheumatoid arthritis, a chronic disease of the joints resulting in stiffness, pain and loss of mobility. Not only is it more prevalent in women than in men but, in addition, the disease appears to advance more rapidly in women.[7]

9.4.2 Biological and social explanations

How can these male : female differences in mortality and morbidity be explained? What is the relative contribution of biologically-determined **sex** and socially-constructed **gender**? This question has given rise to considerable debate and speculation. Several biological explanations have been suggested for the lower mortality rate in females, including differences in the genetic material between males and females resulting in greater resistance to infections in females, or higher levels of oestrogens in females exerting a protective effect against certain diseases, at least before the menopause.[8] Finally, it has been suggested that the biological hazards associated with pregnancy may be one reason why female mortality rates in some developing countries are as high or higher than male rates, and why this may also have been the case in the past in the UK. Widely available contraception and improvements in the safety of childbirth in industrialised countries may have nullified this disadvantage, leading to a fall in female mortality rates.

● In addition to these biological theories, a number of *social* explanations for the gender difference in mortality have been suggested. Can you think of any?

■ First, there are increased risks to men stemming from their higher rates of employment outside the home and in more physically hazardous jobs. Second, there are systematic differences in behaviour between the sexes, which are in part biological but may also result from social pressures operating from childhood or be related to gender differences in the access to resources. These are then manifested in, for example, higher risk-taking behaviour among men: greater use of dangerous drugs, faster driving, or higher smoking rates.[9] In

---

[7] Rheumatoid arthritis is the subject of a case-study in the final book in this series, *Experiencing and Explaining Disease* (Open University Press, 2nd edn 1996; colour-enhanced 2nd edn 2001), Chapter 3. Coping with disability in later life is discussed in *Birth to Old Age: Health in Transition* (Open University Press, 2nd edn 1995; colour-enhanced 2nd edn 2001), Chapter 11.

[8] Evolutionary explanations for the greater longevity of females in most human societies are discussed in *Human Biology and Health: An Evolutionary Approach* (Open University Press, 2nd edn 1994; 3rd edn 2001), Chapter 8.

[9] Gender differences in risk-taking behaviour among adolescents in the UK are discussed in *Birth to Old Age: Health in Transition* (Open University Press, 2nd edn 1995; colour-enhanced 2nd edn 2001), Chapter 6.

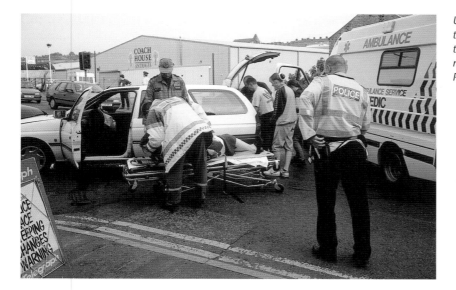

Unlike most causes of death, the mortality rate from road traffic accidents peaks among males aged 15–24. (Photo: Peter Olive/Photofusion)

turn this behaviour feeds through to mortality: for example the higher prevalence of smoking in men is reflected in the higher incidence of cancers of the lung, as shown in Figure 9.3, as well as higher rates of coronary heart disease and of other cancers including those of the mouth and pharynx, oesophagus and bladder.

Other behavioural differences, apart from smoking, that may contribute to the excess of male mortality include the higher consumption of alcohol by men which contributes to the higher incidence of cancer of the larynx and oesophagus, and cirrhosis of the liver. The transmission patterns of HIV also primarily affected men in the first decade of the UK AIDS epidemic, especially among homosexuals and intravenous drug users: only 3 per cent of AIDS cases diagnosed in 1987 were female. However, by 1999 this pattern had changed, with 24 per cent of all AIDS cases diagnosed in that year being female.

Gender differences in behaviour have also been suggested as part of the explanation for the higher mortality from coronary heart disease in men, such as a higher prevalence among men of a so-called 'coronary-prone personality' characterised by aggressive and competitive behavioural traits. However, despite a considerable amount of research in this area, the influence of personality types on the distribution of coronary heart disease (or any other disease) is still unclear.[8]

How might the apparently paradoxical observation of higher *morbidity* rates for some diseases in women be explained? This finding may partly result from the method of measuring morbidity (based on health-service use) and partly from gender differences in attitudes to health care.

● Can you suggest how these two factors might explain some of the gender difference in morbidity rates?

■ First, methodological problems in the measurement of women's visits to a GP may arise as a result of the inclusion of consultations for contraception,

[10] Research on the possible association between personality and heart disease is discussed in *Birth to Old Age: Health in Transition* (Open University Press, 2nd edn 1995; colour-enhanced 2nd edn 2001), Chapter 8.

ante-natal, and post-natal care. Second, women may be more predisposed to care for their health. This would contribute to their higher consultation rate and might also lower their mortality rate. Third, they may also have greater access to health services, because they are less likely to be in full-time employment. Fourth, women have traditionally cared for the health of other members of the family. This may have lowered the consultation rate of men while raising women's own rate, especially if they consult on their own behalf while, for example, taking children to the GP.

The patterns of gender and disease illustrate well the complex interaction between biological, social and life-history factors in determining health status, and as you progress through this chapter you will see gender differences reappearing in many different contexts.

In summary, the key points are:

(1) Male mortality rates exceed those for females at all ages.

(2) Male:female differences in morbidity vary between different disease categories.

(3) Biological factors, such as genetic and hormonal differences, are thought to account for some of the relative health advantages of females (although menstrual and menopausal discomfort is a source of morbidity among women that men do not experience).

(4) Social relations and structures, on average, place males in more hazardous work, and appear to influence their adoption of more health-damaging behaviour.

(5) Some of the apparent differences in morbidity between the sexes may result from systematic differences in measurement or in the use of health services, or perhaps because of inconsistent social attitudes towards women compared with men who report themselves as ill.

9.5 Age

9.5.1 Mortality, morbidity and the cohort effect

In Chapter 2 you saw how, in industrialised countries, mortality rates typically increase with increasing age after early childhood. Though this pattern is true for almost all causes of death in the UK as in other industrialised countries, there are a few interesting exceptions. For example, suicide is much more common in younger age-groups, and deaths from road traffic accidents among males have a peak at 15–24 years of age. This fits the image many people have of reckless young men in fast cars and motorbikes, although we will suggest shortly that this may not be the whole picture. However, there is a second peak in road traffic accidents — among elderly people — which is seldom considered. These deaths are the result mainly of pedestrians being injured by vehicles.

Another exception to the general pattern is HIV/AIDS: 78 per cent of all HIV diagnoses in the UK up to the end of 1999 were made under the age of 40.

For most conditions, the association of morbidity with age follows a similar pattern to that of mortality – the older we become, the more ill-health we experience. This can be seen in the increasing incidence of most cancers with age, shown in Figure 9.11. (These data are for men, but similar patterns are found amongst women.)

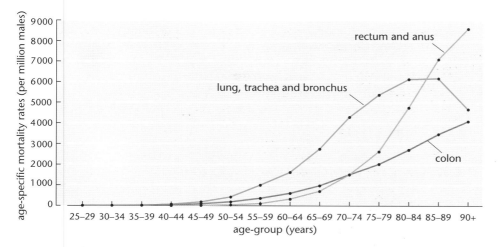

Figure 9.11   *Age-specific mortality rates (per million men in that age-group) from selected cancers in males by age, England and Wales, 1998. (Data derived from Office for National Statistics, 1999a,* Mortality Statistics: Cause 1998, *ONS Series DH2 No. 25, The Stationery Office, London, Table 4)*

● From Figure 9.11, what is the rather surprising exception to this association?

■ The incidence of lung cancer declines after the age of 89.

● Approximately 90 per cent of lung cancers are thought to be due to smoking tobacco. How might you explain the apparent fall in the death rate from the disease after the age of 89?

■ There are three possibilities you may have considered:
   (1) Some men may have survived to later ages because of some form of resistance to the disease.
   (2) All the men who are at risk from smoking all their lives have died of lung cancer (and other smoking-related diseases) by the age of 89, leaving few life-time smokers surviving.
   (3) All the men born more than 89 years ago have some common experiences that make them less likely to develop lung cancer than younger men.

The third explanation, which commands most support, is known as a **birth cohort effect.** A cohort is a group of people who all share a common experience. In the case of a birth cohort the common factor is their year of birth. Such a group tends to share similar life experiences from birth to death. It is known that the prevalence of smoking has varied during this century. Suppose that men who were born during or after the First World War smoked more heavily throughout their lives than men born earlier. In 1998 (when the data in Figure 9.11 were collected) these heavy smokers would have been represented in the birth cohorts of up to ages 80–89 but not older, and would be expected to be suffering from higher lung cancer rates than the older group who had smoked less. The importance of the cohort effect is that it can complicate the appearance of the relationship between mortality and age and lead to misinterpretation of that association. You should bear this in mind when you meet further examples.[11]

[11] The cohort effect in lung cancer among men of different ages in the UK is also explored in the notes associated with the audiotape 'Smoking: A global health problem', recorded for OU students.

World War II soldiers in Italy taking a break. The high prevalence of smoking during this period was reflected in rising lung cancer rates several decades later. (Photo: Imperial War Museum)

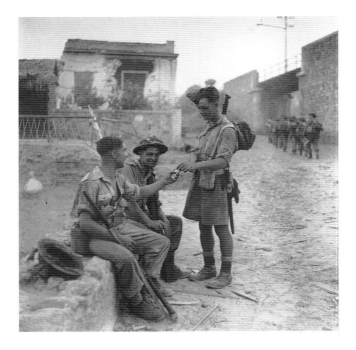

9.5.2 Biological, social and life history explanations

The main reason for the observed age distribution of disease is the biological ageing of the cells, tissues and organs of the body.[12] However, social factors are also thought to influence the pattern. As you will see in the next chapter, the social position of some age-groups (particularly elderly people) means that they are more likely to be exposed to poorer, health-damaging conditions. This may be reinforced by ageist attitudes in society. Apart from biological and social causes, the influence of a person's **life history** — that is, the influence of past events on the present state of health — is particularly important in the context of age. The birth-cohort effect on the incidence of lung cancer illustrates the importance of considering this influence: in that example it was men's tobacco consumption. This is not to suggest that the decision to smoke was an entirely personal choice. In fact, many biological and social factors can influence our 'personal' behaviour.

Another example of such influences may lie behind the high mortality rates in young men caused by road traffic accidents. As we noted earlier, this is often ascribed to the high risk-taking behaviour of young adult males — in particular by those on motorbikes.[13] However, additional factors could include social pressures to exhibit 'macho' behaviour, low income precluding them from car ownership, aggressive behaviour by other road users towards motor cyclists, and time and financial pressure from employers on motorbike couriers.

In summary, the key points are:

(1) Mortality rates increase with age. This is true for almost all causes of death.

(2) Morbidity rates also increase with age.

[12] The biological processes of ageing are discussed more fully in *Human Biology and Health: An Evolutionary Approach* (Open University Press, 2nd edn 1994; 3rd edn 2001), Chapter 8.

[13] Risk-taking among adolescents is discussed further in *Birth to Old Age: Health in Transition* (Open University Press, 2nd edn 1995; colour-enhanced 2nd edn 2001), Chapter 6.

(3) Biological factors (cell and tissue ageing) are largely responsible for this pattern.

(4) The health of some age-groups (particularly elderly people) is adversely affected by their relative social disadvantage.

(5) Health status at any age will be influenced by a person's social circumstances and by their personal life history (their experiences and the past events in their life), as well as their current behaviour (such as risk-taking) or social attitudes towards them.

9.6   Marital status

Like gender and age, **marital status** forms another pervasive personal and social characteristic.

> Marital state is a socially, and generally legally, defined condition, and serves to distinguish between currently married, never married (single) and formerly married (widowed and divorced) people. Although marital state is defined in terms of the presence or absence of a marital partner, it involves more than a personal relationship, for each marital condition is associated with socially sanctioned rights and obligations with regard to children, sexuality, kinship ties, property and domestic and economic services. (Morgan, 1980, p. 633)

This quote from the British sociologist Myfanwy Morgan highlights the social importance of marital status but also the difficulties of determining precisely how to interpret its relationship to health status. By studying marital status, we are in fact attempting to investigate both the effect of a personal relationship on health status *and* the social consequences that flow from it in terms of rights, obligations and resources such as income and housing.

●   What two assumptions do you think there are in using a person's marital status in such investigations? What problems arise from these assumptions?

■   Using marital status assumes that people who are married enjoy the benefits of a close personal relationship; and it assumes that single and formerly married people are not experiencing such a relationship. Both assumptions will be false in a substantial proportion of cases, and the problems arising from these assumptions have increased as the number of people who are cohabiting on a long-term basis has increased.

Partly to avoid such difficulties, some analyses simply report information by 'family type', as you will see below.

9.6.1   Mortality and change in marital status

An association between marital status and mortality was first demonstrated in the nineteenth century, when it was shown that mortality rates were lowest for the married, higher for the single and highest for those widowed or divorced. This has been consistently found ever since. Married people experience lower mortality rates than non-married for nearly all causes of death. The overall age-standardised death rates for married and non-married women are shown in Table 9.3 overleaf.

Table 9.3   Age-standardised death rates per 100 000 women, by marital status, women aged 35–64, England and Wales, 1976–81 and 1986–1992.

	non-manual women		manual women	
	married	not married	married	married
1976–81	358	354	471	620
1986–92	283	305	371	519

Data from Harding, S., Bethune, A., Maxwell, R. and Brown, J. (1997) Mortality trends using the Longitudinal Study, pp. 143–55 in Drever, F. and Whitehead, M. (eds) *Health Inequalities: Decennial Supplement,* Government Statistical Service, Series DS No. 15, The Stationery Office, London, Table 11.5.

The table also distinguishes between manual and non-manual occupational groups, and indicates that, at least in the manual classes, non-married women have significantly higher death rates than married women. The table also indicates that over the period 1976–81 and 1986–92 the decline in death rates was proportionally larger amongst the married groups, resulting in a widening gap between the married and non-married groups over time.

A number of researchers have also explored the relationship between a *change* in marital status and health status. For example, a sequence of studies over several decades have looked at what happens to the surviving partner after their spouse dies. One of the first and perhaps the best known of these studies, published by Colin Murray Parkes and colleagues in 1969, reported **excess mortality** among widows and widowers in the period after their bereavement: they found that the death rate among widowers during the first six months of bereavement was 40 per cent greater than would be expected among married men of that age. The principal cause of death was cardiovascular disease, and the authors suggested that the widowers were quite literally dying of a broken heart. However, subsequent work has produced much less clear-cut results, and many researchers have noted the methodological problems besetting some of these studies, such as the lack of a tightly-defined control group.

Divorce can have a similar effect, though usually during the later stages of marital breakdown rather than at the time of the divorce action. Divorce appears to have a greater adverse effect on men than on women, but, although both bereavement and divorce certainly have an adverse effect on health, there are some circumstances when they could have a positive effect: for example if they follow a period of stress such as a spouse's long terminal illness, or in cases of domestic violence.

9.6.2   Morbidity and family type

The pattern of morbidity in relation to **family type** — which makes reference to marital status but is not exclusively based on it — is shown in Figure 9.12, which reports general practice consultation rates by family type. The figure shows these data for all consultations, and for consultations relating to mental disorders; the figure also shows the statistical significance of these differences.

- How would you summarise the differences shown in Figure 9.12?

- Widowed, separated and divorced adults with and without children generally had significantly *higher* 'any reason' consultation rates compared to the reference group (i.e. married or cohabiting adults with dependent children),

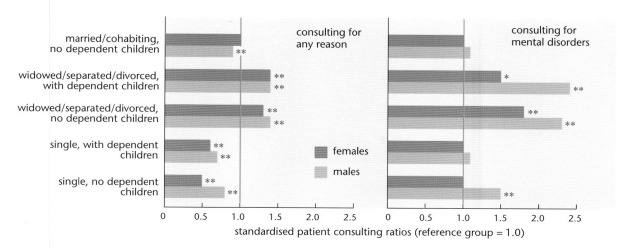

Figure 9.12 *Standardised patient consulting ratios by family type, men and women aged 16–44, England and Wales, 1991–92. (* means a difference significant at the 5% level; ** means a difference significant at the 1% level. Consulting rate for reference group: married or cohabiting adults with dependent children = 1.0). (Data derived from Royal College of General Practitioners/OPCS/DHSS, 1995,* Morbidity Statistics from General Practice: Fourth National Study, *OPCS Series MB5 No. 3, HMSO, London, Table 5G)*[14]

and this was even more pronounced with respect to mental disorders. Single people with or without dependent children generally had significantly *lower* 'any reason' consultation rates than the reference group; consultation rates for mental disorders were similar among single women with and without children, but single men *without* children had significantly higher rates.

Rates of self-reported illness (i.e., rates obtained from household surveys, for example, rather than rates derived from the use of health services) show similar patterns.

9.6.3 Biological and social explanations

How can we explain these patterns of mortality and morbidity across different marital states? Biological explanations may play some role: some of the 'protective' effect of marriage on women's mortality could be due to differential rates of reproductive-system cancers — such as cancers of the breast, uterus or cervix — which are related to personal reproductive or sexual life history to some degree. Several social factors have also been suggested, and these will be discussed in a moment. First, though, it is necessary to consider the process of **marital selection**.

In all the discussions in this chapter, it is assumed that health status is a *consequence* of the biological and social factor under investigation. However, it is possible that the *causal direction* may be the reverse, that is, states of health may influence social status.[15]

● Can you suggest how health may affect marital status?

[14] Note: these are odds ratios for consulting, with each group compared to the consulting rate in the reference group of married or cohabiting adults with dependent children. Thus an odds ratio of 1.2 for a particular group means that their consulting rate is 20% higher than that of the reference group.

[15] Problems in determining the direction of causality are discussed in *Studying Health and Disease* (Open University Press, 2nd edn 1994; colour-enhanced 2nd edn 2001), Chapter 5.

■   People suffering from poor health may, on average, be more likely to remain single, and those bereaved or divorced who suffer poor health may be less likely to remarry than people enjoying good health. Divorce may also be more likely in a marriage in which one partner is often ill, although there will be many exceptions.

Although these selection mechanisms are probably contributory rather than major influences in determining marital status, they are worth bearing in mind and considering for each of the factors discussed in this chapter. (In Chapter 10 we will return to the subject of *social selection* as a partial explanation for disease patterns.)

There are several possible social explanations of ways in which the pattern of health may be influenced by marital status. The social conditions and position enjoyed by different groups will affect their health status: for example, widowed and divorced people will tend to be less well-off financially than the other groups, and couples have certain other advantages such as work-sharing. Emile Durkheim, one of the founders of empirical sociology, concluded in 1897 in *Suicide: A Study in Sociology* that marriage reduced the chances of suicide by almost one-half, owing to the greater social integration of married people. In contrast, the anomalous social position of the single (whether never married or divorced or widowed) in the nineteenth century may have served as a source of stress. Just as you saw in the earlier discussion of the interaction of age and gender with health status, some groups are discriminated against, and in those instances we recognise the existence of ageist and sexist attitudes. Although it is less well recognised, those not married may suffer in similar ways. However, as more and more households fail to conform to the 'ideal' nuclear family, the power of discrimination has waned, just as it has for couples who live together without marrying.

Systematic differences in *health service use* by people of different marital status also need to be considered.

●   Why is it important to do this?

■   Earlier in this chapter we said that differences in morbidity rates derived from health service usage may reflect systematic differences in *illness behaviour* (how people respond to ill-health) within different marital states, and in the response people receive from doctors.

The highest consulting rates for mental disorders, for example, are by widowed or divorced people, with lower rates among married or single people. This is true of both men and women. These may reflect, first, a real difference in the prevalence of morbidity between the groups; second, widowed and divorced people may be more likely to consult their doctor when depressed, anxious, etc., because they have no partner to confide in; or third, doctors may be more willing to label patients' problems as being psychological rather than physical in the knowledge of their marital status, particularly if the person is widowed or divorced.

Finally, the *lifestyles* associated with different marital conditions may contribute to the observed differences. Married people may have a stronger motivation to guard their health for the sake of their partner and dependants, or be more likely to use 'spare' cash for family benefit rather than on (say) fast cars and excessive drinking; the high mortality rates for road accidents and alcohol-induced cirrhosis of the liver among single men would support this theory. Or they may be persuaded to consult a doctor by a concerned partner. The existence of several equally-plausible hypotheses underlines the need for more empirical evidence on the clearly important subject of marital status and health, and in particular the different experiences of men and women.

In summary, the key points are:

(1) Mortality rates are lowest for married, higher for single and highest for those widowed or divorced.

(2) Being unmarried has a greater adverse effect on male than on female mortality. Similarly, divorce or widowhood appears to be more health-damaging to men than to women.

(3) Several social explanations of the apparent 'protective' effects of marriage have been suggested.

(4) Single (never married) people appear to suffer similar morbidity to the married, though the reasons for this observation are unclear.

9.7   Ethnicity and race

Another way in which the population can be stratified is on the basis of **ethnicity** or race. Many people have objected to the term **'race'** as its use in the past has suggested a primarily biological or genetic basis for cultural differences between groups — an assertion that genetic studies do not support.[16] Others have argued that using the term 'ethnicity' implies that health differences arise primarily from cultural variations, and thereby encourages 'victim-blaming'. The term ethnicity is used here, but without prior assumptions about the causes of health differences between different ethnic or racial groups.

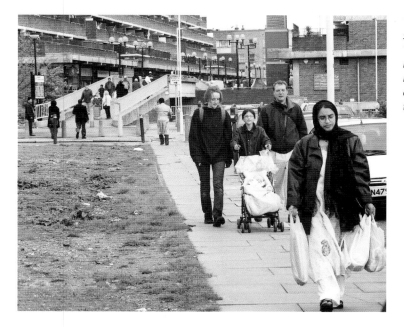

The ethnically-diverse nature of British society is evident on the streets of Whitechapel in London's 'East End': the largest Bangladeshi community in Britain lives among 'cockneys' and families from elsewhere in Asia, the Caribbean, China and the Philippines. (Photo: Mike Wibberley)

[16] There is greater genetic variation between individuals *within* the *same* ethnic group than there is between one ethnic group and another; population genetics are discussed in *Human Biology and Health: An Evolutionary Approach* (Open University Press, 2nd edn 1994; 3rd edn 2001), Chapters 4 and 9.

9.7.1 Mortality rates and country of birth

There are many difficulties in defining and using the concept of ethnicity: for example, is a person's own country of birth, or their parents' country of birth, of more relevance? Despite the ethnically diverse nature of British society, both now and in the past, many routinely collected statistics on health and disease do not provide information on different ethnic groups. However, let us begin by looking at the mortality of migrants to England and Wales by country of birth (Table 9.4).

Table 9.4 Standardised mortality ratios (SMRs) among men aged 20–64 in England and Wales from all causes, by country of birth, 1991–93.

Country of birth	Unadjusted	Adjusted for social class
England and Wales	100	100
Caribbean	89	82
West/South Africa	126	135
East Africa	123	137
Indian sub-continent	107	117
India	106	114
Pakistan	102	110
Bangladesh	137	159
Scotland	129	132
Ireland	135	129

(Data from Harding, S. and Maxwell, R. (1997) Differences in mortality of migrants, pp. 108–121 in Drever, F. and Whitehead, M. (eds) *Health Inequalities: Decennial Supplement,* Government Statistical Service, Series DS No. 15, The Stationery Office, London, Tables 9.4 and 9.5.)

The figures reported in Table 9.4 are *standardised mortality ratios* (SMRs). These express the actual number of deaths in a particular group of people as a percentage of the number of deaths that would be expected if that group experienced the age-specific death rates of the population as a whole (or some specified comparator population). In this case, the comparator population for each group in Table 9.4 is the entire population of men aged 20–64 years in England and Wales, irrespective of ethnic status.

The first data column of the table shows that the unadjusted excess mortality in 1991–93 was highest among male migrants to England and Wales who were born in Bangladesh (37 per cent higher than the average for all men aged 20–64 in England and Wales); next comes Ireland (35 per cent higher) and Scotland (29 per cent higher). But for men born in the Caribbean, mortality levels were 11 per cent *lower* than the prevailing levels in England and Wales as a whole.

However, it is possible that significant social class differences exist in the composition of these ethnic groups, and it would be useful to calculate mortality rates having adjusted for any such differences in social class composition. The final column of Table 9.4 shows what happens to the SMRs once this has been done.

● What difference does adjusting for social class make to the results?

■ In most cases the difference between the mortality rates of minority ethnic groups and the average for England and Wales widens (for example, the excess mortality among men born in East Africa goes up from 23 per cent *before* adjusting for social class, to 37 per cent *after* adjustment).

Table 9.4 shows that, if these minority ethnic groups had a social class composition similar to the England and Wales average, their overall health experience would be even worse than the unadjusted figures initially indicate. (This in turn suggests that, in these ethnic groups, there are *larger* proportions of men in the *higher* social classes — which have a better health experience — than the average for men in England and Wales as a whole.)

At this point you should recall that the ethnic groups in Table 9.4 are defined by *country of birth*.

⬤ What influence might this definition have on the patterns of mortality observed?

■ There are at least three possible influences:

(1) Members of minority ethnic groups born in England and Wales are excluded.

(2) It is difficult to know how long these immigrants spent in England and Wales prior to death, and therefore how much their health experience may have been influenced by their life in England and Wales.

(3) It is possible that the decision to migrate to England and Wales may have been influenced by a person's existing state of health.

All these factors must be born in mind. For example, the first Immigrant Mortality Study in England and Wales (Marmot *et al.,* 1984), showed that almost all immigrant groups had *lower* rates of mortality (all causes combined) than prevailed in their country of birth, suggesting that individuals of above average health tended to migrate. However, more recent work has shown that this is not uniformly true, and that, for example, death rates amongst Irish immigrants to England and Wales are higher than those prevailing in Ireland.

Some clues about these patterns can be sought among the main causes of death. In comparison with death rates for England and Wales as a whole, West and South African immigrants tend to have unusually high rates of cerebrovascular disease (strokes), while immigrants from the Indian sub-continent tend to have high rates of ischaemic heart disease, stroke and diabetes, regardless of their specific country of origin, religion and language. Irish and Scottish immigrant groups tend to have particularly high death rates from accidents and violence. These patterns are complex, but the essential point to note is that social class does not *explain* the ethnic group differences shown in Table 9.4.

9.7.2 Morbidity and use of health services

Table 9.5 (overleaf) shows the self-assessed general health of different ethnic groups in England in 1999. The table shows the age-standardised relative risk of reporting 'very good or good' health, and of having 'very bad or bad' health, where the risk for the entire population is set at 1. So any figure lower than 1 indicates that a group is *less* likely than the whole population to be in that category of health (e.g. 0.7 indicates 30 per cent less likely), and a figure higher than 1 indicates that a group is *more* likely than the whole population to be in that category of health.

Table 9.5 Self-assessed general health by ethnic group, England 1999.

Ethnic group	Age-standardised relative risk of reporting good/bad health (whole population = 1)			
	men aged 16+		women aged 16+	
	very good/good	very bad/bad	very good/good	very bad/bad
Black Caribbean	0.89	1.14	0.83	1.61
Indian	0.9	1.49	0.78	2.2
Pakistani	0.77	2.43	0.71	3.28
Bangladeshi	0.6	3.89	0.61	3.45
Chinese	0.97	1.14	0.91	0.85
Irish	0.89	1.18	0.98	0.92
Whole population	1	1	1	1

(Data from Department of Health, 2000, *Health Survey for England 1999, Preliminary report: Ethnic Health*, DH, The Stationery Office, London, Table 1)

● How does the self-assessed health of the ethnic groups shown in Table 9.5 compare with that of the population of England as a whole?

■ All the ethnic groups shown are *less* likely to assess themselves as being in 'very good' or 'good' health than the population as a whole (all values are less than 1). And almost all the ethnic groups shown are *more* likely to report themselves as being in a state of 'very bad' or 'bad health.

● Using the data in Table 9.5, can you detect any clear differences between ethnic groups or between men and women?

■ People belonging to the Pakistani and Bangladeshi ethnic groups seem to have particularly poor self-assessed health, with a much higher likelihood of being in the 'very bad' or 'bad' categories. There are no clear differences between men and women.

Finally, Figure 9.13 provides some information on use of health services by different ethnic groups.

● What patterns can you identify in Figure 9.13?

■ With the exception of Chinese people, the ethnic groups listed are much more likely to consult a GP than is the case for the population of England as a whole. The highest GP consultation rates are among Indian, Pakistani and Bangladeshi people (particularly Bangladeshi men). The pattern is not so marked for in-patient stays, but is generally slightly greater than the population average, again apart from Chinese men and women, whose rate is much lower.

9.7.3 Biological explanations

What could account for the differences between ethnic groups in mortality, morbidity and health service use outlined above? As in the previous sections on age, gender and marital status, we shall first consider biological explanations. There is a considerable amount of information on the tiny minority of genetic diseases specific

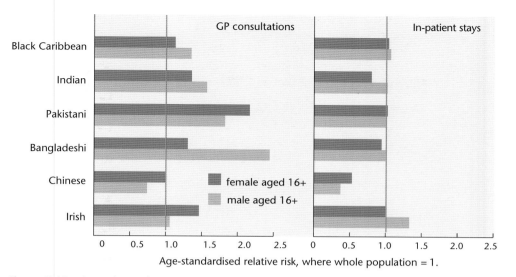

Figure 9.13   *Annual consultations with a general practitioner (GP), and annual in-patient stays in hospital, males and females aged 16+, by ethnic group, England, 1999. (Standardised consulting ratios for each ethnic group compared to the reference group: whole population = 1.0.)* (Data from Department of Health, 2000, *Health Survey for England 1999, Preliminary Report,* The Stationery Office, London, Ethnic Tables 22 and 23)

to certain ethnic or racial groups. These include the blood disorders *thalassaemia* and *sickle-cell disease* (which was discussed in Chapter 3), both of which are predominantly found in black populations, and *cystic fibrosis*, the commonest disease associated with a single gene defect in the UK, which mainly affects white people: in the USA 98 per cent of patients are white.[17] (In cystic fibrosis, abnormally sticky mucus is produced by several organs in the body, particularly the lungs and pancreas, causing blockage and obstruction to normal functioning.)

However, these inherited conditions account for only a small proportion of the ill-health suffered by different ethnic groups. For instance, although there is a significant excess mortality among American blacks compared with white Americans, it has been calculated that sickle-cell anaemia and thalassaemia account for only 0.3 per cent of this excess. Advances in genetics following the publication of the DNA sequence of the Human Genome in June 2000 may well find other examples of diseases with a genetic component that have different ethnic distributions.

9.7.4 Cultural, social and life history factors

Apart from the relatively few biological differences, what other factors could help to explain the health differences between ethnic groups? *Cultural differences* are a frequently cited possibility. For example, there are significant differences between ethnic groups in terms of diet, smoking behaviour and consumption of alcohol: men and women born in the Indian sub-continent generally smoke and drink much less than the average for England and Wales, but there are variations between Muslims and Hindus with, for example, very high rates of smoking found among

[17] The mechanisms by which single gene defects can cause diseases, including thalassaemia, sickle cell disease and cystic fibrosis, are discussed in greater detail in *Human Biology and Health: An Evolutionary Approach* (Open University Press, 2nd edn 1994; 3rd edn 2001), Chapter 4. Thalassaemia and other blood disorders are the subject of the associated TV programme for OU students, called 'Bloodlines' and the audiotape 'Tinkering with nature'.

Bangladeshi men living in the UK. These differences may reflect in part religious adherence, but this cannot explain why immigrant men born in Ireland tend to drink more than average, and Irish and Scottish male immigrants tend to smoke more than average. So cultural differences do explain some of the health differences observed, but many other differences remain unexplained.

Finally, we come to the influence of *social and life history* factors. As you saw above, social class is not a sufficient explanation of the differences shown in Table 9.4, and other factors must play a part. One factor may be racism, which may, for instance, limit employment and housing opportunities. In addition, racist attacks are likely to result not only in physical injury, but also fear and anxiety. Racism can affect not only health status but also the care that members of black and Asian communities receive from health services. In this context, the term 'institutional racism' is usually used, meaning that racist beliefs are accepted as factual evidence for differences between ethnic groups, and these beliefs then become normalised and come to influence and determine the behaviour of the members of that society. The institutionalisation of prejudiced beliefs is not of course confined to racial views, but occurs with views of gender, age and the other factors discussed in this chapter.

In conclusion, it should be noted that social and cultural influences are not independent, and in fact are a good illustration of the kinds of interaction discussed earlier in this chapter. For example, the pattern of health service use shown in Figure 9.13 could be interpreted as showing that although minority ethnic groups consult general practitioners at similar rates to the general population, for a range of reasons including cultural barriers, institutionalised racism and social/economic disadvantages they are less likely to be referred for specialist attention.

In summary, the key points are:

(1) Despite the lack of meaningful routine statistics on the health status of different ethnic groups, there is sufficient evidence to demonstrate the poorer health suffered by certain ethnic minorities living in Britain.

(2) Biological factors are known to account for a very small proportion of the observed differences; most are probably due to a mixture of social, cultural and life history factors, reinforced by the existence of racism.

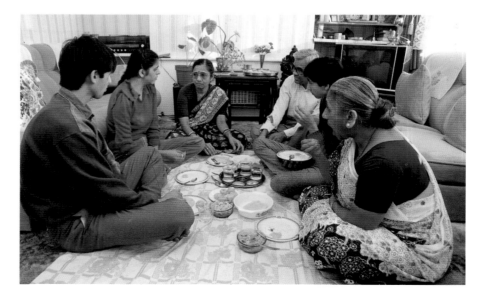

Asians in Britain have distinct dietary patterns, but the relationship between what they eat and their health is not straightforward. (Photo: Mark Power/Network)

9.8 Geography

Variations in mortality rates between different regions of Britain have been noted since at least the last century. Table 9.6 (first data column) shows mortality rates for males in different parts of the UK for 1997, adjusted to take account of any differences in age structure.

Table 9.6 Geographical variations in male mortality in the United Kingdom, 1997, and in morbidity (all adults) in Britain, 1998.

	Age-standardised death rates (per 100 000 population) males	Adults (aged 16+) reporting restricted activity in the 14 days before interview, 1998 %	Adults (aged 16+) reporting a long-standing illness, 1998 %
Scotland	1 184	16	32
North West	1 113	15	36
Northern Ireland	1 093	—	—
Northern and Yorkshire	1 069	15	36
Wales	1 061	21	41
West Midlands	1 041	14	35
UK (mortality)/Britain (morbidity)	1 029	15	33
Trent	1 019	15	34
England	1 007	14	33
North Thames	974	14	30
South Thames	959	13	30
Anglia and Oxford	950	13	29
South and West	935	15	34

Note: Northern Ireland is not included in the General Household Survey from which the morbidity data are taken. (Mortality data derived from Office for National Statistics, 1999, *Regional Trends No. 34*, The Stationery Office, London, Table 7.12; morbidity data from Office for National Statistics, 2000a, *Living in Britain: Results from the 1998 General Household Survey*, The Stationery Office, London, Tables 7.12 and 7.10)

● How would you describe the regional pattern of male mortality?

■ The highest mortality rates are experienced by men in Scotland (1 184 per 100 000, compared to 1 029 across the UK as a whole), the North West of England (1 113 per 100 000) and Northern Ireland (1 093 per 100 000). The lowest mortality rates are in the area of England south of the line between the Severn and the Wash. (This is an example of what is sometimes described as the 'north/south divide' in health experience.)

Geographical variations also exist among morbidity rates for a wide range of diseases. Table 9.6 shows data on the percentage of adults reporting restricted activity in the 14 days before interview or reporting a long-standing illness in 1998.

● How consistent are these differences in morbidity with the mortality differences shown in Table 9.6?

■ There is no clear correspondence. Some regions with an excess mortality also have higher morbidity — for example Scotland and North West England — but the overall pattern is not clear, and the north/south divide is not apparent.

● What features of the data could explain this lack of correspondence between morbidity and mortality by geographical region?

■ First, you may have noted that the morbidity data are not adjusted for differences in age-structure. Secondly, the morbidity data refer to all adults whereas the mortality data were for males only. And finally some of the apparent differences between regions in both sets of data may be not be statistically significant.

Data limitations apart, what are the possible explanations for regional differences in mortality and morbidity rates? The first of these concerns regional variations in climate and geology.

9.8.1 Climate and geology

Climatic and *environmental factors* such as hours of sunshine, humidity and water hardness have been suggested as explanations for some regional variations. For example, it has been shown that the SMRs for malignant melanoma of the skin (the most important skin cancer) are significantly higher in the south of the country than the north: a reversal of the usual 'north/south' pattern. This type of cancer is associated with exposure to ultraviolet light, which is the greater in the south because on average it receives more sunshine of higher intensity. Another environmental feature to have attracted attention in recent years is water quality. It has been established that the death rate from cardiovascular disease is partly associated with regions that have 'soft' water (containing low concentrations of calcium salts), although whether this association has any causal significance is still uncertain.

At a more localised level, the *geological structure* of different parts of the UK can also have an influence on patterns of disease, particularly on the incidence of those cancers associated with radiation. There are some areas where naturally-occurring radon gas seeps from the underlying rock (for example in parts of Cornwall, Scotland, and North Oxfordshire). Houses built in such areas expose their occupants to higher than normal background levels of radiation and, over many years of exposure, these radiation levels may pose a serious threat to health unless preventive action is taken. Indeed naturally occurring radon is second only to smoking as a cause of lung cancer in the UK, possibly accounting for approximately 2 000 deaths each year, or 5 per cent of the total.

9.8.2 Urbanisation and other social factors

Despite all these well-documented influences of the natural environment on mortality, there is *no* evidence that they are the *main* reason for the striking regional variations shown in Table 9.6. However, one feature of the *built* environment with long-established links to the pattern of mortality is the degree of *urbanisation*. The regions shown in Table 9.6 cover huge and disparate areas of the country which include urban and rural environments. In order to measure the degree of urbanisation, it is necessary to look at smaller areas such as local districts or health authorities (these measurement problems have already been encountered in the discussion of developing countries in Chapter 3). When local authorities with excess mortality from particular causes are ranked by SMR, it has been demonstrated that those with the greatest excess mortality are predominantly inner-city areas. This is true of cardiovascular disease — a leading cause of death. It is also true for deaths from lung cancer, pneumonia, bronchitis and stomach ulcer. However, the largest urban area in the UK (London) is in a low mortality and low morbidity region.

Turning to socio-economic factors, it is known that the *social class* composition of the population varies significantly between regions, and also that social class is closely associated with health and disease. However, even when adjustments are made for variations in social class composition, some regions still come out worse than expected, for reasons not fully understood. An analysis of other social variables such as *housing tenure* would reveal similar patterns and lead to similar conclusions: there are regional variations in housing tenure (for example a higher proportion of houses are owner-occupied in the South than in the North), and housing tenure is associated with a range of health indicators including mortality rates. However, there are regional variations in mortality rates *within* each type of housing tenure; for example, the mortality rates for people in rented accommodation is higher in some regions than in others.

A final possible explanation of regional differences in mortality is that people who are attracted from some areas such as the North of England to other regions such as South East England with better employment or other opportunities, are generally healthier and so leave behind a relatively less healthy population. Little research has been conducted on this topic, but while it does suggest that migration has indeed tended to widen regional differences, the overall effect has generally been small. It might also be noted that in some cases people with particular health problems will be attracted to areas of the country where treatment opportunities may be better: for example, of the cumulative total of 32 000 people in the UK diagnosed as infected with HIV by 1999, over 21 000 were reported in the two NHS regions covering London and the South East of England — a proportion far in excess of what would be expected on the basis of the population covered by these health authorities. One explanation is that some people moved to London from other areas of the UK to obtain treatment in large recognised centres, and perhaps also to get more help from support organisations.

In summary:

(1) Mortality and morbidity rates vary between regions, but the differences do not seem to be consistent.

(2) Many of the regional variations in mortality appear to be associated with environmental and social factors (the degree of urbanisation; differences in social class structure; the effect of geographical mobility), but these factors still leave some regional variations unaccounted for.

9.9   Occupation and social class

You have seen that differences in social class structure are one of the factors explaining regional variations in health. Let us now look in more detail at the association between health and occupation or social class. Although occupation and social class are closely related, they are not interchangeable: **occupational mortality** encompasses attempts to measure workplace hazards and other health risks that are *intrinsic* to a person's occupation, whereas **social class mortality** attempts to embrace a wide range of additional factors *extrinsic* to occupation — such as environment, social position or lifestyle — that may influence mortality.

9.9.1 Occupational health risks

Some illustrations of differences in occupational mortality are given in Table 9.7 for the period 1976–89. (These data may seem slightly old, but in fact were published in 1995 in one of the decennial (10-yearly) collections of national statistics; the next set of figures will not become available until 2005.) The long period of time covered by such statistics avoids some of the problems of having relatively small numbers of deaths in particular categories of occupations in any single year.

Table 9.7 Standardised mortality ratios (SMRs) for men aged 15 and over, and women aged 15–59, by type of occupation, 1976–89. (Mortality for each sex in the whole of England and Wales = 100.)

Occupation	SMRs	
	Men	**Women**
glass and ceramic makers	112	104
textile workers	118	114
labourers	117	–
miners and quarrymen	117	–
engineering and allied trades	100	106
clerical workers	93	82
administrators and managers	80	85
professional and technical workers	72	83
all	**100**	**100**

Data from Office for Population Censuses and Surveys (1995) *Occupational Health: Decennial Supplement,* The Registrar General's Decennial Supplement for England and Wales, Drever, F. (ed.) OPCS, HMSO, London, Annex 8.1.

As Table 9.7 indicates, there are substantial variations in the SMR for people in different occupations and, as expected, people in manual occupations tend to experience excess mortality. This may arise from direct risks to health and physical well-being in many manual jobs, which may result in direct loss of life, either suddenly in the form of accidents, or in an attenuated manner through exposure to damaging substances in the workplace over a long period. You may be aware of some examples, such as pneumoconiosis, a chronic lung condition suffered by coal miners.

In addition to specific occupational hazards, many health risks associated with work are of a non-specific nature and arise from *stress*. Stress may arise in a number of ways, but tends to originate primarily from the way in which work is organised. Some examples include low pay (leading to excessive overtime work), incentive payment schemes (speeding up potentially dangerous processes), shift-work (disrupting biological, psychological and social functioning), poor job design (producing boredom and little satisfaction), and bad industrial relations. The effects of stress on health have been demonstrated in terms of accident and sickness absence rates associated with different working practices.[18]

[18] 'Work and stress in adult life' is the title of Chapter 8 of *Birth to Old Age: Health in Transition* (Open University Press, 2nd edn 1995; colour-enhanced 2nd edn 2001). It is also discussed in the OU video associated with this chapter, 'Status and wealth: the ultimate panacea?'.

However, it is possible that the relatively high mortality of men in, for example, the textile industry is a result not only of health hazards directly associated with their occupation, but also the areas they tend to live in, the size and standard of their housing, the quality of their diet, or many other aspects of their lifestyle and environment. One way of separating out the *direct* effects of occupation from those due to *indirect* factors extrinsic to the workplace, is by relating the mortality or morbidity of the workers in that occupation to that of their spouses. This process has suggested, for example, that leather workers are at increased risk of suffering from tuberculosis, chronic rheumatic heart disease and bronchitis — all as a direct consequence of their occupation.

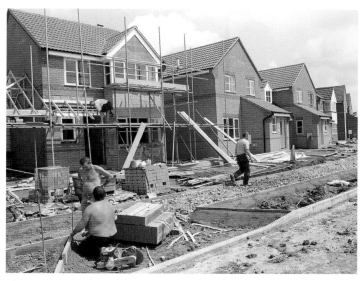

The workers in some jobs have relatively high risks of accidental injury; labourers on building sites have an occupational mortality 17 per cent higher than the national average for all occupations combined. (Photo: Mike Levers)

● Why do you think spouses are a good control group?

■ Spouses share most of the same social conditions as the worker (housing, income, etc.) and the same residential hazards (such as environmental pollutants), but not the working environment.

● For what factors can spouses *not* act as controls?

■ Biological factors relating to sex, and social factors relating to gender, cannot be controlled for by comparing husbands and wives.

Care needs to be taken in making comparisons based on worker–spouse differences. This is well illustrated in studies of the dangers of asbestos. Not only were the male workers at risk of inhaling asbestos fibres, but so were their wives. This was because men took their contaminated clothes home to be laundered by their wives.

In general, and despite the examples given above, it is not thought that factors directly arising from the occupation can explain more than a small part of mortality differences such as those shown in Table 9.6.

9.9.2 Social class and health risks

Risks to health intrinsic to the workplace are only one of many influences on health arising from the circumstances of people's lives. It has become common to group people into social classes based on groupings of broadly similar occupations. One of the most frequently used classifications in the UK is the **Registrar-General's classification of social class based on occupation** (Box 9.1); this groups all occupations into six categories (although they are sometimes combined in various permutations).

Box 9.1 The Registrar-General's classification of social class based on occupation

I   Professional (for example, a doctor or accountant)

II   Managerial and technical/ intermediate (for example, a nurse or teacher)

IIIN Skilled non-manual (for example, a typist)

IIIM Skilled manual (for example, a butcher or electrician)

IV   Partly skilled manual (for example, a postal worker or warehouseman)

V   Unskilled (for example, a labourer or cleaner)

It is generally the case that these *occupational* classes are also referred to as **social classes I to V** in research publications, as in this chapter, but you will also encounter other classifications in this book, for instance that used by the General Household Survey (GHS).

When using these classifications, it has generally been found that the social class of a married woman in employment is *less* predictive of her mortality than is her husband's class, and so it is conventional to assign women their own class if they are single but their husband's if they are married: this is the basis on which the following tables and graphs have been constructed.

Figure 9.14 shows life expectancy at different ages for males and females by social class in 1987–91. The calculations shown in Figure 9.14 are based on national census data and come from a 1 per cent sample of the population of England and Wales — almost half a million people. (Research on this sample has been conducted since 1971, and is known as the Longitudinal Study; we discuss it further in Chapter 10.)

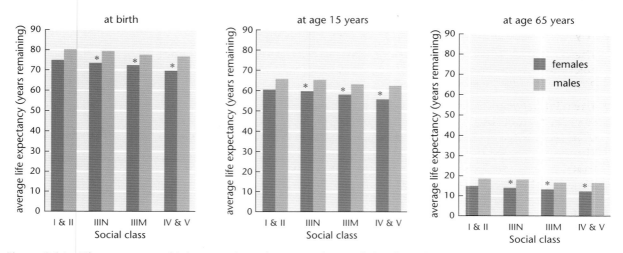

Figure 9.14 *Life expectancy at birth, at age 15 and at age 65 by social class for males and females, England and Wales, 1987–91 (Data from Hattersley, L. (1997) Expectation of life by social class, pp. 73–82 in Drever, F. and Whitehead, M. (eds)* Health inequalities: Decennial Supplement, *Government Statistical Service, Series DS No. 15, The Stationery Office, London, Tables 6.1 and 6.5) (* means a difference significant at the 1% level)*

● First, consider the overall pattern in Figure 9.14. Is there evidence of differences in life expectancy at different ages by social class?

■ Yes, a clear gradient across social classes is evident both in infancy and adulthood and for both sexes. At birth, the difference in life expectancy between the top and bottom social classes is approximately 5 years amongst men and 3.5 years amongst women. This **social class gradient** is sustained throughout adult life, although the differences seem to narrow in older age.

Now look more closely at Figure 9.14, paying particular attention to the sign indicating whether the differences between social classes I and II combined and the other classes are statistically significant at the 1 per cent level (i.e. if, in reality, there was *no difference* in life expectancy between social classes in the population as a whole, then there is only a 1:100 (P = 0.01) chance of recording differences as large as these in the sample on which Figure 9.14 is based).[19]

[19] Significance testing and the circumstances in which the 'null hypothesis' (no real difference) can be rejected are discussed in *Studying Health and Disease* (Open University Press, 2nd edn 1994; colour-enhanced 2nd edn 2001), Chapter 8.

● Given the significance levels quoted on Figure 9.14, to what extent might you now want to revise your initial impression? What can you conclude about the relationship between social class and life expectancy?

■ The figure shows that almost all the differences between social classes I and II combined and the other social classes are statistically significant at the 1 per cent level amongst women, but are not significant at this level amongst men.

However, the *absolute* differences between social classes amongst men are at least as great as they are amongst women, and the overall patterns between the two sexes are consistent. So although the association between social class and life expectancy for men has not passed the most rigorous standard of significance testing, we cannot conclude that there is *no* association. The differences between male social classes may be statistically significant at a less rigorous level of significance (e.g. the 5 per cent level, or $P = 0.05$). It is important to bear in mind the issue of statistical significance, here and throughout this chapter.

Table 9.8 concentrates on differences in adulthood. In addition to showing death rates by social class for men and women separately, it also shows

(1) The ratio between men and women for each social class (the right-hand column, calculated by dividing the male rate by the female rate, e.g. 455 divided by 270 equals 1.69).

(2) The ratio between social classes IV & V together and I & II together for each sex (the bottom row, e.g. 764 divided by 455 equals 1.68). If there were no differences between the top and bottom social classes, the ratio would be 1.0. The ratio of social classes IV & V to I & II, for men aged 35–64, of 1.68 means that the death rate for social classes IV & V (764 per 100 000) is approximately 68 per cent higher than that for social classes I & II (455 per 100 000).

Table 9.8 Age-standardised death rates per 100 000 population by social class, England and Wales, 1986–92.

Social class	Death rate per 100 000		
	Men aged 35–64	Women aged 35–64	Ratio of male : female death rates
I & II	455.0	270.0	1.69
IIIN	484.0	305.0	1.59
IIIM	624.0	356.0	1.75
IV & V	764.0	418.0	1.83
Ratio IV & V : I & II	1.68	1.55	–

Data derived from Harding, S., Bethune, A., Maxwell, R. and Brown, J. (1997) Mortality trends using the Longitudinal Study, pp. 143–55 in Drever, F. and Whitehead, M. (eds) *Health Inequalities: Decennial Supplement,* Government Statistical Service, Series DS No. 15, The Stationery Office, London, Tables 11.4 and 11.7.

● Does the association between gender and mortality vary with social class?

■ The difference between male and female mortality rates is large across all social classes, but there is no clear evidence that the ratio of male to female mortality rates *within* each social class (far right-hand column in Table 9.8) has a strong gradient *across* social classes.

Similarly, the association between social class and mortality does not appear to be strongly influenced by gender (the ratio of social classes IV & V to social classes I & II is 1.68 for males and 1.55 for females). Taken together, this evidence suggests that the 'protective' effect of being female persists almost independently of social class.

Next, Figure 9.15 looks at social class differences in mortality according to some major causes of death.

● In Figure 9.15, what categories of disease show the largest differences in mortality between social classes I & II and social classes IV & V, in each sex? Consider both the *absolute* differences between classes (that is, the lowest subtracted from the highest rate), and the *relative* differences (that is, highest divided by the lowest rate). You should be able to reach conclusions by reading off the approximate value of any bar in the histogram and making rough calculations; exact values are given on page 219.

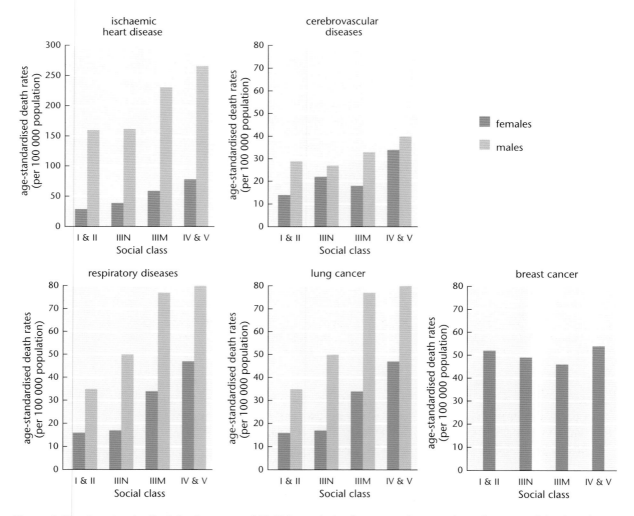

Figure 9.15 *Age-standardised death rates per 100 000 population for men and women by major cause of death and social class, England and Wales, 1986–92 (Data from Harding, S., Bethune, A., Maxwell, R. and Brown, J., 1997, Mortality trends using the Longitudinal Study, pp. 143–55 in F. Drever and M. Whitehead (eds)* Health Inequalities: Decennial Supplement, *Government Statistical Service,* Series DS No. 15, *The Stationery Office, London, Table 11.9, p. 151)*

■ The absolute difference is greatest in ischaemic heart disease amongst men: (160 in social classes I & II, compared with 266 in social classes IV & V — an absolute difference of 106 (266–160) – so if you estimated it 'by eye' at around 100, you have definitely understood the process). The absolute difference is also large in ischaemic heart disease amongst women: 29 in social classes I & II, compared with 78 in social classes IV & V — an absolute difference of 49. However, the relative difference is greatest for respiratory disease amongst men (13 in social classes I & II, compared with 48 in social classes IV & V; dividing 48 by 13 equals 3.6, so the death rate from respiratory disease is 3.6 times greater in the bottom two social classes compared with the top two). The relative difference is also large for lung cancer amongst women. In contrast, mortality from breast cancer is fairly even across social classes — a departure from the normal gradient.

Population surveys of morbidity reinforce the finding from mortality data that people in lower social classes suffer from poorer health than those in higher social classes. An example is total tooth loss. You have already seen its association with age (Figure 9.6); in Figure 9.16 you can see the additional effect of social class.

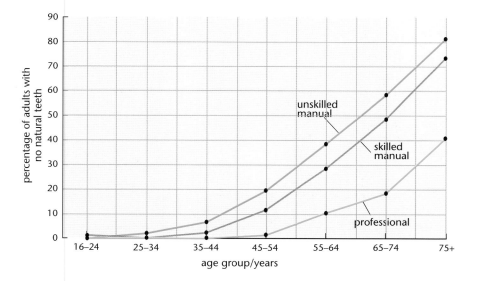

Figure 9.16   *Percentage of adults with no natural teeth, by age and socio-economic group, Great Britain, 1995. (Data from Office of Population Censuses and Surveys, 1996,* General Household Survey 1995, *OPCS Series GHS No. 26, HMSO, London, Table 9.2)*

● At what age is there the greatest difference in the percentage of toothless people between the professional classes and the unskilled manual class? As with Figure 9.15, look first at absolute differences between the three groups at each age, and then at the relative differences.

■ In absolute terms, the difference is greatest in the oldest age-groups (for example, 81 minus 40 equals a difference of 41 percentage points after age 75). In relative terms, the difference is greatest among those aged 45–54 years of age, when 15 per cent of unskilled manual workers have no natural teeth, fifteen times higher than the 1 per cent among the professional classes.

Another example of social class and morbidity comes from the General Household Survey in which, as noted earlier, people are asked to report on their own health status. Figure 9.17 shows rates of limiting long-standing illness for males and females by social class (note that slightly different class categories are used in this survey from those you have seen already in this section), and these data do again suggest quite a marked association between self-assessment of limiting long-standing illness and social class.

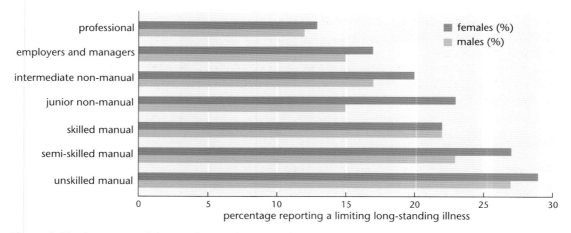

Figure 9.17   *Percentage of the population who reported a limiting long-standing illness by sex and social class, all ages, Great Britain, 1998. (Data from Office for National Statistics, 2000a,* Living in Britain: Results from the General Household Survey 1998, *The Stationery Office, London, Table 7.4)*

How can the social class differences in mortality and morbidity observed in this chapter be explained? A number of explanations have been put forward and they will be discussed in detail in Chapter 10, where some further examples of the mortality and morbidity associated with various occupations and with social class will be given. The consequences for health of unemployment will also be considered there. However, the strength of the association between health and social class is not in doubt, and can be summed up by a quote from the 1998 Acheson Report:

> If all men in this age-group (20–64) had the same death rates as those in classes I and II, it is estimated that there would have been over 17 000 fewer deaths each year from 1991 to 1993. (Department of Health, 1998, p. 14)

In summary, the key points are:

(1) When occupation is used as a proxy for social class, mortality and morbidity rates in lower social classes are higher than in upper social classes. The magnitude of this difference varies with age, being greatest in infancy and childhood, and least in old age. It applies to both sexes, but is generally more apparent in males than females.

(2) The association between social class and mortality and morbidity is present in most specific disease categories, although there are a few exceptions.

(3) Health risks directly arising from different occupations account for only a small proportion of the social class differences described. (Other explanations are discussed in Chapter 10.)

9.10 Conclusion

In this chapter, the contemporary patterns of health and disease in the UK have been described in terms of a wide range of factors, including genetics, life history, environment, and occupation. The patterns that emerge can contribute to our understanding and explanation of the causes of ill-health. Thus, although biological factors may explain much of the age-related pattern, they appear to make a less significant contribution to the patterns associated with the other forms of stratification, such as sex and gender, marital status, ethnicity and social class. In comparison, environmental and social conditions account for much of the observed differences between population groups, with much of the remainder resulting from variations in life histories or culture. The importance and impact of social factors on these patterns is probably best illustrated by the example of inequalities in the health of different social classes — the so-called **social class gradient in health** — and these form the subject of the following chapter.

OBJECTIVES FOR CHAPTER 9

When you have studied this chapter, you should be able to:

9.1 Define and use, or recognise definitions and applications of, each of the terms printed in **bold** in the text.

9.2 Identify the main diseases responsible for the overall patterns of mortality, morbidity and disability in the UK in recent years.

9.3 Describe the association of both age and sex or gender with disease, and review the explanations for these patterns.

9.4 Describe the association between marital status and both mortality and morbidity; the different effects of marital status on men and women; and the social explanations for these differences.

9.5 Outline the main patterns of mortality and morbidity in different ethnic groups, and some possible reasons for these differences.

9.6 Describe the main regional differences in health status in Britain and suggest factors that would explain some of the differences.

9.7 Describe the association between lower social class and higher mortality and morbidity rates, and discuss the contribution of occupational factors to the social class gradient in health.

9.8 Use appropriate examples to illustrate interactions between the factors discussed in this chapter and the need to take account of such interactions when constructing explanations.

9.9 Demonstrate an awareness that reliable interpretation of epidemiological data depends on a good understanding of the data's strengths and weaknesses.

QUESTIONS FOR CHAPTER 9

1   (*Objective 9.2*)

How serious for the health of the population are skin diseases? To answer this, you will need to consider Figure 9.5 and Table 9.2.

2   (*Objective 9.3*)

In 1995, 64 per cent of people aged 75 or over had no teeth, while this was true of only 2 per cent of those aged 35–44 years (see Figure 9.6). Does this mean a further 62 per cent of the younger age group will lose all their remaining teeth over the next 30 or so years? Explain your reasoning.

3   (*Objective 9.4*)

To what extent do death rates by marital status (see Table 9.3) support the argument that those who are married have better health in all social classes? Do you have any reservations about drawing conclusions from these data?

4   (*Objective 9.5*)

How different is the health of minority ethnic groups compared with the population of England and Wales as a whole in terms of morbidity and mortality?

5   (*Objective 9.6*)

Suggest (a) biological, (b) social, and (c) life-history explanations for the regional variation in mortality rates seen in Table 9.6.

6   (*Objective 9.7*)

Overall mortality rates are higher in social classes IV and V than in social classes I and II for both sexes. Is the same class difference in mortality true for all conditions and for measures of morbidity?

7   (*Objective 9.8*)

A major cause of days lost from work is low-back pain. Suggest how age and social class may interact in causing this condition. What might be the limitations of analysing the distribution of low-back pain in relation to only *one* of these dimensions of population structure?

8   (*Objective 9.9*)

The data given in Table 9.5 and Figure 9.13 come from the preliminary results of the *Health Survey for England 1999*, released by the Department of Health in June 2000. This annual survey of a large sample of the population (in a full sample year about 16 000 adults and 4 000 children are included) combines questionnaire-based interviews with physical measurements and the analysis of blood samples. Blood pressure, height and weight, smoking, drinking, general health, and use of services are covered every year. In the population sampled in 1999, which was carefully selected to boost the number of respondents from ethnic minorities, the survey researchers interviewed over 5 000 adults and 3 000 children (aged 2–15 years) from Black Caribbean, Indian, Pakistani, Bangladeshi, Chinese and Irish ethnic groups. The preliminary results are based on the analysis of over 4 000 of these interviews.

(a)   What aspects of the design of this survey tend to give you confidence in its findings about the health of people from different ethnic minority groups in the UK?

(b)   What further information about the methodology and the outcomes would increase your confidence that the results are *valid* and *reliable*? (If you are unsure about the technical meaning of *validity* and *reliability* in survey research, consult *Studying Health and Disease* (Open University Press, 2nd edn 1994; colour-enhanced 2nd edn 2001), Chapter 5, before attempting this question.)

CHAPTER 10

Explaining inequalities in health in the United Kingdom

Study notes for OU students

During section 10.4 of this chapter you will be asked to read an extract from a report by the Medical Services Study Group of the Royal College of Physicians, entitled 'Deaths under 50', which is contained in *Health and Disease: A Reader* (Open University Press, second edition 1995; third edition 2001). The video 'Status and wealth: the ultimate panacea?' is associated with Chapters 9 and 10; we suggest that you watch it a second time at the end of this chapter. The video illustrates the Whitehall Study (discussed in Section 10.4.2 of this chapter), and also the 'programming hypothesis', which links maternal nutrition during pregnancy with the risk of vascular diseases when the baby becomes middle-aged (Section 10.5.5). This hypothesis and the research methods that generated the data on which it is based were discussed in detail in the previous book in this series, *Studying Health and Disease* (Open University Press, second edition 1994; colour-enhanced second edition 2001), Chapter 10, and in the associated audiotape and its notes in the *U205 Introduction and Skills Guide*.

10.1   Introduction

Chapter 9 explored some of the many ways in which mortality and morbidity vary across the population of the UK. In this chapter we look in more detail at how these variations might be explained. We shall refer to many of the dimensions of variation discussed in Chapter 9, such as gender or ethnic group, but will devote particular attention to *socio-economic characteristics* such as social class, occupation, income and housing. There are two main reasons for this. First, partly in consequence of the significance attached to these characteristics, an extensive body of data exists. Second, these factors receive more attention here because other factors such as gender or age are discussed in greater detail in other books in this series.

This chapter considers explanations for inequalities in health under four main headings. It begins by examining the argument that they are mainly an *artefact*, a consequence of the ways in which data are collected and analysed rather than a reflection of a social reality. The second explanation is that people move between social classes on a *selective* basis according to whether they are sick or healthy, thus magnifying any differences that exist. Third, it is sometimes argued that health inequalities arise largely from the *behaviour* of individuals. Finally, a set of arguments is grouped around the idea that health inequalities are primarily a reflection of inequalities in the *life circumstances* and *material conditions* of the population.

10.2   Inequalities in health: fact or artefact?

Figure 10.1 shows trends in male mortality by social class defined by occupation between 1970–72 and 1991–93. Mortality in the figure is measured in terms of European Standardised Rates, in which death rates are standardised to the European population, thus facilitating international comparisons.

● What trend over time in social class mortality differences is revealed in Figure 10.1? We have calculated the combined mortality rates in the bottom two classes (IV and V) in 1970–72 and the combined mortality rates in the top two classes (I and II); then we have expressed these figures as a ratio, and repeated the calculations for the two later periods.

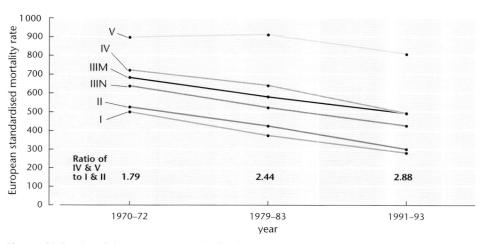

Figure 10.1   *Trends in European Standardised Mortality Rates of men aged 20–64, England and Wales, by social class, using the Registrar-General's classifications, 1970–72 to 1991–93. (Data from Drever, F. and Bunting, J. (1997) Patterns and trends in male mortality, pp. 95–107 in Drever, F. and Whitehead, M. (eds)* Health Inequalities: Decennial Supplement, *Government Statistical Service, Series DS No. 15, The Stationery Office, London, Table 8.6)*

■ The age-standardised death rates have fallen in all groups, but more so in the higher social groups. The differences between the top two and the bottom two social classes appear to have widened, from 1.79 in 1970–72, to 2.44 in 1979–83, and to 2.88 by 1991–93. Death rates in the lower two social classes were almost three times higher than those in the top two classes by the end of this period.

This evidence that the social class gradient in mortality has been apparently widening over recent decades, could be challenged on a number of grounds. Four arguments in particular have been used to suggest that the trend, and to some extent the inequalities themselves, are an *artefact* of the ways in which the data have been collected:

1   The information on deaths and the information on the numbers in each class come from different sources, and errors in either can lead to a numerator/ denominator problem (explained below);

2   Occupations have been re-classified over time into different social classes, making comparisons over time difficult to perform;

3   Published statistics are often based on narrow age-groups containing a small proportion of total deaths, which may not be typical of the entire spectrum of ages;

4   The size of social classes has been changing and the proportions of the population at either extreme of the social class spectrum are quite small, so that the widest mortality differences affect relatively small numbers.

Let us examine these in turn, beginning with the numerator/denominator problem.

10.2.1   The numerator/denominator problem

The main source of information on health inequalities by social class in England and Wales has traditionally been the Registrar General's *Decennial Supplement* which has been published since the nineteenth century. Every ten years, cross-sectional information from the national census on the social class composition of the population, measured using occupation as a 'proxy', is combined with information about deaths by social class during the period around the census. So the 1991 census was combined with data on deaths for 1991–93 to create the *Decennial Supplement on Occupational Health* (OPCS, 1995). Putting together information from different sources in this way carries a number of problems, but one in particular is that to calculate a *rate*, for example a death rate among women in social class V, it is necessary to divide the number of such women who died (the numerator in the fraction) by the number of such women in total in the population (the denominator):

$$\frac{\text{no. of women in social class V who died (numerator)}}{\text{total no. of women in social class V (denominator)}} = \begin{array}{l}\text{mortality rate}\\\text{of women in}\\\text{social class V}\end{array}$$

Errors in the number above *or* below the line in such a fraction can produce misleading results, for example, if occupations are misclassified on death certificates. Some studies have suggested that such problems can increase or decrease occupational class mortality rates by up to 20 per cent (Kunst, 1997). For these reasons, the results of an earlier *Decennial Supplement on Occupational Health* (in 1979–83) were accompanied by a warning that some of the data were subject to serious bias from this and other sources.

One way of avoiding the 'numerator/denominator' problem is to measure mortality not as a rate, but using some relative measure. One option is to use a **proportional mortality ratio**, or PMR, which gives the percentage of *actual* deaths from a particular cause in a population group as a *ratio* of the percentage of deaths that would be *expected* in a standard population. We can illustrate this with a hypothetical example: if, in Great Britain as a whole, 25 per cent of deaths were caused by cancers, but cancers caused 37.5 per cent of deaths in social class V, then the proportional mortality ratio (PMR) for cancers in social class V would be

37.5 divided by 25 = 1.5 (× 100) = 150

To put this another way, in this illustrative example, the fact that PMR = 150 means that there is 50 per cent *more* cancer in social class V than we would expect on the basis of the population as a whole.

However, while PMRs do avoid the possibility of a numerator/denominator problem, they also have limitations. The most serious drawback is that if a particular disease causes an unusually high proportion of deaths, this will necessarily *lower* the proportions dying from *other* causes, and vice versa.

Another way of avoiding the problems potentially inherent in the cross-sectional Decennial Supplements is to follow a cohort of individuals over time. Since 1971 this has been done by the **Longitudinal Study**, in which a one per cent sample of the population of England and Wales (0.5 million people) is being followed over time, and any vital events such as deaths are recorded alongside information on employment and other characteristics. Although the sample contains half a million people, it is still only a small proportion (1 per cent) of the population; when you subdivide further (e.g. into social classes), relatively low numbers fall into the highest and lowest social classifications, and these small numbers may not be representative of the population as a whole. For this reason, the Longitudinal Study has the limitation that, because it is based on relatively small numbers, there may be insufficient information to make sub-classifications such as deaths by age, sex, cause of death and occupation. However, because the sample contains the numerator (those who died in any given period) and the denominator (for example, everyone in social class V at the beginning of the period), and because it can track life events such as spells of unemployment, it has proved to be an increasingly valuable data source for social scientists, epidemiologists and others, and has already produced a vast amount of useful information. You will encounter the Longitudinal Study frequently in this chapter.[1]

Table 10.1 shows some information taken from the Longitudinal Study, which compares mortality by social class between 1976 and 1992. Social classes I and II have been combined, and so have classes IV and V, to avoid any problems related to small numbers.

Consistent with the trends shown in Figure 10.1, mortality has fallen over time in all classes, yet there is clearly a widening of social class mortality differences. For example, the ratio of 1.53 amongst men in 1976–1981 means that death rates were 53 per cent higher in social classes IV and V combined compared to social classes I and II, but by the later 1980s and early 1990s this difference had increased to 68 per cent.

[1] Research based on the Longitudinal Study also features prominently in another book in this series, *Birth to Old Age: Health in Transition* (Open University Press, 2nd edn 1995; colour-enhanced 2nd edn 2001).

Table 10.1   Trends in age-standardised mortality rates per 100 000 people: men and women aged 35–64 by social class, 1976–1992, England and Wales.

Social class	women			Social class	men		
	1976–81	1981–85	1986–92		1976–81	1981–85	1986–92
I & II	338.0	344.0	270.0	I & II	621.0	539.0	455.0
IIIN	371.0	387.0	305.0	IIIN	860.0	658.0	484.0
IIIM	467.0	396.0	356.0	IIIM	802.0	691.0	624.0
IV & V	508.0	445.0	418.0	IV & V	951.0	824.0	764.0
Ratio IV & V : I & II	**1.50**	**1.29**	**1.55**	**Ratio IV & V : I & II**	**1.53**	**1.53**	**1.68**

Data from Harding, S., Bethune, A., Maxwell, R. and Brown, J. (1997) Mortality trends using the Longitudinal Study, pp. 143–55 in Drever, F. and Whitehead, M. (eds) *Health Inequalities: Decennial Supplement*, Government Statistical Service, Series DS No. 15, The Stationery Office, London, Tables 11.4 and 11.7.

● Has the health gradient been increasing steadily over this period for both sexes?

■ No, the gap between upper and lower social classes remained the same for men and closed substantially for women between 1976–81 and 1981–85, but in the period 1986–1992 the gap increased again in both sexes — at least according to the Longitudinal Study data. (The next Decennial Supplement based on this sample is not due for publication until 2007.)

10.2.2 Reclassification of occupations

A second potential artefact explanation for mortality differences arises from the re-classification of occupations that takes place between censuses. This problem however, has long been recognised by official statisticians. One way of dealing with it is by presenting figures on the basis of the old as well as the new classification. Another way of avoiding this problem is to use the same classification of occupations over time so that observed differences cannot be the result of reclassifications. Such exercises have found that trends towards a widening gap in mortality inequalities cannot be explained by changes in the classification of occupations.

10.2.3 Small proportion of deaths

The argument that evidence for health inequalities is sometimes based on a relatively small proportion of deaths occurring in certain age-groups can easily be addressed by looking at differences across a wider range of age-groups. However, as you have seen in the previous chapter (Figure 9.14), a social class gradient in life expectancy exists at birth, but persists through adulthood and is still clear at the age of 65.

Related to the question of small numbers is the possibility that differences in mortality are not statistically significant. For example, Figure 10.2 (overleaf) shows the standardised mortality ratios (SMRs) for six different occupations. It suggests that farm workers, wood workers and administrators all have lower mortality rates than the population as a whole (whose SMR = 100), while paper and printing workers, food, drink and tobacco workers, and textile workers all have higher mortality rates than the population as a whole.

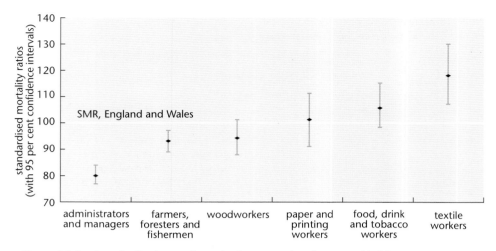

Figure 10.2 *Standardised mortality ratios by occupational group, with 95 per cent confidence intervals among 187 871 males who were aged 16+ in the 1971 Census, calculated from deaths between 1976 and 1989. (Data from OPCS, 1995,* Occupational Health: Decennial Supplement, *The Registrar General's Decennial Supplement for England and Wales, Series DS No. 10, Drever, F. (ed.) HMSO, London, Annex 8.1)*

The figure also shows this information with 95 per cent confidence intervals around each point: that is, one can be 95 per cent confident that the true figure lies within this range.

● For which of the occupational groups can you be 95 per cent confident that their SMRs are significantly higher or lower than the population as a whole?

■ Administrators and managers, and farmers, foresters and fishermen have lower SMRs, and textile workers have higher SMRs, than the average for England and Wales. In the other three occupational groups, the 95 per cent confidence interval crosses the line showing an SMR of 100, indicating that one cannot be certain that the SMR of these occupational groups is in fact significantly higher or lower than the average for the population as a whole.

Statistical significance is less of an issue (although it should always be considered) when entire social classes are being compared, as the numbers involved are large enough to ensure that the confidence intervals are narrow and any differences are demonstrated to be significant by the application of statistical tests. However, this can be a problem when specific occupations are being examined, and for this reason official publications sometimes (but not always!) indicate whether differences are statistically significant.

10.2.4   Changes in size of social classes

Next we turn to the argument that observed inequalities in health may be influenced by changes in the size of different social classes. This argument has two elements: first, that the lowest social classes, which suffer the highest mortality rates, are declining as a proportion of the population, and that some allowance should therefore be made for the falling numbers involved; and, second, that the sizes of the social classes at the top and bottom extremes are relatively small. Table 10.2 shows the percentage of men aged 20–64 in each social class at the 1981 and 1991 censuses.

Table 10.2   Proportion of men aged 20–64 in each social class, England and Wales, 1981 and 1991.

Social class	1981 %	1991 %
I	5.6	6.5
II	22.0	26.4
IIIN	10.8	9.7
IIIM	33.4	29.9
IV	15.3	14.1
V	5.5	4.8

Data from Drever, F. and Whitehead, M. (eds) (1997) *Health Inequalities: Decennial Supplement*, Government Statistical Service, Series DS No. 15, The Stationery Office, London, Appendix B, Table B.4, p. 244. Percentages do not sum to 100%, due to unoccupied or inactive persons who cannot easily be allocated to a social class.

● What changes occurred over this period in the combined size of the three manual classes, compared with the three non-manual social classes?

■ A falling proportion of the population was classified as being in social classes IIIM, IV and V (down over 5 per cent from 54.2 to 48.8 per cent), and an increasing proportion in classes I, II and IIIN (up over 4 per cent from 38.4 to over 42.6 per cent).

Debate tends to focus on the decline in the relative size of the lower social class groups, but the expansion of the top social classes with *lower* than average mortality is also relevant to this discussion. This important point, that measures of inequality have to take into account those with lower than average mortality as well as those with above average mortality, is often neglected. So the effect of changes in the social class distribution of the population on observed mortality differences is far from obvious.

One way of addressing the fact that the proportion of the population at the extremes of the social class spectrum is relatively small is to group social classes, as we did in Table 10.1 (and also in Chapter 9). Another approach is to use alternative social classifications to see if similar patterns emerge. Table 10.3 reports the results of this kind of analysis.

First note that Table 10.3 refers to all men aged 65–74 and is thus less prone to the problems of small numbers of deaths that affect some analyses based on younger age-groups, where relatively few deaths occur. The table classifies individuals according to type of **housing tenure** (that is, whether they live in property they own or property rented from either a private landlord or a local authority), and access to car transport, both of which indicate income and way of life. Using either classification a clear mortality gradient emerges from Table 10.3: for example, the SMR in relation to car access varies from 82 to 121. Moreover, because there are only three status groupings, the numbers within each group are large, contradicting the argument that mortality differences are an artefact based on small and diminishing numbers at the extremes of the spectrum.

Table 10.3   Standardised mortality ratios in 1981–92 of men aged 65–74 in England and Wales, by housing tenure and car access.

Socio-economic indicator	SMR
housing tenure	
owner occupiers	86
private renters	109
local authority tenants	117
car access	
two or more	82
one	91
none	121

Data from Smith, J. and Harding, S. (1997) Mortality of women and men using alternative social classifications, pp. 168–83 in Drever, F. and Whitehead, M. (eds) *Health Inequalities: Decennial Supplement*, Government Statistical Service, Series DS No. 15, The Stationery Office, London, Table 13.5.

This type of analysis also suggests that social class groupings based on occupation may obscure considerable variation in terms of mortality experience *within* social classes. For example, and extending the analysis shown in Table 10.3, the SMRs of men in manual social classes (IIIM, IV and V) aged 65–74 vary from 83 among those in owner-occupied housing with one or more cars, to 122 among local authority tenants with no car. In other words, mortality differences between specific sub-groups *within* social classes can be almost as great as those *between* high and low social classes.

A third approach is to use some measure of health inequality that takes into account the distribution of health across *all* social classes rather than simply the difference between the highest and lowest groups. Figure 10.3 shows such an analysis, comparing the distribution of males aged 45–64 by socio-economic group, and the distribution of males aged 45–64 who have long-standing illness, by socio-economic group.

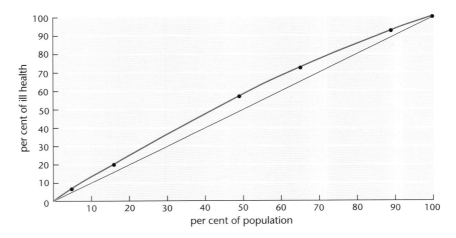

Figure 10.3   *The distribution of males aged 45–64, and males aged 45–64 with long-standing illness, by socio-economic group, Great Britain 1998. (Data derived from Office for National Statistics, 2000,* Living in Britain: Results from the General Household Survey 1998, *The Stationery Office, London, Tables 3.17 and 7.3)*

If health were equally distributed across all social classes, then the unskilled manual social class, containing 5 per cent of men aged 45–64, would also contain 5 per cent of men aged 45–64 who report a long-standing illness. Adding the next social class — semi-skilled manual workers — would take the percentage share of the population up to 16 per cent, and again if health was equally distributed then the percentage share of all men in this age-group who report a long-standing illness would also go up to 16 per cent, and so on. The result would be a diagonal line from 0 to 100 per cent, showing equal shares of population and ill-health. However, if ill-health was *not* equally distributed across the population, the resulting line would depart from the diagonal, and the larger the difference between the actual line and the diagonal, the greater the degree of inequality.

As Figure 10.3 shows, long-standing illness in 1998 in Great Britain was not equally distributed across socio-economic groups in men aged 45–64. The lowest socio-economic groups had a larger proportional share of people with long-standing illness than their share of population, and vice versa in the higher groups. The result is clearly seen in the curved line above the diagonal. These curves are called *Lorenz Curves*, and are a useful summary way of examining inequality across an entire population rather than simply between top and bottom groups. The area between the diagonal line and the curved line can also be measured and expressed as an index number, which provides another useful way of summarising the degree of inequality and how it is changing over time, or how it differs between countries.

10.2.5   Summary

This section has examined the four main ways in which observed social class differences in health might be statistically misleading. In each case the evidence indicates that dealing with the statistical problem does not remove the social class gradient in health; nor does it remove the increasing 'health gap' between top and bottom social classes:

1   The numerator/denominator problem can be avoided by using longitudinal data or proportional mortality ratios (PMRs): both methods indicate the existence of social class gradients in mortality.

2   Problems arising from the re-classification of occupations into different social classes can be avoided by making comparisons over time using the same classification, or by tracking individual occupations: both methods confirm the existence of social class gradients in mortality.

3   Published statistics are often based on narrow age-groups containing a small proportion of total deaths, but social class gradients in mortality are found in all age-groups from birth to old age.

4   The proportions of the population at either extreme of the social class spectrum are quite small, but equally great mortality differences can be found between large groups defined on other socio-economic criteria such as housing tenure or car access. We shall return to these alternative social classifications later in the chapter.

10.3   Social selection on the basis of health

At the heart of the theory of **health-related social selection** is the idea that moves made by individuals into or out of occupations, social classes, or employment are partly determined by a process of 'selection' on health grounds. For example, people in poor health might move into lower, less skilled occupations if their health poses problems to themselves or their employers. Conversely, people in good health may be more likely to move into higher status and more skilled occupations. Note that the theory assumes **social mobility**, i.e. that people can change their social class during their lifetime.

If social mobility were influenced by health, then the lower occupational classes would have a growing proportion of members in poor health and the SMRs for these classes would be pushed *up*, whereas in the higher occupational classes SMRs would be pushed *down* by new class entrants in good health and class leavers in bad health. Thus health differences between occupational classes would exist, not because class position influenced health, but because health influenced class position.

10.3.1   Evidence for social selection

Evidence of health-related social selection has come from a number of studies. For example, one study conducted in the United Kingdom in the 1950s examined the distribution of men with schizophrenia by social class on admission to hospital.

● How might you test the 'null hypothesis' that the social class distribution of these men was the *same* as in the population as a whole?

■ One way would be to compare the social class distribution of males of the same ages among the patients and in the population as a whole.

In fact, the observed number of patients in social class V was roughly twice as high as would have been predicted using this method. In addition, the social class distribution of the patients was quite different from the social class distribution of the *fathers* of the patients (their class of origin). One explanation might be that these males had fallen to the bottom social class *because* they had developed schizophrenia.

Another well-known study conducted over the period 1951–1980 by the medical sociologist Raymond Illsley, on a sample of women in Aberdeen, found that women who were *taller* than other women in their social class of origin (that is, the social class in which they grew up, based on their father's occupation) were more likely to marry into a *higher* social class. As height is influenced not only by genetic inheritance but by health in the early years of life, this suggested that good health in childhood was indeed a factor influencing the upward social mobility of the taller women.

Women who are taller than average for women in the social class in which they grew up are more likely to marry into a higher social class. (Photo: PA Photo Library)

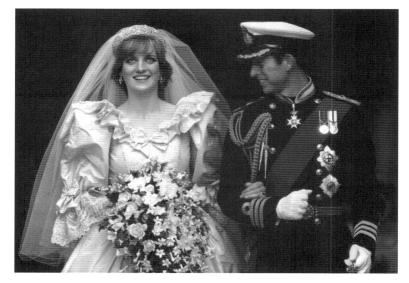

Illsley was able to pursue this issue by using the longitudinal Aberdeen Maternity and Neonatal Data Bank to examine the perinatal mortality rate (PNMR) of the first-born babies of women, again classified according to the social class of their father (their class of origin), and the social class of their husband (the class into which they moved). The PNMR is known to be influenced by maternal health, among other factors. Table 10.4 shows some results from this study.

● What does Table 10.4 reveal about the health of women who were *upwardly* mobile in terms of social class compared with those who were *downwardly* mobile (using the PNMR of their first-born babies as a 'proxy' for maternal health)?

■ Using this indirect measure, the health of women who moved up the social class structure was markedly better than the health of women who moved down. For example, the PNMR for babies born to upwardly mobile women whose fathers were from social class III Manual (that is, who had married men

Table 10.4 Perinatal mortality rate (per 1 000 births) in relation to the social class of the husbands and the fathers of the women whose babies died.

Social class of woman's father	Perinatal mortality rate Social class of woman's husband			
	I–IIIN	IIIM	IV and V	all classes
I–IIIN	17	18	31	19
IIIM	19	26	29	26
IV and V	17	26	33	27
all classes	18	24	31	24

Data from research by Raymond Illsley on the Aberdeen Maternity and Neonatal Data Bank, reported in Wilkinson, R. G. (1986a), Socio-economic differences in mortality: interpreting the data on their size and trends, in Wilkinson, R. G. (ed.) *Class and Health: Research and Longitudinal Data*, Tavistock, London, Tables 9.7 and 9.17.

in social classes I–III Non-manual), was 19 per 1 000, compared with 29 per 1 000 for babies born to women from social class IIIM who were downwardly mobile (that is, who had married men in social classes IV or V).

This study, while demonstrating that differences in perinatal mortality were influenced by social mobility, did not estimate *how much* of these differences might be explained in this way. However, a subsequent re-analysis of the Aberdeen data estimated that no more than 10 per cent of the social class difference in perinatal mortality rates could be accounted for by movements between social classes (Wilkinson, 1986b).

10.3.2 Social selection and unemployment

Another group in which the potential contribution of health-related social selection has attracted much attention has been people who are unemployed. There seems to be little doubt that **unemployment and health** are in some way associated — ill-health, in fact, seems to be a feature of unemployment. For example the Longitudinal Study found that, between 1981 and 1992, the SMR of men aged 25–64 who had been employed at both the 1971 and 1981 censuses — that is, who seemed to have a history of being in employment — was 83 (all men = 100). By contrast, men who had been employed on only *one* of these census dates had an SMR of 127, and men who had been unemployed on *both* dates had an SMR of 194. These data also illustrate the point that the *duration* of unemployment must be considered, and not just employment status at one point in time.

● What alternative interpretations could you place on the evidence that ill-health and mortality are higher among unemployed people than among those in employment?

■ It could be that something about the experience of unemployment causes an increase in ill-health and mortality. However, the direction of causality could be the other way round and poor health could *lead to* unemployment. Finally, there could be some other explanation in which both unemployment and poor health are independently related to some third factor or factors.[2]

[2] Discussion of causal direction and confounding factors in the interpretation of epidemiological and social survey data occurs in *Studying Health and Disease* (Open University Press, 2nd edn 1994; colour-enhanced 2nd edn 2001).

Unemployment is very unevenly distributed across social classes: in 1998 only 7 per cent of the professional group were in 'workless' households, compared to 17 per cent of the skilled manual group and 36 per cent of the unskilled manual group. (A **household** is defined as people living together in the same accommodation, regardless of whether they are related to each other.) With respect to morbidity, the General Household Survey of 1998 (ONS, 2000a) found that 31 per cent of unemployed men and women reported some long-standing illness, compared with 27 cent of employed men and 24 per cent of employed women. The differences between employed and unemployed people for long-standing illnesses defined as 'causing a limitation to normal life' were even greater.

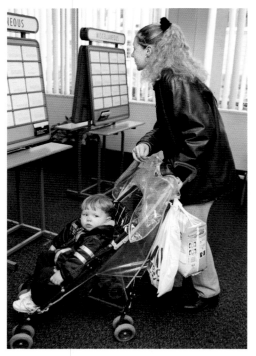

Unemployment has been consistently shown to increase the risk of ill-health and mortality, particularly among people who are long-term unemployed. (Photo: John Harris, Report Digital)

One way of seeing *how much* of the health difference between employed and unemployed people might be attributable to health-related social selection is to follow individuals over time. If selection due to ill-health were a major reason for becoming unemployed, then the observed difference in health between unemployed and employed people at the beginning of the study period should *decrease* over time.

● Can you explain why?

■ Over time, increasing numbers of the originally healthy would become ill, while a proportion of those made unemployed because of ill-health would either die or recover.

However, when researchers tracked the subsequent mortality of men who, in 1971, were seeking work but were not at that time recorded as temporarily or permanently sick, they found that the differences between this group and those in employment *increased* rather than narrowed. Five years later the SMR of the group seeking work was 129 compared with 85 among the employed (all men = 100), but after ten years the SMR of the group seeking work had increased to 146, compared with 92 among the employed group (Moser *et al.*, 1990).

● How would you interpret these data?

■ They suggest that as time passed the health of the group who were initially out of work deteriorated further. This evidence strongly suggests that health-related social selection was not a major reason for the increased mortality among those seeking work.

As with differences between unemployed and employed, so with differences between social classes: if a major reason for the existence of health inequalities between social classes is health-related social selection, then by following a group of individuals over time the original differences should become *less* pronounced as those who were originally ill recover or die, while those who were originally healthy become sick. And again the Longitudinal Study has provided an opportunity to examine this. Turn back to Table 10.1, which shows the death rates from 1976–81 to 1986–92 for a cohort of individuals originally identified in 1971 at the start of the Longitudinal Study.

● Does Table 10.1 indicate a narrowing or widening of mortality differences between these groups over time, and what does this suggest in relation to health-related social selection?

■ As you saw earlier, the table suggests a widening of mortality differences over time, indicating that the influence of social selection on the observed differences between social classes must be minor.

10.3.3   Summary

In theory, social class differences in health could exist for no other reason than health-related social selection: upward mobility among the more healthy and downward mobility among the less healthy. In practice, it is difficult to estimate the proportion of observed social class differences that could be attributed to social selection, but comparisons of groups by class of origin *versus* class of attainment, and longitudinal research, indicate that this proportion must be small. The major explanations for health inequalities between social groups must lie elsewhere.

10.4   Lifestyle and behaviour: a case of self-destruction?

We can now turn to the third possible explanation for health inequalities between social classes: that they arise because there are differences in the health-promoting or health-damaging behaviour of individuals in different social classes. This view is exemplified by a report from the Medical Services Study Group (MSSG) of the Royal College of Physicians, 'Deaths under 50'. (An extract from the report is reprinted in *Health and Disease: A Reader* (Open University Press, 2nd edn 1994; 3rd edn 2001) and Open University students should read it now.) The study is of interest less for the actual data quoted (which relate to the period 1977–78), than for the interpretations placed on the data.

● The Study Group paid particular attention to 98 cases from a sample of 250 patients who died. How did they label the cases, and why?

■ The 98 cases were described as cases of 'self-destruction' because, according to the Study Group, 'the patients contributed in large measure to their own deaths'.

● In attempting to explain the 'causes' of these deaths, what factors did the Study Group emphasise?

■ They emphasise self-poisoning, excessive smoking, drinking and eating, non-compliance with medical treatment, and failure to seek medical help.

● How did the Study Group seek to explain these aspects of individual behaviour?

■ They did this primarily by discussing existing mental illness, reckless or uncooperative attitudes, and a failure to heed health education in general and doctors' advice in particular.

To examine this argument in more detail, let us first look at some of the factors cited by the Study Group.

10.4.1   Evidence for 'self-destructive' behaviour

Tobacco consumption

Smoking may contribute to the patterns of mortality and morbidity that concerned the MSSG and is frequently cited in discussions of 'lifestyle' or behavioural factors. Table 10.5 shows patterns of cigarette smoking in Great Britain in 1982 and in 1998–99. You can see that at both time points a higher proportion of manual workers of both sexes were smokers, compared to the national population, and there is a clear social class gradient.

● What happened to cigarette smoking among men and women in non-manual social classes compared with those in manual social classes between 1982 and 1998–99?

Table 10.5   Prevalence of cigarette smoking among men and women aged 16+ by social class, Great Britain, 1982 and 1998–99.

	Male smokers in each class/%		% Reduction 1982 to 1998–99	Female smokers in each class/%		% Reduction 1982 to 1998–99
	1982	1998–99		1982	1998–99	
professional	20	15	25	21	14	33
employers and managers	29	21	28	29	20	31
intermediate and junior non-manual	30	23	23	30	24	20
skilled manual	42	33	21	39	30	23
semi-skilled manual	47	38	19	36	33	8
unskilled manual	49	45	8	41	33	20
all aged 16 and over	**38**	**28**	**26**	**33**	**26**	**21**

Data from Office for National Statistics, 2000a, Statbase (http://www.statistics.gov.uk/statbase/mainmenu.asp), *Living in Britain: Results from the General Household Survey 1998*, Table 8.7, The Stationery Office, London.

■ Cigarette smoking fell among men and women in all classes, but by different amounts. The fall among men in the professional social class was 25 per cent compared with a decline of just 8 per cent among men in the unskilled manual social class. The pattern among women was similar, with a fall of 33 per cent in the number of women smoking in the professional class, compared with a fall of 20 per cent among women in the unskilled manual class. So the gap between top and bottom classes got *wider* — just like the health divide in overall mortality rates.

The relationship between cigarette smoking and many diseases, especially lung cancers and other respiratory diseases, is now well-established. Smoking is by far the most important cause of lung cancer and, as you saw in Chapter 9, lung cancer is the commonest cancer among men and the second most common cancer among women. The proportion of men in the lowest social class who smoke is three times higher than in the highest social class, and amongst women the difference is almost as great, so it is clear that the different smoking habits illustrated in Table 10.5 account for some of the social class differences in mortality and morbidity.

It is also clear from these data that the historically higher rate of cigarette smoking among men may help to explain some of the gender differences in the incidence of specific diseases. But the *narrowing* of differences between the sexes in smoking prevalence will also have important consequences for gender-related mortality patterns. For example, between 1986 and 1998 the mortality rate for lung cancer among men fell by 32 per cent, but that among women rose slightly (as you saw in Figure 9.3). This pattern of falling smoking rates but rising lung cancer rates is due to a cohort effect, as discussed in Chapter 9: lung cancer is caused by smoking *in the past*, and the increase in lung cancer in women *now* reflects an increase in smoking among women in the past.[3]

Alcohol consumption

Another example of 'self-destructive' behaviour mentioned by the MSSG was excessive drinking. As with smoking, there is strong evidence that excessive alcohol consumption has a number of detrimental health consequences, including digestive cancers, cirrhosis of the liver, fatal road traffic accidents, and psychiatric disorders. Figure 10.4 shows (a) the average weekly intake of units of alcohol; (b) the proportions of men and women by socio-economic group who did not drink at all in the week prior to the survey; and (c) men who drank more than 8 units and women who drank more than 6 units of alcohol during the previous week.

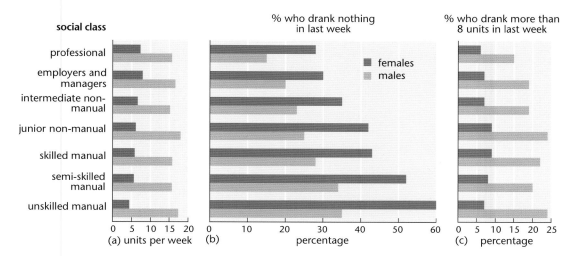

Figure 10.4 *Alcohol consumption by socio-economic group, Great Britain, 1998. (Data derived from Office for National Statistics, 2000a,* Living in Britain: Results from the 1998 General Household Survey, *The Stationery Office, London, Table 9.17 and Table 9.7)*

- Considering the average number of alcohol units consumed each week (Figure 10.4a), how would you describe the social class differences?

- There is no clear gradient across social classes, but some suggestion that average weekly alcohol consumption among women rises in higher social classes.

- Now consider the rest of the information in the figure. How would you summarise it, and what light does it shed on the conclusions of the MSSG?

- The proportion of men and women who did not drink at all in the week before the survey shows a steep gradient across the social classes, with the highest proportion of 'non-drinkers' in the lowest social classes — the reverse of what MSSG would predict. The proportion drinking more than 8 units in the last

---

[3] Cohort effects in relation to smoking and lung cancer are explored further in the audiotape for OU students, entitled 'Smoking: A global health problem'.

week shows the reverse gradient among men (the pattern in women is not clear). Taken together, these two observations suggest that a larger proportion of the higher social classes drink moderately — whereas the lower social classes seem more divided into non-drinkers and heavy drinkers.

This interpretation might have some bearing on mortality gradients across social classes — moderate consumption of alcohol, for example, is now thought to have some protective effect against heart disease (evidence that was not available to the MSSG!). But the overall relationship between alcohol consumption patterns and health differences between social classes is not clear and cannot be used as evidence that the social class gradient in health is due to self-damaging behaviour.

Physical exercise

Another aspect of behaviour that may have health consequences is voluntary participation in physical activities. Figure 10.5 provides some information on participation rates in a sample of such activities in 1996 by social class, and shows that participation is generally higher in higher social classes, and in all cases is lowest amongst unskilled manual workers.

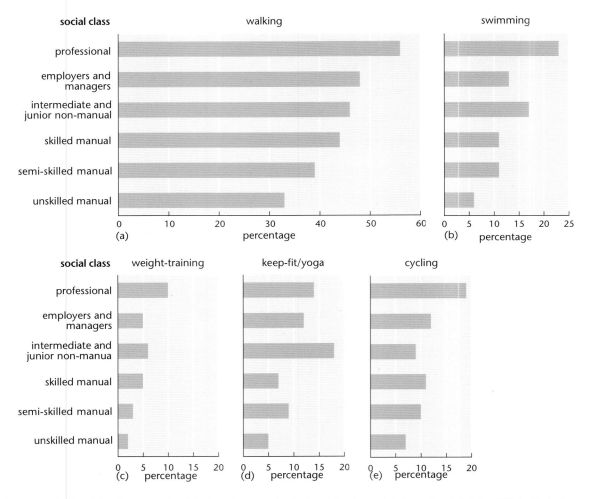

Figure 10.5 *Participation rates of adults in voluntary physical activity, by social class, Great Britain, 1996. (Data from Office for National Statistics, 1998,* Living in Britain: Results from the General Household Survey 1996, *The Stationery Office, London, Table 13.10)*

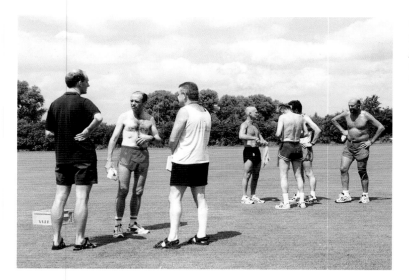

Office workers who run at lunchtime once a week have lower levels of physical activity than manual workers whose job involves standing, walking and lifting. (Photo: Mike Levers)

● Why must we be cautious in interpreting the results of Figure 10.5 as a measure of physical activity?

■ Consider an office worker who goes jogging twice a week, and a farm labourer or factory worker on a production line, who takes no voluntary physical exercise. The voluntary exercise taken by non-manual workers may be much less than the job-related physical activity of manual workers.

Other behavioural factors

Many other aspects of the lifestyle or the behaviour of individuals could be discussed in the present context, including aggressive risk-taking behaviour among young people; differences in the use of contraception; or social class differences in the use of health services and preventive services, such as those for ante-natal care and child health. For example, studies of vaccination rates show clear social class gradients; failure to immunise children appears to be particularly high among groups defined as 'especially disadvantaged', according to composite indicators which include such factors as housing amenities and parental education. The effectiveness of some aspects of preventive health care is hotly disputed, but if we assume at this point that these preventive services do make a positive contribution to health, then the lower use of such services among people who are socially disadvantaged is a factor that must be considered when trying to explain differences in mortality and morbidity.

So, although the relationship between behaviour and health and disease is often far from straightforward, enough information exists to indicate that differences in health-influencing behaviour do contribute to social class differences in mortality and morbidity. This raises three questions:

• how much do they contribute?

• why do such differences in health-influencing behaviour exist?

• what other factors should be considered?

10.4.2 Estimating the contribution of behaviour

One attempt to answer the first question has been going on since 1967 in the **Whitehall Study,** which has been tracking the health of a cohort of almost 18 000 people employed in the civil service in London – ranging from senior professional civil servants to porters, janitors, caretakers and other manual workers in government services. This study found that for almost every cause of death the lower employment grades had higher mortality rates than the higher employment grades. For all causes of death combined, the gap between top and bottom grades was 110 percentage points (that is, the bottom grades had more than double the mortality rates of the highest grades). The gradient was particularly steep for lung cancer and other smoking-related diseases such as bronchitis, and smoking was also much more prevalent in the lower employment grades. This suggested that at least some of the difference between the grades *was* due to smoking behaviour. However, even after all smoking-related causes of death were excluded, the excess mortality among the lowest grades compared with the professional and executive grades remained, being reduced from a 110 per cent excess to an 80 per cent excess.

In the 1980s, the researchers also looked in detail at coronary heart disease, and found a 70 per cent excess mortality among the lowest grades compared with the professional and executive grades. They then adjusted these figures to make allowance for all factors known to increase the risk of coronary heart disease, including smoking, high blood pressure, high levels of cholesterol and blood sugar, and lower than average height — almost all of which were again more prevalent in the lowest grades. These adjustments reduced the excess mortality in the lowest grades from 70 per cent to almost 40 per cent. Thus, well over half (i.e. 40 of the 70 percentage points) of the difference in mortality from coronary heart disease between the lowest and the top employment grades remained, *even* when all known risk factors were excluded (Marmot, 1986). This residual excess mortality cannot be attributed to any known type of health-damaging behaviour.[4]

The same cohort of civil servants was investigated again in 2000 by the same researchers. They found that after more than 25 years of follow-up, employment grade differences still existed in total mortality and for nearly all specific causes of death, and that the main risk factors (such as cholesterol levels, smoking, blood pressure, and diabetes) could only explain around a third of the difference between the highest and lowest grades (van Rossum et al., 2000).

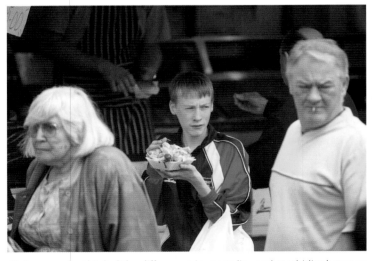

Similar findings have been demonstrated in studies of unemployed people in the United Kingdom, and of American families with low income, pointing to the same conclusion: known risk factors and behavioural differences do explain a *part* of the observed inequalities in health between social groups, but no matter how many such factors are taken into account, substantial inequalities in health remain.

Only around a third of the differences in mortality and morbidity between social classes can be attributed to any known type of health-damaging behaviour such as smoking, heavy drinking, poor diet or lack of voluntary exercise. (Photo: Mike Levers)

4 Professor Michael Marmot, who leads the Whitehall Study Team, talks about its findings in the OU video associated with this chapter, 'Status and wealth: the ultimate panacea?'. The contribution of different risk factors to rates of coronary heart disease are discussed in detail in *Dilemmas in UK Health Care* (Open University Press, 2nd edn 1993; 3rd edn 2001), Chapter 10, which also draws on data from the Whitehall Study.

10.4.3 | Where does self-damaging behaviour originate?

The second question raised by behavioural explanations of health inequalities is where such differences in behaviour originate. It has been suggested that certain behavioural traits and attitudes, which may adversely affect health, are passed on from generation to generation, for example, through child-rearing practices. In this way, health disadvantage may persist despite considerable improvements in education, living standards, and other factors. Figure 10.6 illustrates this argument with reference to patterns of dental attendance.

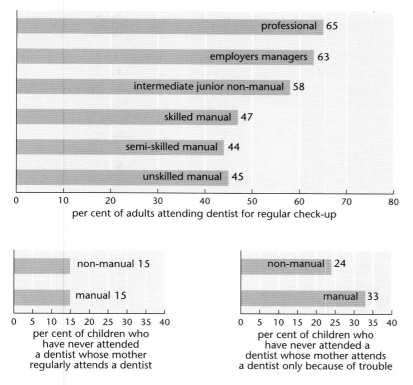

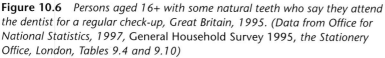

Figure 10.6 *Persons aged 16+ with some natural teeth who say they attend the dentist for a regular check-up, Great Britain, 1995. (Data from Office for National Statistics, 1997,* General Household Survey 1995, *the Stationery Office, London, Tables 9.4 and 9.10)*

The upper part of Figure 10.6 shows the percentage of adults attending a dentist for regular check-ups, by social class. A clear and strong gradient exists, with 65 per cent for adults in the professional class making regular attendances, compared with 45 per cent in the unskilled manual class.

- The lower part of the figure shows how the attendance pattern of a mother may influence her children. Summarise the pattern shown by the figure.

- If the mother is a regular attender, then the likelihood that her children have *never* attended a dentist is quite low — only 15 per cent — and the mother's social group appears to have no influence. But if the mother does *not* regularly attend the dentist for a check-up and only goes because of some kind of trouble, there is a much higher likelihood that her children will never have been to the dentist: between one quarter and one in three will never have done so.

A great deal of research has focused on the mechanisms by which health disadvantage may be passed on from generation to generation — a process often referred to as the **cycle of deprivation**. As one might expect, this suggests that, although there are some relationships between the attitudes and behaviour of parents and those of their children, they are far from straightforward. However, even acknowledging that parental influences play some part, this would only provide part of a transmission mechanism from one generation to another, *not* an explanation of why these differences exist and are related to social class in the first place.

Returning to Figure 10.6, for example, the question of why dental attendance patterns are so strongly related to social class is clearly still of fundamental importance. This raises a particular criticism of explanations of health inequality based on the behaviour of *individuals*: namely that it is unrealistic to examine the behaviour of individuals in isolation from their social and material circumstances. If income, education, housing, access to transport, work environment and other factors all vary across social groups, can individual behaviour be assumed to be unrelated to them? The next section examines these factors and attempts to reach some conclusions.

10.4.4   Summary

It has been argued that higher mortality in some social groups may be related to health-damaging behaviour. It is clear that health-damaging activities such as smoking are more prevalent in social groups with higher mortality, and that potentially health-improving activities such as physical exercise are more prevalent in social groups with lower mortality, although some factors such as high alcohol consumption do not fit this pattern so neatly. There is firm evidence that these behavioural differences do explain part of the differences in mortality between social classes, but that at least 40 per cent of the difference cannot be explained by behavioural differences. More important, however, it is not clear that the behaviour of individuals can be isolated from their social and material environment. This environment forms the subject of the next section.

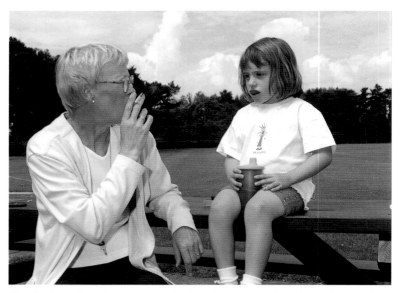

The children of smokers are more likely to become smokers themselves, suggesting one explanation of how health-damaging behaviour originates. (Photo: Mike Levers)

10.5 | Material circumstances

The social and material environment may affect the distribution of health and disease in broadly three ways.

- First, factors such as housing conditions or employment may have a *direct* effect on the state of someone's health: for example, damp housing may lead to chest disease, employment hazards to accidents.

- Second, there may be *indirect* effects: the income associated with an occupation may constrain a person's ability to purchase good housing, adequate nutrition, and so on, or may lead to stresses that in turn make it more likely that a person will smoke or drink to relieve inescapable tensions. Or, the social context of an occupation or a particular social status may encourage or discourage certain types of health-related social behaviour such as smoking or risk-taking.

- Third, the social and material environment may affect a person's *use of health services*, which may in turn affect their health (this point has already been discussed in the previous chapter in the context of interpreting morbidity statistics derived from health-service use).

Evidence of the effect of health *care* on health is considered elsewhere[5]; here we are primarily concerned to examine the evidence on the direct and indirect effects of social and material circumstances on health.

10.5.1 | Occupational hazards

Let us begin with the working environment and health. The different risks to health associated with different occupations are reflected in *occupational mortality rates*, some examples of which were given in Table 9.7 in the previous chapter. These reflect not only the more obvious work hazards, but other aspects of occupation that are likely to be directly related to health and safety at work. For example, manual workers are much more likely to work out of doors, to spend most of the day standing, to have insecure jobs with a high risk of unemployment, to have shorter holidays and much less access to 'fringe benefits', first-aid facilities or toilets. The work may be repetitive and tedious, such as on a production line, or the workplace may be noisy or cramped or poorly lit.[6]

Occupations involve their own specific hazards to health. Industrial accidents and disease, for example, still take a considerable toll. In 1998 over 270 deaths and 30 000 major injuries at work were officially notified to government agencies in the UK. In addition to these, 135 000 injuries were reported in which the person involved had to take more than three days off work to recover (Health and Safety Executive, 2000). It is known that some accidents and injuries which should be reported to the official health and safety agencies in fact go unreported, and that this under-reporting is especially prevalent in relation to less serious accidents. Yet even these 'non-major' accidents might involve the loss of a joint from a finger for example, or concussion resulting in a hospital stay of up to 24 hours. You might like to consider whether you would regard losing a piece of a finger at work as serious or not!

---

[5] *Dilemmas in UK Health Care* (Open University Press, 2nd edn 1993; 3rd edn 2001).

[6] The physical and organisational aspects of work and their contribution to stress among workers are discussed in *Birth to Old Age: Health in Transition* (Open University Press, 2nd edn 1995; colour-enhanced 2nd edn 2001), Chapter 8, which also refers to the problem of defining and measuring 'stress' and its relationship to ill-health.

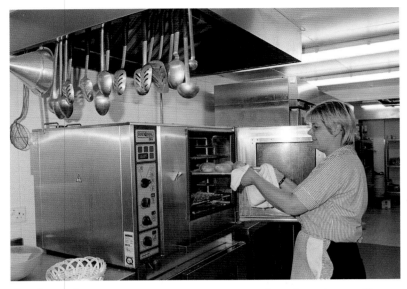

Catering workers frequently suffer injury from cuts, scalds and burns, most of which go unreported. (Photo: Mike Levers)

The Health and Safety Executive has attempted to uncover the likely degree of under-reporting in the official injury figures by commissioning surveys of households and asking questions about workplace accidents and ill-health. In 1991 such a survey indicated that on average more than two-thirds of injuries went unreported in breach of the law, but that the problem was especially bad in some industries: in agriculture, for example, the study found that 83 per cent of accidents which should have been reported went unreported. A repeat survey in 1995–96 found that the levels of reporting of injuries had improved for most industries, but that almost 60 per cent of injuries were still unreported. On the basis of these findings, the number of reported injuries at work may well be around twice the numbers notified.

Figure 10.7 shows injuries to employees reported to enforcement authorities in 1997-98 by industry. All fatal, non-fatal and 'over 3-day' injuries are included, and the figure also shows the actual numbers of injuries in each industry.

● What does the information in the left-hand side of Figure 10.7 convey about the relative danger to workers in these industries?

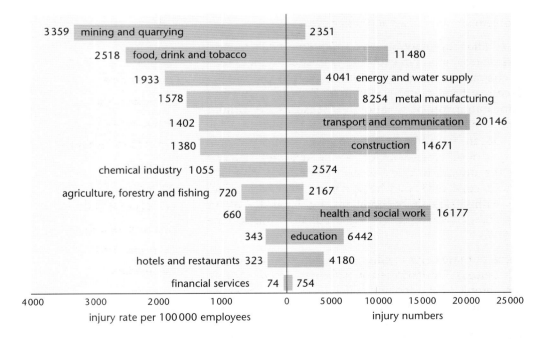

Figure 10.7   *All reported industrial injuries to employees in 1998 by industry: rate per 100 000 employees and total numbers of injuries that year, Great Britain. (Data from Office for National Statistics, 2000,* Annual Abstract of Statistics 1999, *The Stationery Office, London, Tables 7.5 and 9.8)*

■ The patterns are not always what might be expected: the injury rate is much higher in the food, drink and tobacco industry than in the construction industry, and almost as high in health and social work as in agriculture, forestry and fishing.

However, if we focus on the major and fatal injuries, then the most dangerous sectors by far are mining and quarrying and the construction industry; between them, on average 2 workers are killed every week and 13 workers are seriously injured every day.

Well over one-half of fatal injuries are the consequence of falls from a height or of being struck by a moving object or vehicle, but major injuries

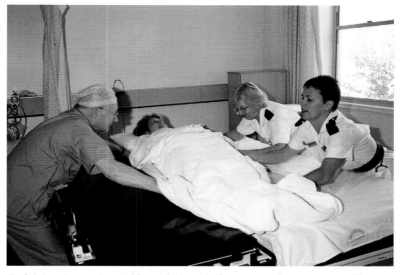

Back injury is a major problem which ends the careers of many nurses. The injury rate *in the health and social work services is almost as high as in agriculture, forestry and fishing, but a far larger* number *are affected. (Photo: Mike Levers)*

are most often caused by slips, trips and falls on the same level. This is one reason why workers in the transport and communications category in Figure 10.7 suffer the highest *number* of injuries, for example to postal workers, especially in winter when paths and steps may be icy. And one-third of all 'over 3-day' injuries are caused by handling, lifting or carrying: this commonly occurs in areas such as retail distribution, but also in health care, where back injuries resulting from the handling of patients are a major problem among nurses and other care staff.

In addition to injury, we must also consider industrial disease resulting from exposure to toxic substances such as chemicals, dust, gases or fumes, or to hazards due to excessive heat, noise or vibration. The main source of information on occupational disease in the United Kingdom is the *Industrial Injuries Scheme* administered by the Department of Social Security, under which individuals are examined to see whether they are sufficiently disabled by the disease in question to qualify for a disability allowance. Benefits may be paid in respect of around 50 'prescribed' diseases or conditions, and Table 10.6 shows the number of new cases diagnosed under this scheme in 1998.

Some of these cases involve poisoning from a variety of substances still found in certain industries. *Pneumoconiosis*, the chronic lung condition suffered by many miners, is included, along with *asbestosis*, a disease caused by inhalation of asbestos fibres. Cases of *byssinosis*, a lung disease found among textile workers and caused by inhaling cotton fibres, have almost disappeared as the industry has declined and new working practices have been introduced. Prescribed conditions which have been

Table 10.6 Incidence of prescribed occupational diseases diagnosed under the *Industrial Injuries and Pneumoconiosis, Byssinosis and Miscellaneous Diseases* benefit schemes, 1998, Great Britain.

Occupational disease	New cases, 1998
vibration white finger	3 033
mesothelioma	590
pneumoconiosis	554
tenosynovitis	415
carpal tunnel syndrome	400
asbestosis	316
dermatitis	271
occupational deafness	258
occupational asthma	222
beat conditions	104
farmer's lung	4
byssinosis	2
others	4 058
total	**10 227**

Data from Office for National Statistics (2000) *Annual Abstract of Statistics 1999*, The Stationery Office, London, Table 9.7.

increasing include *tenosynovitis* (inflammation of the tendons) due to frequent or repeated movement of the hand and wrist, as on an assembly line or in prolonged use of a computer keyboard. Other prescribed conditions include *vibration white finger* (the subject of a legal settlement involving thousands of mine workers in the late 1990s); *dermatitis* (inflammation of the skin) resulting from contact with substances such as mineral oil, soot or tar; *'beat' conditions*, where the hand, elbow or knee may swell as a result of prolonged or severe pressure on the affected area (common among workers using drilling equipment); and *occupational deafness*.

Once again, however, these data do not tell the whole story. First, many people suffer from an occupational disease that is not recognised as being severe enough to qualify for benefit. For example, a survey of GPs in 1989 suggested that around 60 000 people consulted their GPs with occupational dermatitis, although, as Table 10.6 indicates, in 1998 fewer than 300 were recognised as qualifying for benefit. There is no reason to suppose that the number of cases dwindled to these few in less than a decade. Second, many conditions related to occupations are not on the official list of prescribed diseases, for example, *emphysema*, a respiratory disease common among people working in dusty conditions. The difficulty is that diseases such as emphysema may be caused or aggravated by atmospheric pollution or smoking.

One survey of the national population carried out by the Health and Safety Executive in 1995 estimated the overall *prevalence* of work-related ill health by asking people whether they had any illnesses or conditions, in the twelve months prior to the survey, which had been caused or made worse by their work (current or past), and then checking this information against their medical records. This survey indicated that, for example, 170 000 suffered from work-related deafness, tinnitus or other ear conditions; 36 000 from vibration white finger, and 19 000 from pneumoconiosis (Jones, Hodgson and Osman, 1997).

● How do these figures compare with the annual number of these diseases or conditions that are 'prescribed' (Table 10.6)?

■ It should be noted that the survey figures reported above relate to prevalence, while the figures in Table 10.6 relate to incidence. Despite this difference, it is clear that far more people consider themselves (and are considered by their treating doctor) to have work-related diseases and conditions than are recognised for the purposes of receiving benefit.

Another problem in assessing the scale of occupational disease is that the effects of exposure to industrial hazards may take many years to become apparent. The story of *mesothelioma* (a cancer of the chest lining caused by exposure to asbestos) illustrates this point. New regulations to control asbestos were introduced in 1969, but as this type of cancer may take up to forty years to develop, it will be many years before these improvements are reflected in lower mortality rates. The number of cases of the disease recorded on death certificates rose steadily from the 1960s onwards, and since the worst exposures occurred between 1935 and 1970 (many of them during the lagging of ships with blue and brown asbestos in the early years of World War II, and its removal when the hazards became known after the war), the peak of cases is probably still to come. The numbers appeared to stabilise in the late 1990s, but whether this was the beginning of a trend or a temporary pause will not become apparent until at least 2010. Similarly, regulations to control noise levels in the workplace have gradually been tightened, with new controls introduced in 1990, but the legacy of laxer controls will be apparent in the occupational deafness figures for many years into the future.

10.5.2   Income and poverty

Although occupational and industrial hazards do contribute to observed health inequalities between social classes, they account for a relatively small proportion of all ill-health and mortality, and for a relatively small proportion of the differences between social classes. The *indirect* effects of occupation on health inequalities seem to be more important, and the most likely way in which occupation will indirectly exert an influence on health is through earnings, which help to determine the living standards of individuals and other members of their families.

Before looking at the evidence linking income to health, it is worth looking at the distribution of income in the UK. There are wide differences in average weekly earnings before tax between manual and non-manual, male and female full-time workers, and substantial disparities of income also exist within these categories. Figure 10.8 shows a broader picture: the percentage of total income in the UK received by different income bands in the population between 1961 and 1993 (a *decile* is a 10 per cent band).

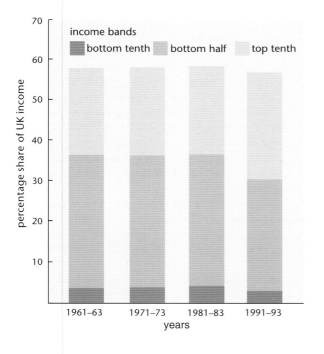

Figure 10.8 *Percentage income shares of the bottom decile, bottom half and top decile income bands in the population, UK, 1961 to 1993. (Note: income here includes salaries, social security benefits, rents, interest and dividends, and is measured net of personal direct taxes). (Data from Goodman, A., Johnson, P. and Webb, S. (1997)* Inequality in the UK, *Oxford University Press, Oxford, Table 3.2)*

● How would you describe the distribution of income in 1991–93?

■ In 1991–93 the poorest 10 per cent (bottom decile) of the population received less than 3 per cent of all income in the UK. The bottom half received about 27 per cent of total income, while the richest 10 per cent (top decile) received 26 per cent, or almost as much as the entire poorer half of households.

● How has the distribution of income changed since 1961–63?

■ Income distribution was fairly stable until 1981–83, but after that date income inequality widened sharply in the UK.

This striking increase in income inequality is one of the biggest social and economic changes to have affected the UK in the last 20 years. One major reason was the policies of the Conservative governments from 1979 to 1997, which reduced taxation on higher incomes and wealth to try to encourage innovation and entrepreneurial risk-taking. Similar policies were pursued during this period in a number of other countries, such as the USA and New Zealand, and later (and to a lesser extent) by several European countries. There is also some evidence that rapid economic changes in industrialised countries in the 1990s and the start of the new millennium, centred around the growth of internet-based commerce, have — at least initially — accentuated income inequalities.

Another way of examining income and its distribution is to attempt to draw a line defining the number of people who are in poverty, which can be conceptualised in three main ways. The first is based on the concept of **absolute poverty**, which simply means lacking the means to survive. Secondly, **relative poverty** has been defined as:

> … the absence or inadequacy of those diets, amenities, standards, services and activities which are common or customary in society. People are deprived of the conditions of life which ordinarily define membership of society. (Townsend, 1979, p. 915)

However, the concept of relative poverty does not escape the necessity of defining the level of resources that is necessary to allow people to live 'as is common and customary in society'.

A third approach adopted in many studies of poverty is to lay down a set of minimum necessities in nutrition, clothing, household goods and so on, then assess whether families or individuals have sufficient income to obtain these minimum necessities. This **subsistence approach** to defining poverty was pioneered in York in 1899 by Seebohm Rowntree, a member of the Rowntree chocolate family, which later set up the Joseph Rowntree Trust for social research. Subsequent studies in this and other countries have been deeply influenced by the concept of subsistence standards, which has also formed the basis for recommending minimum state social security benefits and minimum earnings in a number of countries. In the UK, social security benefits are still implicitly based on a subsistence view, and parliamentary regulations define the items of normal day-to-day living that families are expected to be able to meet from the benefits they receive.

Table 10.7 Proportion of households receiving benefits, Great Britain, 1998.

Benefit	%
family credit or income support	15
housing benefit	18
council tax benefit	23
jobseekers allowance	4
retirement pension	28
incapacity or disablement benefits	15
child benefit	29
any benefit	**70**

Data adapted from Office for National Statistics (1999c) StatBase (http://www.statistics.gov.uk/statbase/mainmenu.asp), based on *Regional Trends 34*, 1999 edition, Table 8.7.

● What is the main problem with using benefit levels to define poverty?

■ Increases (or decreases) in benefit levels have the effect of altering the numbers of people classified as being in poverty.

However, this method does give some rough indication of the number of people on income levels that restrict them to basic necessities. Table 10.7 indicates the proportion of households in Britain in 1998 who were receiving some form of benefit. An extraordinary 70 per cent of all households were receiving one or more of the benefits listed, with 15 per cent of households receiving Family Credit or Income Support, and almost one quarter of all households receiving Council Tax benefit. However, the largest single proportion in the table relates to child benefit, which is paid irrespective of income levels, and similarly receipt of a state retirement pension is not in itself a good guide to wealth or poverty.

An alternative way of assessing the extent of poverty is to measure the number of households living on incomes below some fraction of the national average. Table 10.8 shows the percentage of all households with incomes below one-half of the average for the UK in 1979 and 1992–93, and comparable information for a range of different family types.

Table 10.8 Percentage of family types with incomes below half the contemporary average (mean) UK, 1979 and 1992–93.

	1979	1992–93
pensioner couple	16	25
single pensioner	16	25
couple with children	7	20
couple without children	4	10
single with children	16	43
single without children	6	18
all	**8**	**20**

Data from Goodman, A., Johnson, P. and Webb, S. (1997) *Inequality in the UK*, Oxford University Press, Oxford, Table 8.8.

Overall, the proportion of households living on incomes below half the contemporary average rose from 8 per cent in 1979 to 20 per cent by 1993. But, as the table shows, some family types were much more affected than others by this change. In particular, by 1993 no fewer than 43 per cent of all lone parents were living on incomes below half the average, a very substantial increase on the 16 per cent in this situation in 1979. But even groups who in 1979 could have confidently expected to avoid falling below this low-income threshold — such as single people without children or couples without children — could no longer do so by 1993.

Comparisons over time in the numbers of the poor are complicated by the many changes that have taken place in the social security and tax system. But there can be little doubt that the numbers of poor people on almost any definition increased significantly during the 1980s and into the 1990s.

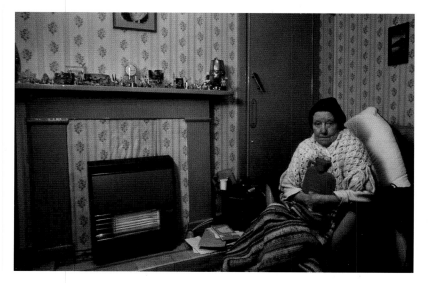

Winter for a pensioner living alone in Hackney, London. In the 1990s, 25 per cent of single pensioners in the UK had incomes that put them below the poverty line.
(Photo: John Sturrock/Network Photographers)

There are many potential reasons why the number of people in poverty increased and inequalities widened in the UK at the end of the twentieth century. Some of the possible candidates include a period of high unemployment, which was partly due to a major restructuring of the UK economy, a large increase in part-time working, the advent of new computer-based technologies and services, ever-increasing international trade and competition, and many other social, political and cultural changes. Extrapolation is always hazardous, but from the perspective of the year 2000 there seemed to be few countervailing factors — apart from a substantial fall in unemployment levels — that might reverse these changes. Consequently, and returning to our starting point, income inequality is likely to play an increasingly important role in explaining health inequalities in the twenty-first century.[7]

10.5.3   Income: cause or proxy?

Although many studies suggest a relationship between income and health, there have been very few attempts to measure the association directly: the usual approach, as noted earlier, is to use social class as a proxy for income, despite the great variations in income levels *within* each social class. One attempt to do so identified 22 specific occupations for which data on income *and* on mortality were available for the years 1951 and 1971 (Wilkinson, 1986c). The occupations were mainly skilled or semi-skilled manual and contained about 2.5 million men. The analysis then examined the relationship between changes in occupation-specific death rates and changes in occupational incomes over this 20-year period.

The results indicated that there was an *inverse* relationship, as would be expected: men in occupations in which incomes rose faster than average appeared to have a lower than average death rate, and vice versa. However, the correlation was weak. This is perhaps not surprising given that those on the lowest income levels, where detrimental health effects are likely to be strongest, are seldom in an occupation at all. Again, this leads to the conclusion that although income, occupation, or composite groupings by housing tenure and car access may be more refined ways of classifying a population than social class alone, they are essentially indicators of a *way of life* that influences health in a multitude of different ways, rather than being important influences on health in their own right.

Another hypothesis that has given rise to heated controversy proposes that the *degree* of income inequality in any society affects the health of the society *as a whole*, independently of the actual levels of income of particular groups. This hypothesis, labelled the **Wilkinson hypothesis** after its main proponent, Richard Wilkinson, asserts that inequality is itself a risk to health. His research shows that those who live in a more unequal society in terms of income distribution have a higher probability of death than those who live in a more equal society, regardless of whether you are at the top or bottom of the income gradient.

It is possible to think of circumstances where inequality might be a health hazard — for example, the close proximity of rich and poor might engender crime and violence, and it has also been suggested that large income inequalities may increase levels of frustration which in turn may adversely affect behaviour and health. Further, it has been argued that *toleration* of high levels of income inequality in a society is a sign of a society that is not prepared to invest in its **social capital** — that is, its norms and mechanisms of civic participation, trust, mutual aid and reciprocity — with resultant damage to health for all, including the better-off.

[7] A comparison of different strategies for tackling poverty occurs in *Dilemmas in UK Health Care* (Open University Press, 2nd edn 1993; 3rd edn 2001), Chapter 11, which also evaluates the potential impact of alleviating poverty on inequalities in health.

However, the detailed mechanisms on which the Wilkinson hypothesis rests are not always clear: why, for example, should higher property taxes on wealthier home-owners in London have any direct bearing on the likelihood that someone in Tyneside might die from heart disease? Until such mechanisms are clarified, links between income inequality and health must be viewed as associations rather than as causal connections.

10.5.4   Housing and the built environment

One way in which income may influence living standards is shown in Figure 10.9, which contains information from a survey conducted in 1996 on the relation between socio-economic group and **housing standard** in households where the oldest person is aged 75 or over. The proportion of houses in disrepair in all socio-economic groups may strike you as surprisingly high, and may reflect lower incomes among pensioners. However, a social class gradient is also in evidence, with almost one third of those in the lowest socio-economic group living in housing defined as 'poor' by the Department of the Environment.

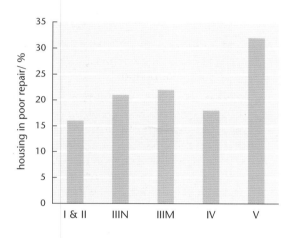

Figure 10.9 *Standard of housing in relation to socio-economic group, in 2 398 households where the eldest person was aged 75 and over, England, 1996. (Data from Department of the Environment, 1999,* English House Condition Survey 1996, The Stationery Office, London, Table A7.31) *(Social class is assigned to a household on the basis of the current or last occupation of the (usually male) 'head of household'.)*

Concern about the relationship between housing conditions and health goes back many years. In the 1920s, T.H.C. Stevenson, a key figure in the development of the Registrar-General's classification of occupations, looked at the relationship between infant and child mortality and tenement size, and found clear associations between the child mortality rate and the number of available rooms, which he used as the index of overcrowded conditions. These are illustrated in Figure 10.10 overleaf, Stevenson's original hand-drawn graph. The different lines on the graph relate to duration of marriage: the greater the duration of marriage (and therefore presumably the older the mother and/or the larger the family), the higher the child death rate in that tenement size.

Since Stevenson drew his graph, housing standards in the UK have been immensely improved. Millions of homes have been demolished in slum clearances, and by 1996 over a third of the British housing stock had been built after 1964 (although some of these are alienating and low-quality houses and flats). However, our knowledge about the relationship between housing and health is still limited. Attention has focused on aspects such as lack of amenities, presumed to be associated with accidents when children have no protected place to play, and with overcrowding, which may increase the risk of infection among children for example. Damp housing has been suggested as a cause or exacerbating factor in respiratory

Figure 10.10 *Diagram drawn by T.H.C. Stevenson to show the relationship between child mortality, tenement size and duration of marriage, based on data from the 1911 Census (from Fox, J. and Goldblatt, P. O. (1982) OPCS Longitudinal Study 1971–5, Socio-Demographic Mortality Differentials, Series LS, No. 1, HMSO, London, Figure 5.1. p. 65)*

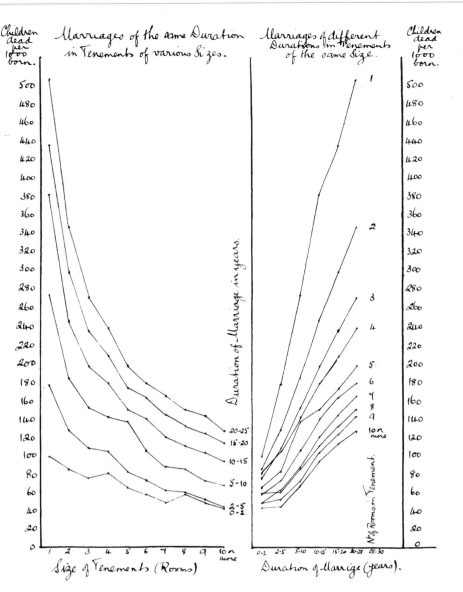

diseases. Structural defects such as poor wiring may put children at particular risk.[8] The psychological and practical difficulties associated with high-rise flats or isolated housing estates may also adversely affect the health of those who live in them, particularly women or children or elderly people at home.

One factor that is related to the state of repair, amenities and habitability of housing is the type of *housing tenure*. (Some evidence on this was presented earlier in Table 10.3, and a social class gradient was found.) The Longitudinal Study has also provided data on mortality in relation to housing tenure. When the researchers looked at mortality patterns by cause of death, they found that the clearest association between type of housing tenure and mortality rates was for respiratory diseases and lung cancer. But a significant association between type of housing and mortality rates existed for almost *all* causes, and not just those that might be directly related to housing conditions.

[8] The contribution of housing defects, both in design and repair, to accident rates among children is discussed in *Birth to Old Age: Health in Transition* (Open University Press, 2nd edn 1995; colour-enhanced 2nd edn 2001), Chapter 5, and in an associated TV programme for OU students.

● What does this suggest about the association between housing tenure and health?

■ These findings suggest that housing standards may be an important influence on mortality in their own right, but housing tenure is essentially an indicator of a more general way of life that may influence mortality.

It would clearly be desirable to be able to measure housing conditions more accurately than just by the type of tenure. However, there is one group that has grown substantially during the 1990s in which the connection may be more direct: the **homeless**. People defined as homeless include all those evicted from homes because of mortgage repossessions or failure to pay rent, and those housed in temporary accommodation by local authorities, as well as those who are sleeping in hostels for the homeless or 'sleeping rough'. In the *English House Condition Survey 1996* (Department of the Environment, 1999), no fewer than 6 per cent of all households said that they had some experience of homelessness in the previous decade. It is known that homelessness is associated with many forms of ill-health. Homeless women are three times as likely to be admitted to hospital with problems while pregnant, and their babies are three times as likely to be of low birth-weight, compared with those of other women. Children living in temporary accommodation are much more likely to miss immunisations and routine health checks, and are more likely to be involved in accidents.

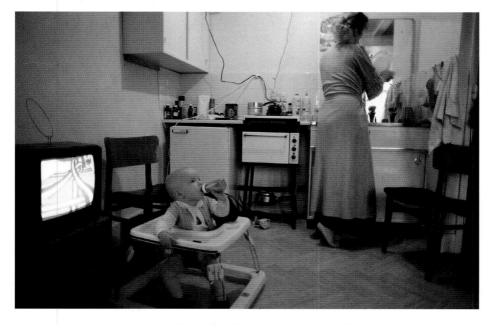

Homeless families living in temporary accommodation experience substantially increased risks to their health. (Photo: John Sturrock/Network Photographers)

From a research perspective, it is often hard to prove that homelessness *causes* ill-health, as many other factors may be involved. For example, some surveys have found a high prevalence of mental disorders among those living in hostels or sleeping rough, but this is partly because a growing number of homeless people are from mental hospitals that have been run down and closed.[9] Despite these difficulties, the association between homelessness and health is sufficiently strong to have made housing a growing public-health issue.

[9] The closure of long-stay mental health hospitals in the 1980s-1990s and shortcomings in the provision of community care for former patients are discussed in *Caring for Health: History and Diversity* (Open University Press, 2nd edn 1993; 3rd edn 2001), Chapter 7.

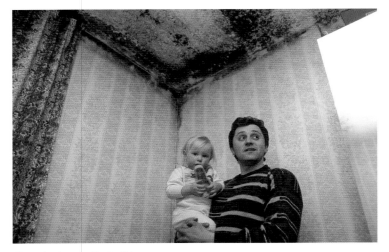

Chronic damp affects this house occupied by a family in Tower Hamlets, London. (Photo: Michael Abrahams/Network Photographers)

In interpreting the relationship between housing and health other factors also need to be considered. For example, the health problems associated with damp and cold are a result not only of a house's condition, but of the ability of the occupants to maintain and heat it adequately. In 1998, the average household in the UK devoted around 4 per cent of its disposable income to fuel, light and power, equivalent to around £13 per week. However, those on lower incomes spent significantly *less* than the average on fuel, light and power — around £10 per week — although this represented a higher *proportion* of their income — over 6 per cent (*Social Trends 30*, 2000b, Table 6.7). As a result, although relatively small numbers of people (200 in 1998) are recorded as dying each year because of very cold conditions in their homes, far higher numbers may be adversely affected by cold and damp conditions at home.

There is also some evidence that the configuration of houses, street layouts and so on can have health implications. For example, a detailed study of differences in health between Middlesborough and Sunderland found that the mortality rates of child pedestrians in road traffic accidents in 'low income' local-authority housing estates in Middlesborough was over three times higher than in comparable estates in Sunderland. The researchers suggested that the layout of the estates they had surveyed in Sunderland was safer for pedestrians (Phillimore and Morris, 1991).

However, the same research has emphasised that these fairly obvious differences in housing and other conditions are not the whole story, and that people in apparently identical circumstances can experience quite different health outcomes. One possibility is that these are related to the constant changes in local economies, the rise and fall of industries, employment, prosperity, confidence and uncertainty, and the ways in which people respond to these changes. The health consequences of these responses would be subtle but might be far-reaching.

To illustrate the kind of mechanisms that might be involved, it is worth considering studies of severe threats to survival such as famines, when all the informal arrangements for mutual insurance and social support are thrown into doubt:

> … their failure in times of widespread calamity is in fact well documented: in times of famine the ordinary rules of patronage, credit, charity, reciprocity, and even family support tend to undergo severe strain and can hardly be relied upon to ensure the survival of vulnerable groups (Drèze and Sen, 1989, p. 74).

This is sometimes referred to as the breakdown of the **moral economy**, with its informal social ties, habits and values, and the concept may offer some insight into the health differences between apparently very similar communities. However, the evidence also suggests that, although the moral economy may be strained to breaking point in the advanced stages of famines, it may well be *reinforced* in the earlier stages or in the face of less severe stresses. And finally, we must be cautious in moving between the extreme circumstances of a famine and the relative health differences found between social groups in developed countries.

10.5.5 Food and nutrition

Families living on different incomes display many clear differences in addition to housing costs in their patterns of expenditure, and one area of particular importance is expenditure on food. For example, in 1998 the average household in the UK devoted about 17 per cent of its income to food. However, those on *lower* incomes devoted a much *higher* proportion of their income to food: for example, those in households with the lowest 20 per cent of disposable income devoted almost a quarter (23 per cent) of their expenditure to food, compared to just 14 per cent of expenditure on food in the households with the top 20 per cent of disposable incomes (*Social Trends 30*, 2000b, Table 6.7). Detailed studies of individual households have found that low-income families often perceive their food expenditure as their most flexible commitment, which is often used as an emergency fund to 'even out' fluctuations in income and to meet emergencies (Kempson, Bryson and Rowlingson, 1994).

Finally, there is evidence that the composition of diet varies substantially between different income groups. Figure 10.11 shows trends in the consumption of fats and fruit between 1975 and the 1990s, by different income groups.

● What differences exist between different income groups in fat and fruit consumption?

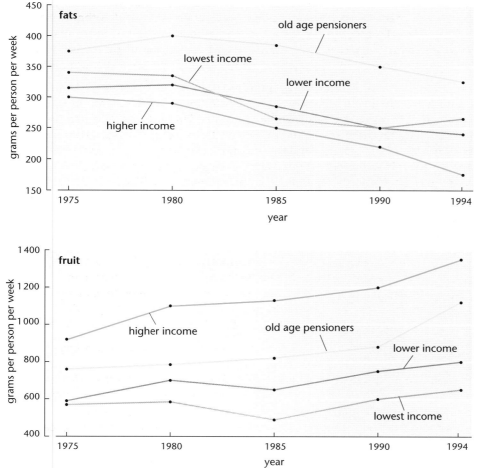

Figure 10.11 *Fat and fruit consumption per week (grams per person) by income group, United Kingdom, 1975–1994. (Source: Ministry of Agriculture, Fisheries and Foods, and Charlton, J. and Murphy, M. (eds) (1997) The Health of Adult Britain 1841– 1994, Volume I, The Stationery Office, London, Figures 7.3 and 7.5)*

■ In all groups the general trend since the 1970s has been for fat consumption to decline and for fruit consumption to increase. However, higher income groups have moved to much lower levels of fat consumption than other income groups, and to much higher levels of fruit consumption.

The health consequences of very different patterns of diet and food consumption are not easy to predict, as Chapter 11 will show, but it is clear that amongst low-income families the opportunity to *choose* a particular diet can be severely restricted. And it is also clear that inadequate nutrition in early life may have very long-lasting effects. For example, infants whose growth and development have been restricted by a prolonged shortage of food are more prone to infection and may never reach the height they would otherwise have attained (a topic we explore further in Chapter 11).

Since the late 1980s, particular interest has been generated by the work of a group of epidemiologists, historians and statisticians at the University of Southampton, led by Professor David Barker (O'Brien, Wheeler and Barker, 1999). This group has developed the so-called **programming hypothesis**, which suggests that inadequate maternal nutrition during pregnancy adversely affects the development of fetal blood vessels, which in turn increases the risk of coronary heart disease and stroke when the baby reaches late middle-age.[10] And since maternal nutrition is adversely affected by low income, the effect of these nutritional factors during fetal life could contribute to the observed social class gradients in morbidity and mortality.

● What is the main reservation about whether fetal programming is *causally* associated with vascular disease in later life?

■ The programming hypothesis cannot rule out the possibility that individuals whose early growth and development was affected by inadequate nutrition were also exposed to *other* aspects of social and material disadvantage, not only in childhood but throughout their lives. The cumulative effects of poor circumstances over many years may have a greater influence on their mortality and morbidity.

The programming hypothesis is still the subject of much debate, but scientific experiments on the effects on the development of laboratory animals of restricted nutrition during fetal life seem to support its conclusions, and it continues to gain ground. Perhaps in the future we can expect to see interventions against cardiovascular and perhaps other diseases redirected from early adult life to the nutrition and care of pregnant women and infants right at the beginning of life.

10.6 Conclusion

A theme running through this chapter, and indeed the book as a whole, is that by exploring the social and economic system and its patterns of inequality, the distribution of health and disease becomes more readily understandable. The material in this chapter has shown that although (a) artefacts of the ways in which data are collected and (b) social selection do account for a small proportion of the

---

[10] Professor Barker talks about this research in the OU video associated with this chapter, entitled, 'Status and wealth: the ultimate panacea?'. The programming hypothesis and the research methods that generated the data on which it is based are discussed in greater detail in *Studying Health and Disease* (Open University Press, 2nd edn 1994; colour-enhanced 2nd edn 2001), Chapter 10.

observed inequalities in health between social groups in the UK, recurring patterns of social and economic inequality are systematically associated with the social class gradient in mortality and morbidity. Cumulatively, these social and economic inequalities are an important part of the explanation for the observable inequalities in health. However, it seems clear that health differences may also be present when social and economic circumstances seem very similar, and there can be very long lags between a factor exerting an influence and the health outcome, as the 'programming' hypothesis suggests.

In apportioning relative weights to factors associated with ill-health, emphasis is too often placed on one particular type of variable rather than acknowledging the *interactions* between them. Many of the 'behavioural' or 'lifestyle' category of explanations for health inequalities are influenced by environment and social context, diet is influenced by low income, and so on. Attitudes to health-influencing activities such as regular dental care may reflect individual outlook, which may be influenced by parental attitudes, all of which may be related to availability, accessibility or quality of care. The same variety of explanations is seen in public perceptions of why people are poor. Some suggest individual characteristics such as laziness and lack of will-power as the reason, whereas others suggest social injustice and the abstract workings of society.

Chapter 11 concludes this book with a detailed study of the relation between food and health, which exemplifies and explores many of these themes. But perhaps an appropriate point on which to finish this chapter is to note that concern with how inequalities can be explained is not just idle academic curiosity: different explanations have very different implications for policies to reduce inequalities in health. Picking an informed route through these various explanations is therefore central to choosing and designing effective health policies.[11]

OBJECTIVES FOR CHAPTER 10

When you have studied this chapter, you should be able to:

10.1 Define and use, or recognise definitions and applications of, each of the terms printed in **bold** in the text.

10.2 Identify different ways in which inequalities in health can be measured across social classifications, and comment on trends over time in social class composition and health inequalities between social classes.

10.3 Outline and evaluate the various artefact explanations of health inequalities in the United Kingdom.

10.4 Discuss the potential contribution of individual behaviour to contemporary patterns of health and disease in the United Kingdom, and describe methods by which this contribution has been evaluated.

10.5 Outline ways in which the social and material environment may affect the distribution of health and disease, stressing interactions between factors.

[11] The dilemmas inherent in designing policies to reduce health inequalities by reducing poverty are discussed in *Dilemmas in UK Health Care* (Open University Press, 2nd edn 1993; 3rd edn 2001), Chapter 11.

QUESTIONS FOR CHAPTER 10

1   (*Objective 10.2*)

Drawing on data presented in Figure 10.1 and Table 10.1, summarise the general trends in health inequalities between social classes in the UK from the 1970s to the 1990s. Explain why the combination of these two sets of data increases confidence in the conclusions you have drawn.

2   (*Objective 10.3*)

The proportion of the population in the lowest social classes with the poorest health experience has been declining. Do you think this suggests that health inequalities must have declined also?

3   (*Objective 10.4*)

To what extent might patterns of smoking and alcohol consumption contribute to social class inequalities in health?

4   (*Objective 10.5*)

Explain why occupation is a useful basis on which to classify people into social classes for the purpose of evaluating inequalities in health. How much of the 'health divide' between social classes can be directly attributed to occupation?

5   (*Objectives 10.4 and 10.5*)

Compare the following two quotes from a Royal Society for the Prevention of Accidents (ROSPA) booklet. What view of the underlying causes of industrial accidents does each of them take?

> Accidents do not happen, they are caused; horseplay and tomfoolery, carelessness and thoughtlessness, lack of concentration, lack of respect for oneself and others, familiarity, drinking, fatigue, haste, working conditions, irritability and boredom. (quoted by Kinnersley, 1974, p. 197)

> The 'attitude of the worker to safety' is no more the cause of industrial accidents today than it was in the days when little children were mangled in unguarded machinery in the cotton mills. Machines, buildings, and arrangements of work are still designed to the cheapest specifications that will produce goods at the greatest profits. Engineering design concentrates on the product and excludes the operator until the last moment. Safety, health and last of all comfort are treated as bolt-on goodies. (Kinnersley, 1974, p. 195)

CHAPTER 11

Food, health and disease: a case study

Study notes for OU students

This chapter uses the case-study approach you have already met in Chapter 4 on Bangladesh, but this is a much longer exploration of the many complex issues to do with food production, the influence of diet on health, and the impact of modern agricultural methods on the environment. It takes both an evolutionary and an historical approach to examine the origins of the human diet and its progression to the types and amounts of food we eat today. The health implications of contemporary diets in the developed and developing world are discussed in the context of environmental sustainability and climate change. In Section 11.5.2, we refer to an article by Paul Epstein entitled 'Climate and health', which appears in *Health and Disease: A Reader* (Open University Press, 3rd edn 2001). You could usefully read it at that point in this chapter if you have time; it is set reading for Chapter 10 of the next book in the course, *Human Biology and Health: An Evolutionary Approach* (Open University Press, 3rd edn 2001).

11.1   Introduction

In Chapter 4, the case study of Bangladesh, we aimed to enhance your understanding not only of the health profile of that country and its underlying causes, but also to illustrate the more general truth that the 'causes' of states of health or of disease are always parts of a web of interconnected factors. This final chapter is also a case study, but this time the focus of the case is 'food' — a particularly complex aspect of the health environment. In approaching the web of interactions that has food at its centre, we are casting our gaze over a vast territory.

- Suggest some of the ways in which food might interact with health in individuals, populations and at the global level.

- You probably thought first of the nutritional components of food (e.g. vitamins, fat, protein, fibre) and how they affect the health of individuals. The reliability of scientific knowledge about nutrition also needs consideration, given the ever-changing advice about what we should, or should not, eat. The amount of food energy consumed relative to that expended on physical activity is another important factor, with obesity at one end of the spectrum and starvation at the other extreme. Variations in the diets of different populations, the security of their food supply and the entitlement to food (Chapter 7) of different sections of society, all fit into the 'food web'. You may also have thought of food safety issues, for example the BSE crisis, *E. coli* food-poisoning outbreaks or salmonella in eggs. Finally, the global dimension raises important questions about the changing nature of food production methods and their impact on the environment, which in turn has implications for global climate change, population and environmental sustainability, and the health not only of our own species but of all life on earth!

We cannot hope to do justice to all these issues in a single chapter, but we will attempt to give you a greater understanding of some of the key debates and the policy implications of different approaches to 'feeding ourselves' and 'feeding the world'.

11.1.1 Interdependencies between countries

By this stage in the book, you have built up a general picture of the improved health and chances of survival experienced by virtually all human populations during the twentieth century. These changes have resulted in greater longevity, faster growth rates and larger body size (a point we return to in the next section). However, it will also have become clear that such changes have been more rapid and extensive in some countries than in others, with the result that there are now quite substantial differences in health between human populations alive today in different parts of the world. One interpretation (which Chapter 8 has already undermined) is to say that such disparities are just a reflection of countries being at different stages of economic and social development. According to this analysis, the disparities should disappear — given sufficient time — as the poorer countries acquire more wealth and distribute it more equitably amongst their populations. Although there is some truth in this view, it sets aside some important issues.

First, few people now believe in the rather simple picture of global development as a more or less inevitable procession, in which nations pass *independently* in sequence along a common pathway, each one repeating the same stages on their way to the same goal. Instead, it is now understood that the development process itself is shaped by **interdependencies between countries**. For example, the movements of people across national boundaries can undermine, or nullify the effectiveness of local programmes for the control of infectious disease agents or their vectors. Perhaps even more serious for the future, it is increasingly clear that individual countries through the effects of their agricultural and manufacturing processes on the global environment, are becoming interdependent in a new way — one country's discharges become part of everyone else's burden of pollution.

Second, it is very difficult to disentangle the relative impact on the health of populations of two factors: the introduction of medical and other techniques for controlling or curing diseases, and the effects of improvements in the material and social conditions of life. The two are inextricably interconnected. Moreover, the interactions are not confined to events *within* each country, but are influenced by interconnections *between* countries. For example, the international trading of foodstuffs is becoming an increasingly important component of the economic growth of all countries. However, for low-incomes countries, attempts to increase GNP by growing 'cash crops' for the global market may result in simply reducing their self-sufficiency in food. Failure by a country to invest in a balanced production so as to secure and sustain a supply of food for its population which is both affordable and safe to eat, tends to result in rising levels of malnutrition and food-borne diseases. But then again, much of the income from international trade is often needed to repay the interest on loans from the richer countries, which may have been spent in part on the health system. So it is not a simple matter of hard work and sensible policies for a poor country to 'progress' towards attaining the characteristics of the developed world.

This leads to a third observation: the conditions that prevailed in the nineteenth century, when today's developed industrial economies (for example, England) started their 'journey' through the demographic and epidemiological transitions, no longer exist. Events have moved on at breathtaking speed.

● List some major differences in the conditions facing today's developing countries, compared with the situation when England began industrialisation.

■ Among many possible answers are the growth in communications technology; the rise in huge multi-national businesses, including those involved in food production and processing; global trading in commodities, currencies and shares; a massive rise in the burning of fossil fuels; an increase in extreme weather conditions due to climate change; the development of high-technology medicine and genetic engineering; and a world population which has already passed six billion.

Thus, even if we retain the imagery of nations developing along a common pathway, what must be done for those at the rear of the development 'procession' who may never reach the goal because those who preceded them have already 'trampled the ground'? Moreover, it seems unlikely that any country — whatever the level of income achieved so far — can continue indefinitely along a development pathway in accord with the expectations of the past. A continued improvement of health in the lowest income countries — and even maintaining the levels already achieved in those with the highest — may be critically dependent upon a better understanding of the ways in which economic, social and environmental factors interact to sustain not only the health of the human population, but also the integrity of the environment itself.

Before we move on, it is important to emphasise that the focus on food is not made with the intention of implicating food supply as the single, or even principle, cause of the differences in health status between the populations of countries having low or high average incomes. As in the case of Bangladesh in Chapter 4, it is the *interconnectedness* between nutrition and other factors that determines the outcome. Indeed, we could have chosen a quite different starting point, for example a particular kind of disease pathogen, or social class, or housing, or public sanitation, or gender. In any of those cases, the end result would have been a description of the same web of causes.

11.2 Hunger and malnutrition: the normal lot of humans?

Was it correct, as John Boyd Orr said when he became the first Director General of the UN Food and Agriculture Organisation (FAO) in 1947, that two-thirds of the world's population then suffered some degree of hunger or deprivation throughout their lives? Was it correct to say that by 1970 the proportion had fallen to nearer one-third and by 1990 to one-fifth? (FAO, 1996, p. 44). Is it still declining in the twenty-first century?

These apparently straightforward questions turn out to be quite difficult to answer. Perhaps the first thing to say is that if such levels of hunger and malnutrition have been the normal lot of humankind, then in terms of *biological fitness* the human species has nonetheless up to now been outstandingly successful. (As you saw in Chapter 5, to a biologist fitness means the successful transmission of genes to future generations; that is to say, the ability to survive long enough to reproduce and to protect that investment sufficiently to ensure that the offspring also have a chance to reproduce.)

We now have a larger total **biomass** (i.e. the sum of the body weights of all people now alive) than that of any other mammal with the possible exception of the cow, which owes its present population size (about 1.3 billion) almost entirely to human livestock farming. Perhaps more significantly, there has — during the past hundred years or so — been a sustained increase in *reproductive fitness*. Not only does each generation produce a larger *number* of individuals who survive to contribute to the ancestry of future generations, but also a greater *proportion* of all those born survive to do so. To accept that this is so in no way weakens the moral issues raised by the existence of *any* degree of serious hunger, particularly when that could be avoided by greater equity in food entitlement without significant loss to anyone else. But it does suggest that if chronic hunger does still afflict a large proportion of the world population, it is not severe or extensive enough to impair the biological fitness of the *species* as a whole.

In Chapter 5 we noted that, in addition to Malthus's idea of 'positive checks', there are other biological/evolutionary processes through which a population may regulate its density, rather than simply having a maximum size imposed upon it by some limiting factor in its environment (e.g. food supply). Many animal species are known to regulate their numbers at levels somewhat below the maximum that could be sustained by the available food supply and there is no reason to suppose that humans lack the capacity to do the same. This ecological perspective emphasises the capacity of humans in traditional societies to make adjustments to their reproductive capacity so as to sustain an equilibrium with their natural environment. However, this leaves us with an account of the human condition that differs markedly from many other descriptions of the contemporary world, in which much of the existing population is said to be constantly beset by hunger.

The most likely explanation of the apparent discrepancy between the ecologist's view and that of the international development assistance agencies lies in the meaning they attach to the word 'hunger'. We need to be very careful to use this word and others like 'starvation' in a consistent way. The scientific definitions of these terms are not necessarily the same as when they are used colloquially, so we must spend a little time establishing the sense in which they will be used in the rest of this chapter.

That emotive word **hunger** has no scientific definition and there are no agreed methods for measuring it. Moreover, according to circumstance it has more than one common implication: for some people at some times it is a signal of desperation; for others it simply expresses a keen healthy appetite. Compare the likely implications of a complaint of 'hunger' by a child in an Ethiopian peasant family, with those of a similar plea made to almost any British parent!

Almost as problematic is **starvation**. The precise meaning is a sustained deficit of energy intake below energy expenditure. Because the first law of thermodynamics operates for people as well as for machines, this must mean a continuous loss of body weight. Although people do die from starvation caused by food shortages in some countries and some circumstances, prolonged starvation is quite rare except in the middle of famines, even in poor countries, and when death does occur it is frequently as much due to infectious disease as to lack of available food.

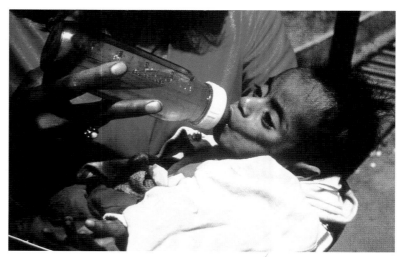

Young children are particularly vulnerable to fatal infections when their immune defences are disrupted by prolonged malnutrition; South Sudan, 1994. (Photo: Thierry Gassman © CICR)

Another term we must be clear about is **adaptation**, which refers to the anatomical and biochemical features of an individual organism, which enable it to survive and reproduce in its *current* environment. However, in a population of organisms, such features vary slightly amongst the individual members, so that if the environmental conditions change, for example in terms of food supply, some of those individuals will be better adapted than others to cope with the new environment. Those individuals will in turn reproduce offspring with similar attributes, which will thus become more common in the population.

As you will see, one of the most effective adaptations humans use in order to survive in situations with differing levels of food supply is to change average body size. But it is important to be clear that if we refer to the populations of poor countries, with their smaller average heights and weights, as being adapted to different (i.e. lower) food intakes than those of richer countries, we are not excusing the continued existence of inequity. The conclusion is not that the causes of the different health 'problems' experienced by people living in high as compared to low income countries are simply the outcomes of eating different *quantities* of food — too much in the one and too little in the other. As you will see, it makes no more sense to say that people in poor countries are generally smaller in size than those who live in richer countries *because* they have been unable to eat as much food all their lives, than it does to say that they eat less food *because* they are smaller. Neither proposition, taken on its own, helps us to understand how the differences arose: moreover, as a basis for intervening in that process, such simplistic diagnoses have so far led only to frustration.

11.2.1 Attempts to measure the adequacy of food supplies

Most of the statements about the extent of world hunger which have been made during the past fifty years (including Boyd Orr's) have resulted from attempts to measure the adequacy of food supplies reaching the populations of whole countries. In Chapter 7, we described data on *annual food-energy supplies per capita*, as well as some of the technical problems that limit the reliability of such information. However, given such an estimate, laboratory measurements on a range of human subjects can be used to determine the minimum levels of energy and nutrients that would be required in a country's food supply — given equitable distribution — in order to avoid malnutrition.

Comparisons of food supplies with population requirements suggest there has been a continuing decline in the proportion of the world's population who are experiencing hunger. However, there is controversy about whether this decline is real, or is simply due to under-reporting the size of the food supply in the past, which makes more reliable recent estimates 'appear' to have gone up. Another possible source of error is the complexity of the mathematical models used to estimate changes over time in the distribution of food amongst the populations.

Since, for these reasons, it is difficult to establish whether limitation of food supply has been a 'positive check' (as Malthus would put it) to the health and growth of populations, can we perhaps find evidence of the converse? Have there been situations in the past in which populations have experienced *improvements* in health and survival, which could be attributed to improved quantity or quality of available food? If so, it would be reasonable to conclude that they had previously been undernourished.

● What contribution did the work of Thomas McKeown make to this hypothesis?

■ As you saw in Chapter 6, McKeown argued that the improved food supplies available to the population of England from the beginning of the nineteenth century were the principal cause of the steady decline in mortality from infectious diseases, which (for most causes) pre-dated any medical advances in treatment or prevention.

However, you will also recall that the same data led the historical demographer Simon Szreter to challenge McKeown's hypothesis. The problem, of course, is that unlike a laboratory experiment, changes in a population's food supply in real-life are always associated with changes in economic and social factors, which also have implications for people's behaviour, standards of living and hence health. As we said at the outset, the contribution of food to health is enmeshed in a web of interconnecting causes, and cannot be disentangled as a single factor.

In summary, we can distinguish a number of factors related to food, which have played a part in generating geographic differences between human populations in terms of life-span, body size and by implication, general health. Although these differences have developed and widened over time between countries whose paths of economic development have diverged, food seems generally to have played a complementary (as opposed to an initiating) role in these trends. The people of the industrialised world have become taller and heavier over the past two hundred years. As a result, their food requirements have increased and as you will see in the next section, these have been met by increasingly intensified agricultural production. We can predict the same sequence of events for people living in middle or low-income countries, as their life expectancy and physical stature undergoes the same trend, provided they achieve a sustained improvement in their standards of living and general health provision.

Evidence that food *supply* ever has been, or is now, a constraint to health and performance of the great majority of people in middle and low-income countries, is at best inconclusive. Moreover, at a global level, supplies have so far more than kept pace with population growth. For example, in the period from 1970 to 1990, world average *per capita* dietary energy supply increased by 11 per cent, from 2 440 to 2 720 kcal per day, despite an increase of about 2 billion in the number of people (Food and Agriculture Organisation, 1996, p. 11).

Of course, as you saw in Chapter 7, the existence of food surpluses at global or national level does not in any way ensure that at the local level, individuals or households will have sufficient entitlement to meet their basic food needs. There have always been and still are significant numbers of people who have to exist at the very margin of survival. For them, a quite small, or even temporary adverse change of circumstances may make the difference between continued subsistence at bare adequacy and the onset of actual starvation — with death or permanent damage to health an inevitable outcome if the adversity is not relieved. Because of the fragile nature of their food entitlement, such people are often the first and always the worst affected by domestic stresses, warfare, natural disasters, or famines — from whatever cause.

11.2.2   Food energy needs of human societies: body sizes and workloads

In Chapter 5 we traced the changes in social organisation and control over natural resources which have taken place in the human population from prehistory up to present times. Table 11.1 attempts to summarise the consequences for life-span and body size of the human species' increasingly effective exploitation of the environment. An 'archaic' society represents a major part of human evolutionary history—the past 1 million years perhaps — during which the physiological and biochemical adaptations to our present omnivorous dietary pattern took place. Such a society would have consisted of hunters and gatherers of food and would also have made use of the very early phases of agriculture: virtually every able member would have been physically engaged in getting food. Such people exist today in only a few limited areas, for example the Yanomani Indians of South America or some tribes in New Guinea.

Table 11.1   Population averages for different types of societies. (Daily energy requirement is the amount of food energy an average individual would require to support biological needs, e.g. growth, maintenance, repair and reproduction, and physical activities, e.g. hunting, food gathering and socialising.)

Characteristics of population	Type of society		
	archaic	transitional	industrial
average expectation of life at birth	31 years	51 years	76 years
average age of population	19 years	23 years	38 years
average height of population	118 cm	135 cm	153 cm
average weight of population	27 kg	33 kg	55 kg
average daily energy requirement	**1 500 kcal**	**1 830 kcal**	**2 200 kcal**

(kcal is defined on p. 76) Data for the 'archaic' group are based on a synthesis of forest-living tribes in Brazil and Papua New Guinea from Velazquez, A. and Bourges, H. (eds) (1984) *Genetic Factors in Nutrition*, Academic Press, London and New York; Malcolm, L. A. (1974) Ecological factors relating to child growth and nutritional status, in Roche, A. F. and Falkner, F. (eds) *Nutrition and Malnutrition*, Plenum, New York; and Rappoport, R. A. (1968) *Pigs for the Ancestors: Ritual in the Ecology of a New Guinea People*, Yale University Press, New Haven. The transitional and industrial data are based on Bangladesh and the UK respectively.

'Transitional' refers to societies currently in the process of the demographic and epidemiological transition: a significant fraction (about a half) of such a population will be physically active in producing the food needed by the whole. Transitional societies include many Asian and most African countries, which have predominantly young, fast-growing populations, even though birth and death rates are now falling. 'Industrial' refers to societies such as that of the United Kingdom, which have largely passed through the demographic and epidemiological transition, and are close to stability of population in terms of numbers and age structure. A very small fraction (about 1 in 20) will be economically active in the direct production of food.

The physical characteristics in Table 11.1 are intended to give an impression of the age, size and life expectancy at birth, of the population average in each type of society (both sexes combined). In practice, the daily energy requirement would have varied quite widely in archaic societies, according to the ecology of their habitat and the amounts of energy expended in hunting, gathering or exploiting it in other ways for food. The figure for daily energy requirement in the table is chosen to represent the average needs of a hunter-gatherer living in an 'easy' situation, similar to that of contemporary coastal tribes in New Guinea or the

Yanomani Indians of the Venezuelan and Brazilian rainforest. The New Guinea tribes-people can meet their food energy needs with an input of only an hour or so of gardening work a day; the Yanomani spend little more than this daily on hunting and gathering. As a consequence, the food energy needs of these archaic peoples are determined mainly by their average body weight, rather than their workloads.

The equivalent value for the 'transitional' people assumes a fairly high workload typical of a complex well-organised society, sustained by relatively non-mechanised agriculture, such as the Bangladeshi farmers described in Chapter 4. Even if some animal power is used, a substantial part of the daily food needs of such people has to be directly re-invested in the form of strenuous work done on the soil and the crops, for example, ploughing fields with an ox-drawn plough, planting rice seedlings by hand, lifting and carrying heavy loads including irrigation water, and threshing grains. The food energy needs of such people are more influenced by their workloads than by the body weights of the workers.

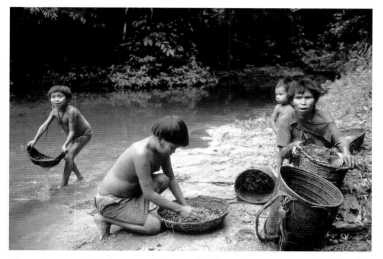

These Yanomani Indians need to spend only an hour or two a day hunting or gathering food, such as shellfish from the Orinoco river, to meet their food energy requirements. (Another photograph of a Yanomani family appears in Chapter 5.) (Photo: Mark Edwards/Still Pictures)

● How do you explain the greater average energy requirement of the members of the industrial population, even though most of their occupations are highly mechanised and need very little energy for muscular work?

■ Their larger average energy consumption is a reflection of two factors: they consume more calories to sustain their body weights, which are greater than archaic or transitional peoples at all ages; and the industrial population as a whole has a higher energy requirement because the majority are adults (who need more calories), whereas children predominate in the other societies.

Although it is clear that the amount of food energy that could possibly be extracted from any particular natural environment must exert some influence on the numbers, ages, body sizes and food consumption levels of the population that lives within it, there is nothing to suggest that these characteristics are determined in any simple way by that maximum food availability. The rates of energy expenditure of an average individual living at any of the three stages of the evolution of human society represented in Table 11.1, can best be understood as the result of an equilibrium between the human population and the wider ecology of the biological system of which it is a part.

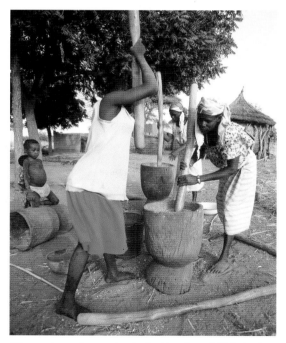

Women pounding maize in Burkino Faso,1998. In the rural communities of most developing countries, people expend a lot of energy to grow, harvest and extract nutrients from their crops. This heavy workload is a major determinant of their food energy requirements. (Photo: Mark Edwards/Still Pictures)

11.2.3 Changes in body size: malnutrition, infection, or adaptation?

Since it seems to be so difficult to assess the adequacy or otherwise of the food available to past or present populations, why not simply observe the effects of food deprivation directly, i.e. measure people's **nutritional status?** Only a few years ago, it was usual for international nutritionists to refer to measurements such as weight or height in adults, or the rates of increase of these parameters in children, as direct indices of nutritional status. Individuals below certain critical 'size-for-age' limits were classified as 'malnourished'. The implication was that body size (in particular of children), could be used as a direct measure of the amount of food available to them as individuals, or to the households or communities in which they lived.

However, this view has changed over the past few years, to the extent that many health scientists now prefer to speak simply of assessing child *growth*, or of **anthropometry** ('human-measurement'), thus avoiding altogether the use of the terms 'nutritional status' or 'malnutrition' as the common direct cause of smallness.

How has this important change of views come about?

Critical periods

Studies from birth onwards of the patterns of growth of children have shown that certain **critical periods** of growth and development are of special importance. Growth is affected by any environmental stress (including a lack of nutrients), during the later stages of intra-uterine life and in the first two years or so after birth — up to about the age when weaning is complete in pre-industrial societies. During this period, there is also a capacity to 'catch up' on any lost growth, provided the stress is reversed.

However, as the end of this critical period is approached, the ability to recover fully is reduced. The result is that a child who suffers repeated episodes of stress through and beyond the second year of life may end up with an accumulated short-fall — in height and to a lesser extent weight — which is permanent. (You may wish to look back at the photograph in Section 2.4.4 of Chapter 2, which illustrates this point.) Not only that, the deficit is 'carried over' into the next phase of life in the form of a modified set of 'instructions' for the mechanisms by which the body achieves its final adult size. These altered instructions, even in the absence of further stress, result in an adult who is shorter (and correspondingly lighter) than he or she would have been without the stresses during infancy. It has been found that although this process of *stunting* and *wasting* can be reduced by improving the health environment of mothers and small children, after the age of around two years relatively little further can be done to reverse its effects, even by intensive feeding treatments.

The curve of growth in height shown in Figure 11.1 illustrates how this process might operate. A girl whose length as a baby follows the average of the normal range (the smooth curve labelled 50th centile), suffers a series of setbacks to growth. She catches up again at first, but after the age of two years further illness causes growth to fall away towards the lower end of the normal range (the dotted curve labelled '3rd centile'). Finally she becomes an adult whose height growth finishes at the lower end of the normal range.

Infectious diseases of early childhood, such as diarrhoeal or respiratory tract infections, not only affect growth directly, through the toxins they produce in the body, but also act indirectly through reduced appetite. If growth is severely affected,

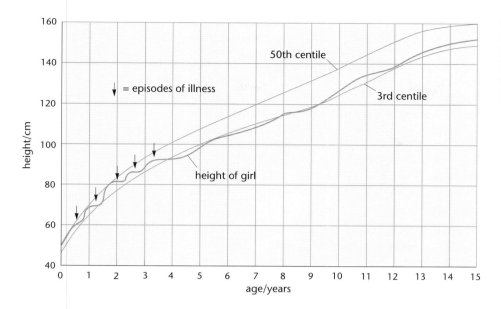

Figure 11.1 *Effect of early illness on growth in height. The arrows indicate repeated episodes of illness (Data from P. Payne)*

from whatever cause, there may also be damage to the immune system, which defends the child from infections — increasing the likelihood of further severe illness. Thus, whatever the nature of the initiating event, (disease or inadequate food), the outcome is likely to be the same: a self-reinforcing sequence of growth checks, with any remaining deficit in height after about two years being followed by a life-long pattern of smallness.

● Explain why, given these effects on health, we need to be very cautious about drawing conclusions regarding the adequacy of food supplies in a country on the basis of people's *current* body size.

■ Adults are as likely to be the size they are because they were stressed in some way by their environment *in the past*, as because of food deprivation in the present. In addition, the source of those past stresses is most likely to have been a series of infectious disease episodes, sometimes complicated by lack of available food.

Does being smaller matter?

Obviously, then, populations with large numbers of small adults are ones in which, *in the past*, many young children have suffered a good deal from infectious illness and perhaps also from a shortage of food. These circumstances may have been compounded by a lack of care and attention, including parental care and other resources such as medical treatment, which might have minimised the impact of illness. But can we say any more than that? For those that did survive, does being somewhat smaller than the average as an adult *matter*?

To ask this kind of question is by no means to imply that the process of illness and deprivation, which results in children becoming permanently smaller, could simply be regarded as either inevitable or acceptable. At the time it happens, it means that the children affected are living in a socially and materially deficient environment. Moreover, if deprivation is very severe, it carries a high risk of death at the time. And even if the child does survive, there may be adverse effects on psychological development and on the capacity to withstand further illnesses. The Canadian nutritionist George Beaton has summarised all this as follows:

> The primary conclusion that I have come to is that it is not *being* small that matters. Rather, it is *becoming* small that is critically important. It is that mix of environmental forces that leads to growth failure that also has consequences in other aspects of development and may have long term sequelae for population development. The corollary to this conclusion is that the current emphasis on growth promotion, should be seen as an attack on *constraints to growth and development*. The real objective is not to make people bigger. (Beaton, 1989, p. 37)

There are fascinating parallels between this account of the significance of poor environments on children in less developed countries, and the discussion in Chapter 10 of the 'programming' hypothesis. This implies that the kind of environmental deprivation that results in smallness at birth or infancy could account for the higher risk of serious heart disease and strokes among socially deprived adults in the UK. Kent Thornburg of the Oregon Health Sciences University, summarises the life-time consequences of continued social deprivation in wealthy and otherwise 'developed' countries, in a way that resonates with George Beaton.

> Being born small is a powerful risk factor for heart disease. It's equal to, if not more powerful than, other risk factors like lifestyle (quoted in *New Scientist*, 17 July 1999).

Of course, if health and social services aimed at improving mother and child health are implemented and if they prove to be effective and universally available, then the next generation when adult, will probably be taller and proportionally heavier than their parents. These will go on in their turn to have somewhat larger babies than they were themselves, and so on until an upper limit of size is reached. This explains the increases in adult size which have been seen in the offspring of Asian migrants to the United States and the slow upward trend in average height which occurred in Europe over three or more generations during the nineteenth and early twentieth centuries.

Becoming larger will imply higher food energy needs for human populations in the future. In the meantime, however, being small does quite usefully reduce overall food requirements. The upper part of Table 11.2 shows the body weight, from 6 months of age up to adulthood, of an average European girl. The lower part of the table shows that of a girl who is typical of many rural Asian populations.

● Comparing the weights, what pattern do you see?

■ They start to diverge sometime between 6 months and one year.

Below the values for weight for each girl, you will see those for the three components of **daily energy requirements**: *maintenance*, which is the energy cost of just staying alive, with no energy used for physical activity or growth; *growth*, which is the energy needed to synthesise and store new tissue; and *activity*, the energy cost of moving the body and other objects around. The table shows the daily energy requirement of each girl, which is the sum of these three. The next row of values is for the total energy needed, added up for all the days these two girls have lived up to the particular ages at the top of each column.

Table 11.2 The effect of reduced growth on energy needs from 6 months to 25 years in an 'average' European girl and her rural Asian counterpart.

age/years	0.5	1	5	10	25
European girl					
weight/kg	7.2	9.5	17.7	35.2	57
energy needs/kcal					
maintenance	360	620	890	1140	1370
growth	80	50	25	70	0
activity	220	320	580	700	850
total per day/kcal	660	990	1495	1910	2220
lifetime total/kcal	**94900**	**245500**	**2606000**	**5166600**	**16472000**
Asian girl					
weight/kg	7.2	9	14	22.5	43
energy needs/kcal					
maintenance	360	590	700	790	1032
growth	80	20	20	30	0
activity	220	300	460	490	710
total per day/kcal	660	910	1180	1310	1742
lifetime total/kcal	**94900**	**238200**	**1764000**	**4036000**	**12390000**
Energy saved by smaller body size of Asian girl					
per day/kcal	0	80	315	600	478
lifetime/kcal	**0**	**7300**	**296000**	**1130600**	**4082000**

Data from P. Payne, previously published as Table 11.2 on p. 170 of the 1993 edition of this book.

The two rows at the bottom of the table show the amounts of energy 'saved' as a result of the smaller size of the Asian as compared with the European girl at each particular age. The daily savings are simply the differences between the daily rates. While the children are very young, the energy savings are relatively small: at one year, the difference is 80 kcal a day. If you look back at the Bangladesh family profile in Chapter 4, you will see that the total needs of that family were between 7.8 and 10 *thousand* kcal each day. Even that very poor family would hardly be likely to notice a saving of 80 kcal a day. However, the daily savings do become more significant as the girls become adult, as the bottom row in the table shows. The cumulative differences (that is, the daily savings added up over the 25 years) are very substantial: by the time she reaches the age of 25, the Asian woman has used more than 4 million kcal *less* energy than her European counterpart. This would be sufficient to feed another younger sister up to the age of 10.

11.3 Food supply and food entitlement: origins of the diet of industrialised countries

So far, we have been looking at what is arguably the most basic function of food: its role in providing a source of energy, not only for the growth and maintenance of the body, but also for the physical work needed to produce that food in the first place. Our next step in unravelling the interconnections between food and health is to look at how the economic and social changes resulting from the agricultural and industrial revolutions affected both the quantity and the composition of the diets of the people who lived through these great transitions.

11.3.1 The industrial revolution: from peasants to workers

Only some twenty years after Malthus published his first essay in 1800, William Cobbett, a journalist, political pamphleteer and enthusiast for all kinds of country pursuits, was writing his account of 'rural rides' around the English countryside. Cobbett was an enthusiastic agent of agricultural development, and he tells story after story of innovation and change, of new techniques and the adoption of new crop varieties and more varied patterns of production.

He also saw what he considered to be a complete refutation of Malthus' theory: namely, evidence of *de-population* of the countryside at the same time that food production was expanding. On being told that the census figures showed a 40 per cent increase of the total population between 1801 and 1821 (look back at Chapter 6, Figure 6.1), he wrote, 'A man that can suck that in, will believe, literally believe that the moon is made of green cheese'. What angered him was that relatively few of the peasants were receiving the benefit of expanding agricultural production. Writing about the food and wool produced in Somerset, he describes how:

> The infernal system causes it all to be carried away. Not a bit of good beef, or mutton, or veal and scarcely a bit of bacon is left for those who raise all this food and wool … and the canal that passes close by it … Devizes … is the great channel through which the produce of the country is carried away to be devoured by the idlers, the thieves and the prostitutes, who are all tax-eaters, in the Wens of Bath and London. (Cobbett, 1830, pp. 316–17)

Cobbett's detailed accounts of the economy of individual farms and cottage households give us a starting point for understanding what these changes must have meant for the nature of the food entitlement of working-class households. As far as rural life was concerned, Cobbett was obviously an idealist, but his careful listing of what he called a 'fair share' of the produce of the labour of a family of five is probably a reasonable account of the largely self-sufficient food provisioning of labourers' households that he had known as a child:

> In order to come at the fact here, let us see what would be the consumption of one family; let it be a family of five persons; a man, wife, and three children, one child big enough to work, one big enough to eat heartily, and one a baby; … and this is a pretty fair average of the state of people in the country. (Cobbett, 1830, pp. 305–8)

If we make some 'guestimates' about what the body sizes, ages and work outputs of the members of this family are likely to have been, we can use the same method on which the values in Table 11.2 were based, to estimate that the family would have needed to expend something between 12–13 000 kcal per day. You might remember from Chapter 4 that the peasant family of five in Bangladesh consumed and expended about 10 000 kcal per day. All but the youngest members of both families would have worked hard and long. The members of Cobbett's family, though not as big as contemporary Britons, would have been taller and heavier than the Bangladeshis, which largely accounts for their higher energy requirement.

Table 11.3 shows the amounts of staple foods which could have been available to a rural British family of five persons in around 1800 in an average week. In addition, the family would also have had some vegetables and fruit in season from their own garden (which Cobbett does not mention). On this estimate, the week's food would indeed have provided the five of them with about 13 000 kcal per day (12 960 actually).

Table 11.4 shows the amounts of basic grains for bread-making, brewing and feeding to pigs, together with several sheep which the household would have needed to keep over a year, in order to ensure their weekly food supply. Using contemporary prices, Cobbett calculated the *annual income* that would have been needed had the family been dependent on a cash wage: £62 6s 8d.

Table 11.3 Staple foods consumed over a week by a rural British family of five persons in around 1800.

Food	Quantity	Energy/kcal
bread	35 lb (15.9 kg)	34 000
bacon	14 lb (6.4 kg)	41 000
mutton	7 lb (3.2 kg)	7 700
beer	10.5 gallons (47.7 litres)	8 000
total		**90 000**

Data from P. Payne, previously published as Table 11.3 on p. 172 of the 1993 edition; based on Cobbett, W. (1830) *Rural Rides*, reprinted 1967 by Penguin English Library, Penguin, London.

Table 11.4 Quantities and costs of basic commodities needed for provisioning a British family of five for a year in around 1800.

Commodity	Quantity	Cost in 1800		
		pounds	*shillings*	*pence*
wheat	3 quarters, 6 bushels	10	10	0
barley	22 quarters, 3 bushels	37	16	8
sheep	7 carcasses	14		
total		**62**	**6**	**8**

Data from P. Payne, previously published as Table 11.4 on p. 172 of the 1993 edition; based on Cobbett, W. (1830) *Rural Rides*, reprinted 1967 by Penguin English Library, Penguin, London.

Cobbett acknowledged that few labouring families could achieve even half of this income in the 1820s. How then did the rural labourers manage to live? His book, *Cottage Economy*, published in 1823, gives a vivid impression of the complex structure of food entitlement. A substantial part depended upon rights of access to land and forest, for producing their own food and fuel. That access might be wholly or in part through 'common' rights, or as land rented, or in lieu of a portion of wages. Wages themselves would commonly be paid partly as cash and partly in kind. Although small-scale rural industries still provided some money through employment of women and children, by 1820 these were already declining because of competition from the new factories.

Entitlement to cash and resources, however, was only the starting point of food provisioning. In addition, the labour component of preservation and preparation — salting, smoking, baking and brewing, to say nothing of growing vegetables and fruit — was of major importance for maintaining food security. The degree of self-sufficiency this gave was essential, not just as a way of minimising cash expenditure, but as a necessary hedge against widely fluctuating prices and wages from season to season and, because of variations in the weather, from year to year.

Comparing diets in 1800 and 1900

Some eighty years later (around 1900), a survey of the food expenditure of 2 000 urban working-class families, representative of the whole country, was carried out by the British Board of Trade. Table 11.5 shows the weekly purchases of families averaging five members, and earning just over £1 per week (the lowest of five income-bands), 70 per cent of which was spent on food.

● What do you think are the important differences between the list in Table 11.5 and Cobbett's peasant family's diet of the previous century?

■ First of all, the much greater variety of items, several of which (sugar, rice, tea, cocoa) were imported, and many others were bought in a pre-prepared form (bread, bacon, cheese, currants etc.). A much higher proportion of the energy comes from wheat flour and potatoes, and in addition sugar appears as a new source of significant amounts of energy in the diets of working people. Beer, which provided nearly 10 per cent of the cottager's energy, has been replaced by tea (although, quite possibly, drinking alcohol in any form was simply not regarded any more as a part of the 'diet', and anyway might not have been admitted to). Meat, and especially bacon, had become a secondary source of energy. Bearing in mind also the likely trends in the *composition* of these meats, the proportion of energy from fat was probably much lower by 1900 than it had been a century before.

● Those are the more obvious qualitative changes. According to Table 11.5, what was the average daily food *energy* supply of the British family in 1900? How does it compare with that of Cobbet's cottagers, and how would you account for the difference?

Table 11.5 Staple foods consumed over a week by a poor urban British family of five persons in around 1900.

Commodity	Quantity/in lb (kg)	Energy/kcal
bread and flour	28.4 (12.7)	34 500
potatoes	14.1 (6.4)	5 440
rice, oats	2.5 (1.1)	3 960
sugar	3.9 (1.8)	7 200
meat	4.4 (2.0)	6 320
bacon	1.0 (0.5)	3 250
milk	6.9 (3.1)	2 015
cheese	0.7 (0.3)	1 230
butter	1.1 (0.5)	3 700
currants	0.4 (0.2)	480
fruit and vegetables	not known	not known
tea, coffee, cocoa	0.6 (0.3)	900
total		**68 995**

Data from P. Payne, previously published as Table 11.5 on p. 173 of the 1993 edition; based on Burnett, J. (1966), *Plenty and Want*, Nelson, London.

■ The energy supply per day in 1990 was just over 9 800 kcal (68 995 divided by 7 days). This is much lower than that of Cobbett's cottagers (12 960 kcal per day), but is consistent with what we know about the lower demands made by industrial employment for sustained physical work, as compared to agricultural labour. In addition, much of the energy the cottage family had to expend in producing, processing and preparing their own food had, by 1900, already been supplied by others before the family purchased it.

What is interesting about the *entitlement* to food in 1900, compared with 100 years before, is its relatively simple pattern. Virtually everything to do with food acquisition in 1900 depended upon a cash wage. The development of the urban supply system had already much reduced the need for the production, preservation and home processing of basic ingredients.

11.3.2 The modern British 'shopping basket'

By the middle of the twentieth century, the process of transformation of employment from rural labouring to industry had become almost total. By 1980, only about 1 per cent of the UK population worked *directly* in agricultural production, although a much greater proportion — perhaps as much as 30 per cent — were employed in some aspect of processing, packaging, promotion, distribution or sale of food. Table 11.6 brings the sequence of family diets closer to the present day, with a weekly shopping list of an average urban household of five people from the majority white population, living in the 1980s.

Table 11.6   Foods consumed over a week by an average British family of five persons, 1983.

Commodity	Quantity		Energy/kcal
	oz	kg	
white bread	110	3.12	7 270
brown bread	45	1.27	2 840
flour	30	0.85	2 704
cakes, biscuits, cereals	95	2.69	9 430
sugar and sweets	65	1.84	7 370
poultry	35	0.99	1 490
beef and veal	35	0.99	1 686
mutton and pork	40	1.13	2 490
bacon and ham	25	0.71	2 340
sausages	15	0.42	1 270
other meats	40	1.13	1 130
fish	25	0.71	710
cheese	20	0.57	1 700
milk	25	14.2	9 240
butter	20	0.57	4 190
margarine	20	0.57	4 140
fats and oils	15	0.43	3 820
eggs	20	1.40	2 060
vegetables: fresh	140	3.97	1 190
: frozen	85	2.41	1 080
potatoes	210	5.95	4 520
fruit: fresh	100	2.84	1 304
: canned and frozen	40	1.13	290
tea and coffee	15	0.43	1 190
jams, pickles, sauces, spreads	50	1.42	3 680
total			**79 170**

Data from P. Payne, based on calculations of the average food consumption per person in 1981, derived from the National Food Survey Committee (1983) *Household Food Consumption and Expenditure, 1981: Annual Report of the National Food Survey Committee*, HMSO, London.

The daily energy intake works out at a little over 11 000 kcal, which is close to the rate we would expect to find in a rural Bangladeshi family having the same age and sex structure as the British family.

● How do you explain this surprising similarity?

■ Every member of the British family would be taller and heavier than their Bangladeshi counterpart, so they need more calories for growth and maintenance of their body mass, but fewer calories to meet the activity component because they lead a relatively much more sedentary urban life.

Figure 11.2 emphasises the increased *variety* of the 'modern' diet. A comparable photograph of a full year's food for the family in Cobbett's cottage would probably show it quite as large in bulk (except for the lack of packaging), but consisting of only about a dozen items. What differs above all, however, is that by the 1980s most of the economic 'value added' (and, as you will see later, the energy inputs) occurred during the stages *after* the agricultural production of the raw materials, and *before* the foods reached the larder.

You have now seen four contrasting examples of family energy budgets (three here and one in Chapter 4), selected from different locations, historical times and types of livelihood. The intention has been to illustrate households typical of their class: they were not chosen to present either the best or the very worst off, but typical families who, in terms of food supply, had at least the means of survival. That being so, they *must* have been able, over time, to balance the energy expended in pursuing their livelihoods against that obtained from the food they ate. Had those balances been struck at different levels, they would themselves have had to be different people — larger or smaller, or leading different kinds of lives.

Since 1980, some other trends have become apparent. The UK household food purchases found in the *National Food Survey 1998: Annual Report on Food Expenditure, Consumption and Nutrient Intakes* (MAAF, 1999), suggest that a comparable family was consuming about 9 700 kcal per day. The survey also found that some 30 per cent of this intake was eaten away from the home, in the form of meals and snacks

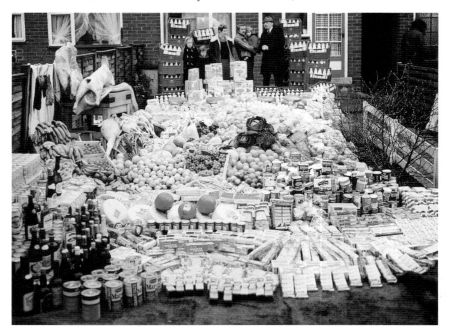

Figure 11.2 *Food for a family of five for a year — the average diet in Britain in the 1980s. (Photo: Andrew Davidson/Camera Press)*

at work and during leisure hours. The reduction in energy intake since 1980 is believed to be a response to the minimal levels of energy needed to support the increasingly sedentary pattern of urban life.

11.3.3 Trends in composition of the British diet

Earlier, you saw how historical studies have led to speculation about the possibility that better availability of food might have contributed to the decline in mortality in the British population during the eighteenth and nineteenth centuries. Similarly, there has been speculation of a reverse possibility, namely that the more recent adverse trends in disorders such as high blood pressure, coronary heart disease, dental caries, diabetes, obesity, etc. might be connected with changes in the composition of foods and diets over the same period. We return to the scientific evidence for such claims later in the chapter; first we must identify the dietary trends in more detail. In particular, the proportions of animal fat, sugar, salt and fibre in the British diet have come under scrutiny.

In looking at such possible associations, we must remember that the older studies (of the kind described above) provide only slender evidence on which to base any quantitative analyses of *national patterns* of diet. Strictly comparable values for the supply of different foods and sources of energy and nutrients — in the form of national food balance sheets — are available only from 1939 onwards. This means that studies of trends and patterns over longer periods of history can only rely on relatively anecdotal evidence.

Taken together with recorded studies of other special groups of people (for example in institutions), trends in family diets in Britain suggest some interesting conclusions. For example, even the relatively poor throughout the nineteenth century expected to eat quite a lot of meat. Records of the amount of meat going onto the market in 1880 imply that about 20 per cent of dietary energy was derived from animal sources ('animal sources' includes meat, eggs, milk, butter and cheese). By 1910, it had risen to 25 per cent — well on the way to the 30 per cent of the 1980s.

Along with uncertainty about the *quantities* of food in the national diet in the past (and of course about its social distribution), there is also doubt concerning its chemical composition. For example, the average proportion of *fat* in meat has probably declined significantly since the nineteenth century because of changes in animal husbandry. It is not necessarily correct therefore to think of previous generations as eating less animal fat than we do today. Indeed, Cobbett's cottagers may have been deriving some 42 per cent of their energy from fat — closer to today's average. The pigs kept in 1820 would have been much older and bigger when they were slaughtered and would have been *very* much fatter. Cobbett's advice about fattening a pig, in his book *Cottage Economy*, was to keep it until it was well into its second year and to:

> … make him *quite fat* by all means. The last bushel (of food) even if he sit as he eat, is the most profitable. If he can walk two hundred yards at a time, he is not well fatted. Lean bacon is the most wasteful thing that any family can use. The man who cannot live on *solid fat* bacon, well fed and well cured, wants the sweet sauce of labour, or is fit for the hospital. (Cobbett, 1823, pp. 121)

Evidently, the main purpose of keeping pigs at that time was not, as it is today, to produce lean meat as cheaply as possible, but was rather to store energy as fat and to preserve it for use throughout the year, by curing and smoking.

The increase in consumption of *refined sugar*, is a much clearer case. This began with the introduction of cane sugar from the plantations of the West Indies around the middle of the eighteenth century. Later this was replaced by beet sugar and more recently has been complemented by glucose syrups made by breaking down starch extracted from cereals such as maize. The consumption of sugar has increased fivefold in 150 years from about 20 grams per head per day around 1850 to its present 104 g (accounting for about 18 per cent of dietary energy).

Another change has been in the levels of consumption of *salt*. Throughout most of history, salt has been expensive. In addition to mining it, the manufacture of salt was an early component of industrial development. Since this process involves evaporation of large quantities of sea water, it is very energy demanding. Salt production played a significant part in the deforestation of northern and eastern Europe in the seventeenth and eighteenth centuries, and was a major user of the peat whose excavation created the Norfolk Broads. With better technology and the introduction of cheap sources of fossil fuel, the price of salt has fallen considerably over the past 150 years in relative terms. It now takes only one-fifth of the time for the average worker to 'earn' one kilogram of salt as it did in 1840. Not surprisingly, the overall consumption of salt has greatly increased and now averages about 12 grams per day, 5 g of which are added in cooking or at the table, with another 5 g consumed in traditional foods such as bread and 2 g in processed foods.

Finally, there has been a steady decline in the amount of *vegetable fibre*, partly because much less fruit and vegetables are consumed than in Cobbett's day (even though the variety has greatly increased), and partly because the increased processing of foods prior to sale has removed much of the original fibre.

11.3.4   Food preservation and its consequences

One further aspect of these historical changes relates to the risk of serious illness due to spoilage and contamination of food by micro-organisms. The last 150 years has seen great changes in the use of processes and storage methods designed to prevent food-borne infections. Cobbett's cottagers would have made use of four basic methods of preserving their food: *drying, smoking, salting* and *pickling*. All of these were seen as integral to the food production process and depended directly upon the knowledge, skills and physical labour of the household. For example, they threshed, dried and stored corn grown on their own land, and smoked and salted bacon from their own pigs. (The large quantity of salt required was probably their most expensive food-related purchase.)

● How do you think preservation methods had changed by the end of the nineteenth century? What further methods had been developed by the end of the twentieth century?

■ By 1900, preservation methods included freezing for bulk transport of meat (Figure 11.3), and the use of sugar and vinegar as well as salt for preservation and pickling. Also at about this time, low-cost packaging of foods intended for mass marketing began, in particular the use of glass bottles, as a means of delaying spoilage. During the twentieth century, deep freezing, drying (e.g. spray drying and vacuum freeze-drying) and irradiation of foods became commonplace. One of the most conspicuous aspects of modern preservation methods has been the use of plastic materials for packaging, together with the almost universal availability of refrigerated and deep-frozen storage in the home.

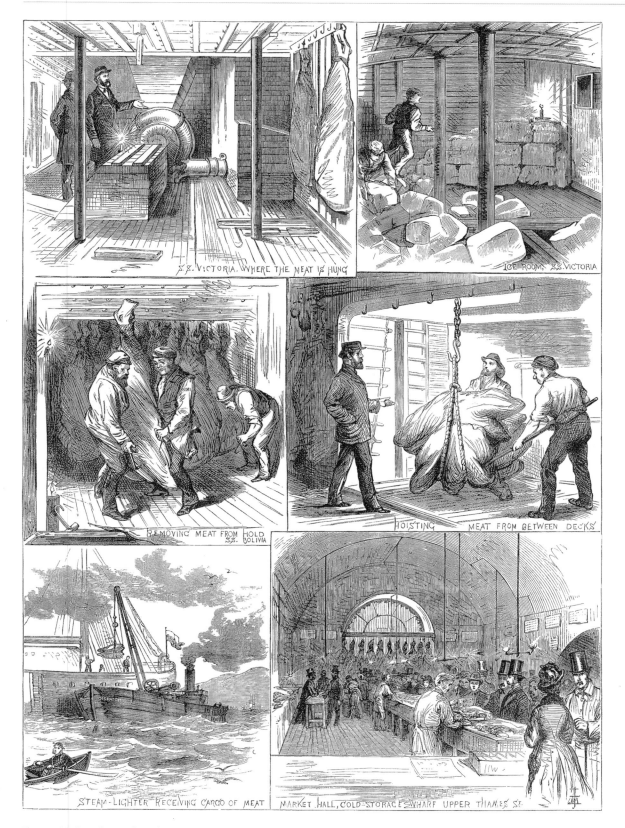

Figure 11.3 *The trade in frozen meat was flourishing at the time of this drawing in the Illustrated London News of 3 March 1877. (Source: The Mansell Collection)*

In terms of public policy, all of these developments have necessitated a parallel growth in the imposition of regulations and inspection for two main reasons. The increase in 'shelf-life' brings with it an increased risk of bacterial or chemical contamination during food production. And the use of additives for preserving, flavouring, colouring, texturing and extending foods, and the chemical composition of materials used for packaging, have the potential to affect the consumer's health.

In conclusion, all the changes in the British diet since the 1800s have resulted in very large increases in the amounts of energy used in growing, transporting, processing and storing food. Globally, food production now consumes vast amounts of energy in the industrialised countries and there is clear evidence that the developing world is rapidly moving in similar directions. Most of this energy is derived from non-renewable sources and this has serious implications for the 'health' of the global environment. The next section takes a closer look at this issue.

11.4 The energy costs of food production

11.4.1 Energy inputs to different kinds of farming

In his book *The Ecology of Agricultural Systems* (published 1982), the geographer Timothy Bayliss-Smith gives an analysis of the amounts of energy needed for food production at different stages in the development of agriculture. Table 11.7 shows three examples, which can be related to the three types of society, archaic, transitional and industrial, which were described earlier (Section 11.2.2). The last column in the table shows the ratio of 'food energy output' relative to the 'energy input' required to produce that food. The first row of the table gives the energy values for an archaic system, a tribe of people who cultivate food gardens in New Guinea. The second row is for Fyfield Manor Farm in Wiltshire in1826, the year it was visited by William Cobbett. You can also think of this as representing the transitional production systems upon which a major part of the developing world's population still depends. The bottom row shows values derived from the energy budget for a mainly arable farm in the south of England in 1971. The column headed 'labour productivity' refers to how many days of food supply for one person, an agricultural worker could produce in one day of agricultural labour.

Table 11.7 Labour and energy productivity of agriculture.

	Labour productivity *days of food per work day*	Energy input (kcal) from: *humans*	*animals*	*machines*	Ratio of food energy output : energy input
New Guinea, 1980	1	100	0	0	14 : 1
Wiltshire, 1826	7	77	21	2	40 : 1
S. E. England, 1971	200	0.2	0	99.8	2.1 : 1

Data from P. Payne; based on Bayliss-Smith, T. P. (1982) *The Ecology of Agricultural Systems*, Cambridge University Press, Cambridge.

● Look closely at Table 11.7. How has labour productivity changed over time and how was this change achieved? What happened to the *efficiency of energy conversion*, i.e. the ratio of energy outputs to energy inputs?

■ The increase in labour productivity means that, by 1971, one man was able to produce enough food in each workday to feed 200 people for a day, compared with between 1 and 7 people fed per man-day in archaic and transitional societies. (With subsequent intensive production methods the figure today would be nearer 1 000). The increase up to 1826 was achieved partly by using horses to supplement human effort, but the really large increase was achieved in the twentieth century by using machines, which almost entirely replaced human and animal power. The increased productivity, however, has been bought at the cost of *much lower* efficiency of energy conversion. In 1971, one unit of 'energy input' produced only 2.1 units of 'food energy output', whereas in 1826 it produced 40 units.

For the twentieth-century farm, we have to count as part of the inputs not only the fuel used by machines, but also the energy for manufacturing and transporting fertilisers, herbicides and insecticides. In 1971, each full-time agricultural worker in the UK was backed by non-agricultural energy inputs equivalent to 11.2 tons of oil fuel per year. The reasons for this are apparent from Figure 11.4 overleaf.

The process of counting the energy cost of food production does not stop there. The ratio of 2.1 units of 'food energy output' for each unit of 'energy input' on a contemporary farm applies only to growing *grain*. Meat products contribute some 30 per cent of the total dietary energy of the human populations of high-income countries. Meat is now mainly produced by feeding pigs, poultry and beef-cattle on specially-grown feed crops, which are themselves the outputs of arable systems operating at a conversion efficiency of 2.1 : 1. Since the animals themselves convert their food energy into meat with an average efficiency of only about 50 per cent, the ratio of energy conversion from 'plant fodder energy input' to meat output is nearer 1:1. In addition, the energy cost of the animal production process as a whole has to include that of maintaining breeding stock. The result is an overall conversion ratio, which (though it varies greatly from species to species) is on average about 1 unit of 'meat energy output' for every 5 units of 'plant fodder energy input'.

Even these values only include energy expended as far as the farm gate. To assess the energy efficiency of the whole system, we have to include the processing, preservation, storage and transport of the foods on their way from farm to the plate. Modern supermarket provisioning involves complex systems of factory processing, packaging and storage. Colossal supermarkets necessitate long-distance bulk transport, often followed by the use of personal car transport by individual purchasers. The energy costs of all of these factors are so variable as to be hard to represent meaningfully in a single value. However, one current estimate for the USA says that although one farm worker can now produce the food needed by upwards of 1 000 other people, every kcal of food energy consumed requires on average a total expenditure of 9 kcal of energy input to produce it (Pierce, 1990, p. 267).

Figure 11.4 *Rising labour productivity and falling energy productivity in English agriculture in the twentieth century.*
(a) Ploughing with horse-power in the 1920s.
(b) Potato planting using a three-row Robot Potato Planter in 1948.
(c) A petrol-driven Forage Harvester at Brill's Farm, Limpsfield, Surrey in 1959.
(Photos: © Museum of English Rural Life, University of Reading)

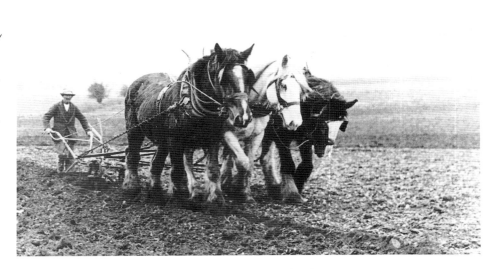

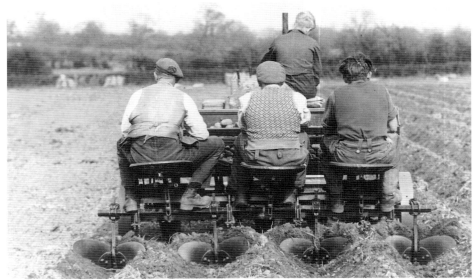

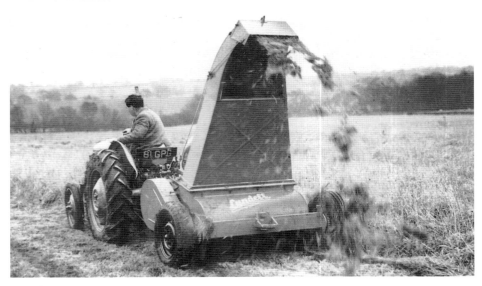

11.4.2 Impact of food production on the environment

The food production systems of high-income countries now account for nearly 20 per cent of their total energy consumption. This energy is mostly derived from coal and oil and is, of course, *solar energy* trapped deep in the earth in the form of carbohydrates in plants that grew millions of years ago. At first sight, this source of energy seems no different from the situation in 1826, which also involved trapping solar energy in fodder plants, feeding these to horses and using their muscle power to supplement human labour. The difference is in the *rate* of recycling of *carbon*. In 1826, the same amount of carbon was directly exchanged back and forth between horses and plants. By contrast, carbon released from burning fossil fuels brings suddenly back into the ecosystem all the carbon that was withdrawn from it millions of years ago, when the plants were laid down as sediments in the earth. Burning fossil fuels results in a *net increase* in atmospheric carbon dioxide.

In addition to carbon dioxide, the huge populations of ruminants kept for meat and milk production, also excrete carbon in the form of methane, a gas that has an even greater 'greenhouse' effect than carbon dioxide. Although less intensive, food production in middle and low-income countries also produces greenhouse gases: the green algae, which live in rice paddies and contribute to their fertility, are a significant source of methane. In this way, the food production and distribution systems of both developed and (to a lesser extent) developing countries are now substantial contributors to climate change. (A short article entitled 'Climate and health' by Paul Epstein appears in *Health and Disease: A Reader* (Open University Press, 3rd edn 2001). Open University students could usefully read this now; it is set reading for Chapter 10 of the next book in this series, *Human Biology and Health: an Evolutionary Approach* (Open University Press, 3rd edn 2001), but it is just as relevant here.)

11.5 Food and health: the growth of scientific knowledge

In addition to sources of energy, foods contain many other substances, which although essential for life, are needed in relatively small quantities. Many of the diseases that have always afflicted human populations are now known to have been caused by diets, which were deficient in these **micro-nutrients.** Much of the story of the development of nutrition as a science, has been about the discovery of these food components, the description of their nature and functions in the body, and the consequences for health of failing to eat enough of them. It is now time to look at the current state of knowledge revealed by this research, and the extent to which deficiency diseases are still a major cause of suffering and death in the poorer countries of the world.

11.5.1 The discovery of micro-nutrients

By the eighteenth century, many of the diseases that we now know are caused by the lack of some essential substance in the diet of the sufferer, were accurately described by physicians, and long before their connection with food was recognised.

● Can you think of some examples of these diseases and the micro-nutrients we now know would have prevented them?

■ *Scurvy*, which is caused by a lack of vitamin C; *anaemia*, a shortage of red blood cells commonly due to iron deficiency; *rickets*, a malformation of the bones in children, resulting from insufficient vitamin D; and *goitre*, a disfiguring enlargement of the thyroid gland, often accompanied by cretinism in children, the result of a low intake of iodine.

Before the nineteenth century, **scurvy** was a daunting prospect for anyone undertaking a long sea voyage. It undoubtedly caused the deaths of many hundreds of sailors and explorers. In 1753 the Scottish physician James Lind published his *Treatise on the Scurvy*. This showed that fatality could be prevented simply by a daily ration of vegetables or lime-juice. This prescription was so effective that, whereas Anson in 1740 had failed to circumnavigate the globe largely because half his crew died of it, Cook in 1774 succeeded without the loss of a single man from scurvy.

Despite this very practical success, Lind's theory was not popular. He believed that scurvy was caused by the *absence* of something in the diet — an idea that seems perfectly reasonable today, but which his contemporary medical colleagues found totally unacceptable. They were quite sure that diseases were always caused by the *presence* of something bad — a poison, a miasma, or worms. Nonetheless they did accept the remedy and fresh food, or at least preserved lime-juice, quickly became obligatory on naval ships — but rejected the theory. Lind, who tried without success to produce scurvy in groups of volunteers by deliberate experiment, finally lost faith in his own idea and died disillusioned. We now know that scurvy is the result of a lack of vitamin C. However, it takes about six months of a very plain and boring diet to produce scurvy in previously healthy adults, so Lind's volunteers probably either got out of the window at night or had friends who came visiting, bringing a few titbits!

In 1912, the Polish-American biochemist Casimir Funk proposed the modern, general theory of essential nutrients and coined the term **vitamins** to describe the existence in foods of a collection of vital substances and a matching set of deficiency syndromes, which result from the absence of any one of them.

Today, **deficiency diseases** are very uncommon in industrialised countries, not so much because we can cure or prevent them by taking tablets (although many people do 'dose' themselves in this way in the often mistaken belief that you can't have too much of a good thing). These conditions have disappeared simply because a sufficiently diverse range of foods, both fresh and well preserved, are continuously available *and affordable* for enough of the time, by the vast majority of people. However, as Table 11.8 shows, micro-nutrient deficiencies — particularly of iron, iodine and vitamin A — produce one of the starkest contrasts between the health of people living in the developed and the developing countries.

Table 11.8 Numbers of people suffering from nutritional deficiencies worldwide, 1998.

Micronutrient associated	Impact of disease	Numbers affected
iron	impaired immunity; reduced physical and mental capacity; increased maternal mortality	2 billion people, mostly women and children under 5; in the lowest income countries, 50% of pregnant women are iron-deficient
iodine	goitre, dwarfism, reduced IQ	760 million, all ages
vitamin A	blindness; impaired immunity	100 million, mostly children under 5

Data derived from United Nations Children's Fund (1998) *The State of the World's Children*, Oxford University Press, Oxford.

These huge numbers are of course a reflection of the interactions between many causal factors: poor diets, the heavy burden of communicable disease, poor living conditions and lack of education — all of which characterise extreme poverty. However, medical research has shown clearly that increased intakes of these micro-nutrients alone can prevent or at least ameliorate some of the worst of these impacts. For example, increasing the intake of vitamin A by young children can reduce the chance of dying before the age of five by between 20 and 50 per cent. It is also clear that although the deficiencies themselves are *preventable*, if they are left untreated, many of the consequences (blindness, learning disabilities, etc.) are *irreversible*.

There is now a downward trend in the numbers of people affected by deficiency diseases over time — very slow in some countries, faster in others. However, even where the prospects are good, it may take decades before measures to prevent or reduce this suffering become available everywhere. Furthermore, there is controversy about the best means to supplement diets with the missing micro-nutrients.

Since at least the 1950s, public health advisors have advocated that although deficiency diseases can be expected to disappear in the longer-term, when living standards rise, governments should take interim measures to counter them by distributing tablets, injections or specially-fortified foods. Others argue that although these substances themselves are cheap, the same cannot be said of the large human and institutional resources needed for the transport, management of distribution, supervision and monitoring of such mass interventions. These kinds of resource are very scarce in poor countries; indeed, their scarcity is as much a part of the poverty of a nation as is the lack of money. The costs and benefits of programmes for distributing micro-nutrients have to be compared with those of other projects, some of which might contribute as much or more to social and economic improvement in the longer term.

A controversial new option hit the headlines in the late 1990s, which could increase the widespread availability of micro-nutrients in the short to medium term, without the large resource costs involved in direct distribution. Advances in biotechnology meant that **genetic modification (GM)** could be used to introduce into staple food crops the capacity either to synthesise missing vitamins, or to concentrate nutritionally important mineral elements such as iron from the soil. In 1999, the first such GM strain was revealed to the media. 'Golden rice' is a rich source of β-carotene – a precursor of vitamin A. It was created by transferring from daffodils the genes responsible for producing β-carotene, which incidentally gives the flowers their orange/yellow colour.

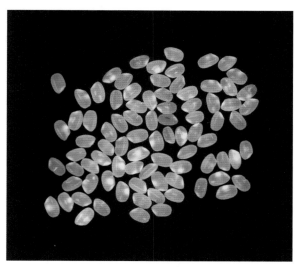

White rice has no natural β-carotene. Diets in countries where rice is the staple food are severely deficient in vitamin A, unless supplemented by vegetables, which may be impossible to grow locally, or are beyond the purchasing power of the poorest in the society. In addition to the 100 million people — mainly children — who are blinded by vitamin A deficiency (Table 11.8), the WHO estimates that a further 250–500 million people worldwide suffer some health risk from it. Golden rice poses a dilemma for those in the developed world who oppose all GM crops. Two biotechnology

Golden rice and its white 'parent', to which three genes that result in the synthesis of β-carotene were added. (Photo: Institute for Plant Sciences, Swiss Federal Institute of Technology, Zurich. Courtesy of Zeneca Ltd.)

companies have agreed that, after safety trials concluding in about 2003, golden rice will be provided free to rice farmers in low-income countries. Profits are expected to come from marketing it as a 'health food' in the developed world.

11.5.2 Research priorities in nutrition

By the middle of the twentieth century, nutrition had become a quantitative experimental science. A very important feature of its development was the growth of research on farm animals. As you have seen, the industrialisation of agriculture demanded increasingly intensive methods of meat production. The drive for increased economic efficiency and the fast growth of the industry, generated very high levels of both public and private investment in research on agricultural animals, far greater than that which has ever flowed directly into research on human nutrition.

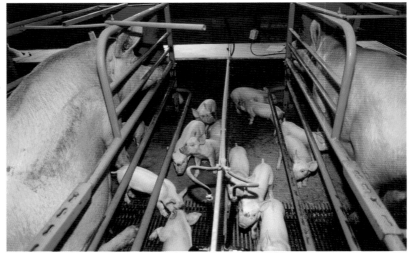

A pig farm in Middlesborough, UK, 1998. Research on intensive methods of meat production, particularly of pigs and poultry, led to large increases in yields in the 1980s; but public opposition to 'factory farming' became widespread in Britain and detailed legislation on farm animal welfare was enacted in 1999 and 2000. (Photo: Mark Edwards/Still Pictures)

Although the cross-fertilisation between human and animal experimentation has brought benefits to both sides, it is important to recognise that the objectives and hence the methods of the two are very different. Research on animal production is essentially aimed at maximising the rate of return on investment. The problem is how to feed the 'production 'units' — be they pigs, chickens or cattle — so as to generate the greatest value of meat (or milk or eggs) for each unit of value spent on food. The research programme is, roughly:

(a) Find out the chemical nature of as many as possible of the nutrients that are essential for *growth* in a particular species;

(b) Of all these nutrients, find the relative proportions in the diet that give the maximum *rate* of growth;

(c) Get as close to that growth rate as possible, using the cheapest foodstuffs and chemical additives available.

The economics of commercial production are such that large-scale producers control virtually every aspect of the animal's environment and behaviour, and use selective breeding to maximise efficiency of energy conversion and minimise variation between individuals. In practice, this has meant concentrating research on the species, breeds and age ranges that have the greatest potential for fast growth. The research strategy adopted is essentially to try to measure the effects of changing the levels of single nutrients, one by one, while holding the influence of all the others as constant as possible. The number of different vitamins, minerals, fatty acids and amino acids (the building blocks in proteins) shown to be essential for some aspect of vital functions now stands at around 50, with some variation between species.

This animal research strategy implies the need for a level of detailed and precise quantitative knowledge about the nutrition of a few varieties of farm animals, which is far beyond anything we could reasonably expect to find out about humans. Moreover, this scientific knowledge is only relevant to the performance of creatures living under the most rigidly controlled environmental conditions. It was against this background of nutrition as an increasingly exact science, that it came to be accepted during the 1950s to 1970s that this kind of approach could be applied to assessing the nutritional adequacy of diets eaten by people in poor countries, and lead to strategies for relieving the extent of starvation and malnutrition.

11.5.3 The 'great protein fiasco'

When this extension of nutrition research methodology to developing countries got under way, there was already a great deal of interest in **protein foods**, partly because these were known to be of crucial importance for animal production, and also because of the wide differences in protein intakes between rich and poor people. During the 1950s to 1970s, the protein contents of a wide variety of the foods and diets from developing countries were measured, using tests based on animal growth — and found to be deficient in comparison with the amounts of protein then considered to be necessary for health.

At about the same time, physicians became very interested in *kwashiorkor*, an illness seen in small children in some poor countries. This is a condition in which the child, typically between the ages of 1 and 3 years, becomes listless and fretful, loses its appetite, develops a dry and flaking skin and a reddish tinge to its hair. Unlike the much more common problem of severe loss of weight, or prolonged failure to grow, these children look chubby and well covered, although in fact this is deceptive — the chubbiness is actually water, rather than normal flesh.

Although kwashiorkor occurs in a number of countries with differing traditional diets, it was first described in the Western medical literature in the 1940's by Cecely Williams, a doctor working in the Children's Hospital in Accra. Later, she used the Côte D'Ivoire word *kwashiorkor*, which describes the result of abrupt weaning onto maize gruel of a child whose mother has a new baby. Cecely Williams herself never suggested that this disease *was* due to a lack of protein. However, maize flour does have a lower protein content than most weaning foods used in Europe and North America, and these observations started off what came to be called the '**great protein fiasco**'. Beginning with the idea that the symptoms of kwashiorkor were the specific signs of protein deficiency, the theory rapidly became extended so that *all* the children of the poorest countries who were small and in poor health were believed to be suffering simply because their diets were deficient in protein.

In contrast to the reception of Lind's ideas about the cause of scurvy, the protein theory was eagerly embraced because it seemed to explain a lot of observations on both humans and animals. It was also attractive in other ways. Industrialised agriculture could produce protein-rich crops such as soy beans, and protein-rich 'waste' products such as the residues after oil has been extracted from seeds like cotton. In addition, there were increasing surpluses and wastes from the meat, dairy and fish production industries of the industrialised countries. Finally, in the days of cheap mineral oil (before the price rises of the late 1970's), there was even

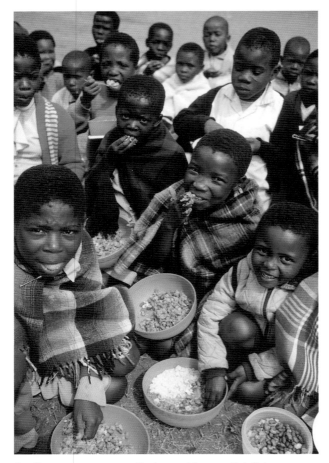

Feeding programmes routinely provide essential dietary energy to children in many developing countries. The high-carbohydrate school meal given to these children in Lesotho by 'Save the Children' provides the bulk of their daily energy intake. (Photo: Liba Taylor/Panos Pictures)

a prospect that yeasts or bacteria could be grown in bulk in continuous fermenters, using petroleum as a substrate, to form a cheap new source of protein. Better still, since these protein concentrates could be added at low cost to existing staple foods, in the same way that vitamins and minerals are added to bread and breakfast foods in rich countries, there would be no need to wait for land or income to be redistributed. The poor could be cured of the physical symptoms of their poverty, without having first to make them richer.

The 'fiasco' came when contrary evidence built up to the point where more people rejected the theory than supported it.[1] Further studies throughout the 1960s and early 1970s seemed to show two things: first, that the diets associated with kwashiorkor were not only low in protein, but in other nutrients as well and, most significantly, they were very low in *energy*. Second, that the young test animals (rats) used to measure the quality of the protein in the diets of poor countries had much higher needs for protein than human children. New committees of different 'experts' had in the meantime lowered the protein requirement figures appropriate for humans, so that by these new criteria most diets in countries affected by kwashiorkor seemed to be more adequate in protein than in energy. Finally, the 'cure' did not seem to work: fortifying diets with additional protein often did nothing to improve health and growth, whereas children given extra dietary energy in the form of carbohydrates and provided with better medical services, often did better.

There is still no agreement about what *does* cause kwashiorkor, although there are plenty of theories, including: psychological deprivation; the measles virus; dietary deficiencies of zinc or of essential fatty acids; and, most recently, toxic substances in foods produced by microscopic fungi. As to the causes of more widespread poor growth and health of children, you will remember from the discussion earlier in this chapter that the most recent view is that the primary cause may have as much to do with infectious disease in early life, as with diet.

Besides giving us a good example of a paradigm shift, this episode in the history of the growth of knowledge about human nutrition was an important demonstration of the way established power groups of professional scientists can determine — for a while at least — not only which ideas should be taken as the basis for policy, but also the priorities for ongoing research. From the beginning of the protein theory to its final abandonment — a period of some 15 to 20 years — a substantial diversion of resources for nutritional research and development took place. The beneficiaries were nutritionists, food scientists and plant breeders, rather than the poor.

[1] Thomas Kuhn's theory of paradigm shifts in scientific and medical knowledge is discussed in *Medical Knowledge: Doubt and Certainty* (Open University Press, 2nd edn 1994; colour-enhanced 2nd edn 2001), Chapter 3. The great protein fiasco is a revealing example of the theory in action.

In the field of international nutrition at least, the episode did have some lasting effect. Over the years, the reports of committees of experts on nutritional requirements have steadily become longer and more packed with technical details about the scientific basis of the recommended values. Moreover, since the protein fiasco, they have also become progressively more circumspect about what use can be made of data on dietary values. Primarily, they tell us about the *minimum* quantities of energy and nutrients that groups of people are *likely* to be eating, *if they are healthy*. But they cannot be relied on for determining to what extent *existing* poor health in a population is the result of insufficient quantity or quality of food supply. Never again, it seems, is the world going to be switched from apparent adequacy to widespread malnutrition from lack of protein (or any other nutrient) and back again, simply at the stroke of a pen in the report of a technical committee. The 'new' paradigm regards the problem of disease in human populations as inherently complex, variable and circumstantial, and not likely to be solved simply by more accurate research on nutrient requirement levels.

11.5.4   Food and the diseases of affluence

Given the history of change and uncertainty about the role of food as a determinant of health, what confidence can we have that any of the ideas now current about eating and health are a valid basis for policy in the United Kingdom and other industrial countries? Are we likely to see a 'great fat fiasco'? Is there just something intrinsically difficult about human nutrition as a subject for research, so that we cannot expect anything other than constant changes of 'fashion'? We have to remember that, although human nutritionists can draw general conclusions about the nature of some fundamental processes from studies on other mammals such as rats or pigs, humans are inherently much more difficult to research.

● Can you suggest some reasons why this is so?

■ Humans are:
   (a) Very slow growing: a farmer, faced with a piglet growing at the rate of a human baby, would very quickly dispose of it as a runt;
   (b) Very long-lived: the pig goes to the slaughter-house less than a year old (but already weighing more than an adult man);
   (c) Very variable and unpredictable: humans are exposed intermittently to a large variety of physical and biological stresses, and because of their wide-ranging patterns of behaviour, some individuals have levels of food consumption twice as high as others of the same age, sex and size;
   (d) Because of ethical or financial considerations, humans are not available for 'experiments' or for diet intervention trials except to a limited extent, and then only under conditions differing from those of normal life.

In addition to being difficult subjects to deal with, there is no single objective measurement of the benefits *versus* the costs of a particular human diet which can be used as a basis for a reference standard. As a 1991 Department of Health Manual on Dietary Reference Values admits, 'there *is* no definition of optimum health'. Instead, there is a rather broad concern to identify the consequences for health or disease of deficiencies or surpluses of any of the thousands of single chemical entities or complex substances that occur in human diets. The overall objective of this venture is to extend the length and 'quality' of life.

For each individual human, the extent of the *interactions* between nutrients, diet, infectious diseases and genetic constitution may be so great that there simply is no ideal diet that would give the best possible outcome for the *individual*, regardless of circumstances. It is even less likely that we shall ever be able to describe the perfect average diet for a *population*. However, the increasingly detailed knowledge of human genetics arising from the Human Genome Project is likely to identify a small number of conditions in a few specific individuals for whom dietary change could lead to substantial health benefits.

Thus the official advice that once emphasised the importance of getting at least the *minimum* requirements of a whole list of individual nutrients (vitamins, minerals, protein, etc.), while cutting down on starches, sugar and fat, has given way to a more cautious advocacy of the benefits of a moderate or **prudent diet**. The prudent diet is based on a rather loose consensus between nutritionists about what are the upper (or lower) limits for the consumption of particular nutrients or types of food, which would minimise the lifetime risk of coronary or arterial disease, cancer, obesity, intestinal problems, tooth decay and other common health problems. The consensus about the guidelines for prescribing such diets shifts from time to time according to both public and professional views about what is considered to be scientifically reliable, economically feasible and socially acceptable. Not surprisingly, the guidelines also vary widely from one country to another.

11.6 Rational choice: the costs and benefits of prudent eating

There is no particular reason to suppose that today's scientific paradigms will be much more resistant to attack than yesterday's. Indeed, since the growth of knowledge owes more to successful *disproof* of false ideas than to attempts to 'verify' the ones we happen to find attractive, we hope you will go away after reading this book and set about trying to prove us wrong. However, we need now to review the perceptions of nutritional problems, and the theories about causes and remedies, which are current among nutritionists and health professionals. This will enable us to reflect on the basis of present policy proposals and speculate about what might be considered as options in the future. We start with the consequences of eating too much of everything.

11.6.1 Energy intake and obesity

It is said that, at any one time, some 25 per cent of the UK population is trying to lose weight. Even if the motivation of many of these weight-conscious people is more related to cosmetic or psychological considerations than to any specific health problem, this is still a high level of popular concern. As distinct from how a person feels about her or his appearance, the term **obese** can be given a more objective meaning when expressed as a **Body Mass Index (BMI)**. This can be calculated as the body weight in kilograms, divided by the square of the person's height in metres.

For example, an adult woman weighing 60 kg and 1.6 m tall, would have a BMI of

$$60/(1.6)^2 = 23.4 \, \text{kg/m}^2 \text{ (kilograms per square meter)}$$

An adult man weighing 68 kg and 1.7 m tall would have a BMI of

$$68/(1.7)^2 \text{ or about } 23.5 \, \text{kg/m}^2.$$

All adults over the age of 16 years, regardless of age or sex, are classed as obese if their BMI exceeds 30 kg/m^2.

● How heavy would the two people just described have to be, in order to be classed as technically obese?

■ The woman would have to weigh 30 × (1.6)^2 = 76.8 kg, and the man would weigh 30 × (1.7)^2 = 86.7 kg.

Judged by this criterion, obesity is becoming increasingly common around the world. In the UK in 1980, samples of people aged 16 years and over had 6 per cent of males and 8 per cent of females with BMIs greater than 30 (Rosenbaum *et al.* 1985, p. 115). By 1997, these proportions had risen to 17.0 per cent and 19.7 per cent (Department of Health, 1997). There is similar evidence of rising levels amongst the urbanised populations in all countries.

Obese people suffer not only psychological trauma and social discrimination, but also from increased risk of illness and death from a number of causes: heart disease, stroke, breast cancer, arthritis, diabetes, not to mention the discomfort and sometimes actual pain in the joints resulting from carrying the extra weight. There is also evidence, for some at least of these conditions, that getting down to *and sustaining* a lower weight reduces those risks. The problem however lies in the word 'sustaining'.

Losing weight

As you might guess from the huge volume of both lay and professional writing on the subject, weight loss can be and quite often is accomplished by a quite extraordinarily diverse range of methods. Besides diet regimes far too numerous to list, there are now drugs that suppress appetite, others which stimulate the metabolism to 'burn off' calories, or impede the digestion of fat, thus reducing the amount which is absorbed into the body. There are synthetic fat substitutes which pass straight through the intestine without contributing any calories. People can have their jaws wired-up to prevent eating solid foods, and there is the final recourse — surgery. The most common outcome of all these strategies is a repeated cycle of successive loss and then recovery of weight. The underlying problem remains, of finding a way of *staying* lighter for life, or at least for a useful length of time.

If we take as a reasonable criterion of success for a course of any of these treatments, that an initial weight reduction should be succeeded by at least five years at a stable and reduced weight: then, according to the clinical psychologist Kenneth Brownell, a person has a better chance of being cured of most forms of cancer, than of obesity (Brownell, 1982). Simply suggesting to people that they should diet in order to avoid *becoming* overweight, or change their diet if they do, is of little avail.

Becoming obese

There is no convincing evidence that some kinds of food are *intrinsically* more 'fattening' than others. Calories on the plate, whether they come from fat or carbohydrate or protein, get converted to body fat with the same efficiency. What may be significant about fats and oils (either animal or vegetable), is that they pack a lot of calories into a small volume, so that whatever mechanism the body uses to control appetite, it is more easily overridden by meals with a high fat or oil content.

As to the causes of obesity, it *has* to be the case that a person who is obese got that way because *at some time* in their development they had a greater excess of energy intake above expenditure than a non-obese person of the same age. However, it does not follow that they will go on continuously eating more than they expend

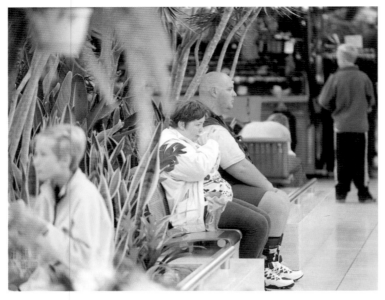

So-called 'fast food' can pack as many calories as a 'square meal' into a much smaller volume; consuming more calories than are used up in physical activity inevitably results in weight gain. (Photo: Mike Levers)

when they have reached adulthood. Just as in the case of under-nutrition, it was important to distinguish between the state of 'being small' and the process of 'becoming small', so it may be more helpful to study *how* some children get to be progressively more overweight for their age than others, than it is to study adults who are already obese.

One team of nutritionists from London University, conducted serial measurements of children, starting from the age of four years and repeated through to adolescence. The results are interesting. First of all, the obese child's family is important. As compared to children whose parents are of average weight, children of obese parents are usually taller and heavier at all ages. They reach sexual maturity at an earlier age and often go on to become obese adults (Griffiths *et al*, 1990).

The chances of the children becoming obese are greatest if both parents are obese, somewhat less if only the mother is, less still if only the father is. This looks very much like an inherited trait and, although we cannot rule out some effect of the passing on of eating behaviour from parents to child, it has also been shown that identical twins, separated very soon after birth and reared apart, remain closely similar in height (though much less so in weight) throughout subsequent life. At least 25 per cent and perhaps as much as 80 per cent of the determinants of obesity are either genetic, or in some other way transmissible from parents at a very early age.

A second and very important finding is that young children of obese parents eat *fewer* calories than those of average-weight parents, despite their faster growth rate.

● How do you think they manage to do this and still become obese?

■ Although they take in less energy, they also expend an even lower amount. In particular, they use less energy when they are at rest (the maintenance component of requirements in Table 11.2). It is the *difference* between intake and expenditure that decides the amount of energy stored in the body as extra weight, not the absolute amounts consumed.

It seems that one of the things which distinguishes obese from normal weight people, is that they are more *efficient* than the average person at storing energy in a form which is readily available for use at some future time. This might explain why the genes that predispose to obesity are so common in the population, despite the seeming disadvantages to health. In the more distant past it could have been very important — in order to cope with the uncertainties of hunting and scavenging — to have been able to store fat in times of food surplus and thus perhaps to use it to survive during a later hungry period.

The epidemic of obesity

So, if efficient fat storage was a survival characteristic in the past, why are we facing what a report of the World Health Organisation (WHO, 1997) described as a global *epidemic* of obesity? The answer seems to begin with socio-economic changes. In all countries, regardless of average incomes, the levels of obesity are increasing along with urbanisation and industrial mechanisation. Moreover, although in the past people in higher incomes or occupational classes were much less prone to obesity than the poor or lower skilled, the rising trend over time is affecting the newly prosperous as well as the not-so-badly off. Surveys have shown that obesity correlates with the possession (and numbers of) TVs, videos, domestic machines and the extent of car use. As to the biological causes, it is *not* just a simple matter of indulging appetite — on the contrary, in the UK at least, at the same time as the number of overweight people is increasing, food energy consumption is on a downward trend.

The UK *National Food Survey for 1998* (Ministry of Agriculture, Fisheries and Food, 1999) showed that on an overall population basis, people are eating on average about 260 kcal *less* per day now than they were ten years earlier. The reason for this is almost certainly a physiological response to reduced physical activity. However, although people have adjusted their energy intakes downwards, it seems they have not done so accurately enough to compensate for their increasingly sedentary life styles. Diets with a high proportion of energy from fat, regardless of its animal or vegetable origin, could well be making that adjustment more difficult. Although the *National Food Survey* showed that the proportion of energy derived from fat and oil in the food eaten at home is declining very slightly over time (it was still 39 per cent in 1998), for people in the age range 20–65 years, one third of all food expenditure goes on meals eaten *outside* the home. When we Britons 'eat out', the dishes we choose have a much higher fat content (averaging 50 per cent of total energy) than the meals we eat at home.

The prognosis for the future is pretty bleak. Although smaller in magnitude, the same pattern of change — lower activity, lower energy intakes and higher body weights in relation to height — became evident during the 1990s in British children of primary and secondary school ages. Moreover, as we said earlier, obese children are more likely to become obese adults.

11.6.2 Dietary fat

Fat is certainly the most notorious example of a diet component that people in developed countries in the late twentieth century have generally been advised to avoid, particularly the kinds of fat that occur in meat, eggs and milk (the *saturated* fats, so called because of their low ability to combine with other molecules). Besides coronary heart disease (CHD), high levels of fat intake are suspected of contributing to cancers of the breast, colon and prostate, as well as having some association with overweight and high blood pressure. These suspicions began with the discovery of associations revealed by comparisons between different populations. Taking data from seven countries, the American epidemiologist Ancel Keys showed in 1980 that those with the highest average fat content in the national food supply were also the countries that experienced the highest mortality from CHD. However, attempts to conduct similar analyses between groups of people *within* single countries (for example, grouping people by region, or by social class) have generally failed to show significant associations between degenerative diseases and fat intake.

The explanation for this outcome might simply be that the differences between the highest and lowest levels of fat eaten by different groups of individuals living in the *same* country are always much smaller than those found between samples from the populations of several different countries. Different national food patterns, cultural traditions, kinds of work and leisure, as well as socio-economic circumstances, will all work so as to *widen* the range of fat intakes and mortality rates observed in any multi-country study. It is much easier to show that a relationship exists between two variables when both vary over a wide range, than when one or both of them doesn't vary very much.

However, because there were indeed large cultural, social and environmental differences between the seven countries that Ancel Keys studied, we might suspect that some of *these* factors (rather than the levels of dietary fat) were contributing directly to CHD mortality. For example, the Cretan men in the study had low rates of CHD mortality *and* low intakes of saturated fat (they did eat a lot of olive oil, which is a good source of unsaturated fats); but they were walking 15–30 kilometres daily to work their fields in the hills!

It is difficult, perhaps impossible, to disentangle the features that contribute to the high expectation of life among Cretan men, but it cannot simply be attributed to their diets. (Photo: courtesy of Simply Travel Ltd.)

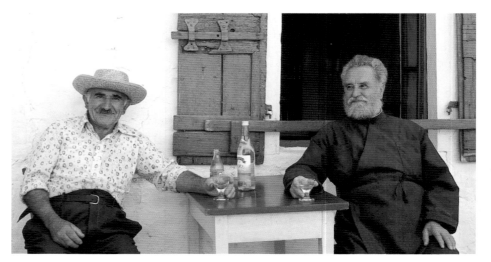

Many of the industrial countries have collected longitudinal data which show a decline over time of CHD rates, paralleled (usually *after* a time-lag of ten years or more), by falling consumption of saturated fats. In the UK, deaths of males from CHD began to decline quite rapidly in the 1970s, closely paralleling the decline in smoking and small changes in dietary fat content.

Cholesterol

Cholesterol, a fatty component of all animal cells and hence of a good many foods, was regarded in the 1980s as the most dangerous of all dietary constituents. This view was based on another association: individuals with high concentrations of cholesterol in their blood do suffer more often from CHD. However by the end of the twentieth century, cholesterol in the *diet* was no longer considered to be particularly important because there is very little relationship *for most individuals* between the amount of cholesterol a person eats and the resulting level of cholesterol in the blood. Current research suggests that it is the blood level of so called **low density lipids (LDL-cholesterol)**, rather than total cholesterol, which is strongly associated with the risk of CHD. Lowering the LDL level depends entirely on increasing the *proportion* of dietary fat which is polyunsaturated, rather than simply reducing total fat intake.

Risk factors for CHD

What started out as the fairly simple proposition that eating too much animal fat is a specific cause of CHD, seems to become more qualified and more complicated with further research. (This is reminiscent of what happened to the belief that in low-income countries all child malnutrition was caused by insufficient dietary protein.) This is partly because epidemiological studies of any kind can only show *associations*: by themselves, they cannot identify *causes*. We still have very little understanding of what really 'causes' coronary heart disease. All that can be said with any confidence is that various **risk factors** have been identified, i.e. factors that seem to be associated with different levels of heart disease in different countries.[2]

● Can you think of some factors other than animal fat intake, which are said to be associated with CHD?

■ Smoking, excessive alcohol, levels in body tissues of free radicals (substances that promote damaging oxidation within cells), low exercise levels, being overweight, high blood pressure (hypertension), psychological stress, genetic susceptibility, simply 'being born small', and being born a male (in all populations, men seem to be much more at risk of CHD than women). Of all these, smoking in particular is widely regarded as having by far the greatest potential effect on the chances of dying from CHD.

Apart from the wide range of possible risk factors, several things are interesting about this list. First, many of the risk factors *are associated with each other*. This could happen in different ways. For example, risk factors such as smoking, high alcohol consumption, and eating lots of meat and cream might be *independent* causes of CHD risk, but tend in practice to be associated statistically because all of them are related to something else — like income. Or they may all belong to a set of behavioural traits in the culture or popular lifestyle of a country or a geographic region. Alternatively, some risk factors might turn out to be linked by a *causal sequence* — perhaps being overweight gives rise to hypertension, which is associated with high blood cholesterol, which is associated with CHD.

Eating less fat

In order to try to pin down the extent to which dietary fat is an *independent cause* of CHD, there have been a number of large-scale intervention trials in which people have been persuaded to reduce their intakes of total fat — and especially of saturated fat — for long periods (5–7 years). In all cases, there has been some reduction in coronary death rates. But reducing total fat intake has been worthwhile only when the subjects were pre-selected as being at high risk of CHD: for example, when they already had blood levels of cholesterol at the top end of the range (remember, that high cholesterol concentration in the blood is a reliable indication that a person is at risk). Intervention trials using *normal* members of the population have found either that reduced rates of death from CHD were offset by increased deaths from other causes, such as cancer (or suicide!), so that there was no overall improvement in survival, or that the untreated control group improved to the same extent as those who were persuaded to change their eating habits. A comprehensive switch to a different pattern of diet might help to postpone death from CHD, but it might simply leave us to die shortly from something else instead.

[2] Coronary heart disease is the subject of a case study in another book in this series, *Dilemmas in UK Health Care* (Open University Press, 2nd edn 1993; 3rd edn 2001), Chapter 10.

It has been a recurrent theme throughout this book that the health experience of adults may be influenced by adverse events or circumstances when they were very young — perhaps even while they were still in the womb. You will remember the discussion in Chapter 10 about the hypothesis of health 'programming'.

● If this theory is correct, what would you expect to see happening to death rates from CHD over time in countries like the UK, and why?

■ They should show a steady decline, because of progressive improvements in antenatal care, maternal nutrition and the health in early childhood of today's middle-aged people, who experienced better standards of living and health services when they were very young.

Moreover, we would expect this to happen irrespective of any changes due to *current* diet or to the *lifestyle* of those adults. We should also expect to see differences in incidence of heart disease between migrant groups who have resided in the UK all their adult life, but who were born in countries having lower standards of living and health services. We do in fact see both of these things: no doubt epidemiologists will still be arguing about what caused the apparent epidemic of CHD and what made it decline, long after it has actually done so!

11.6.3 Salt, sugar and protein

Three other components of diet have also attracted much attention in terms of their possible adverse impact on health.

Salt

There is a minimum physiological requirement for salt, but this appears to be no more than about 4 grams per adult per day. On average, an adult in the UK consumes about three times this amount daily. Salt is believed by many to be a prime candidate for causing hypertension — specifically of the kind that increases with age and has no other obvious physical cause. Reducing salt intake does lower blood pressure in those people who already suffer from hypertension. However, in people whose blood pressure is within the normal range, only those who have a genetic sensitivity to salt respond in this way — about 10 per cent of the population. In addition, useful reductions of blood pressure require salt intakes to be reduced to less than one third of the population average (of about 12 grams per day), which for many people is both inconvenient, because of the need to avoid very many of the common processed foods — and unpleasant.

Sugar

Sugar has been consumed in such dramatically increasing amounts over the past 150 years, that it is not surprising that it is a prime suspect as a cause of diseases that have also risen over the same time. Nutritionists distinguish between 'intrinsic' and 'extrinsic' sugars: intrinsic sugars form part of the natural cellular structure of animal or plant tissues, whereas the extrinsic part comes as free (and immediately available) sugar, which has been extracted from natural sources. Extrinsic sugar has been accused of either initiating or exacerbating obesity, heart disease, diabetes and of course tooth decay. At the very least, its critics describe it as a source of 'empty' calories, meaning that apart from energy it brings nothing else with it to the diet in the way of nutrients or fibre.

Of all of these accusations, only that relating to tooth decay has seriously 'stuck'. Even then, the role of extrinsic sugar is probably best understood as a facilitator of a complex decay process, in which several other factors are involved — some environmental, but also behavioural. Tooth decay is caused by the action of bacteria in the mouth, which produce acid (hence dissolving away the enamel layer) and mineral deposits known as plaque, which get in the way of the saliva that would otherwise protect the teeth from acid. Intrinsic sugars (e.g. in strawberries) and extrinsic sugar (e.g. white granular sugar) in the diet are *equally* potent stimulators of this process. However, the critical factor is probably the length of time that sugar stays in the mouth. Obviously, this will tend to increase with greater intake, but just as (if not more) important, is the timing and the form in which sugar is eaten. Sweets between meals and sweetened drinks (which often also contain acids) are the main culprits, rather than total daily sugar intake. Even then the impact is moderated by oral hygiene, whether by direct cleaning, or subsequently eating other foods, or taking drinks of the kinds that clean the mouth. Another moderating factor is the application of fluoride, either on an individual (dentist or in toothpaste) or a community basis through water fluoridation.

Protein

One of the most consistent associations found in studies of diets of different populations and social groups is that as income increases, so does protein consumption — particularly the proteins of animal origin: meat, fish, dairy products, eggs. As you will see later, this has quite serious implications for the problems of meeting future world food requirements. This leads to the question are the very high protein intakes in industrial countries responsible for any of the diseases of affluence? Comparisons between populations have suggested that high intakes of red meat are a risk factor for colo-rectal cancer, and in 1997 the World Cancer Research Fund suggested that '... if eaten at all, red meat intake should be restricted to less than 80 gm' (per day).

However, since then, long-term studies of diet and health in particular groups such as nurses, vegetarians and vegans, have not only failed to support this advice with evidence, but have indicated the exact opposite. Red meat may have a *protective* effect in respect of cancer of the stomach and oesophagus (Hill, 1998), and high total protein (either animal or vegetable) intakes are associated with lower blood pressure. On this verdict, as in other aspects of the nutritional value of proteins, 'the jury is still out' at the start of the new millennium.

11.6.4 Protective foods

In the UK, as in other developed countries, as anxiety about the risk of becoming vitamin deficient has declined somewhat, so interest has increased in the importance of eating more of some foods (or components of foods) which are believed to play an active part in preventing or postponing the onset of degenerative diseases.

● You have just seen one example — the possibility that red meat could help to reduce the risk of certain kinds of cancer. Can you suggest any others?

■ You might have thought of the following: dietary fibre, antioxidants and *moderate* amounts of red wine.

Fibre

A proportion of what is left in the gut after a meal has been digested and absorbed, is a mixture of carbohydrate materials coming mainly from the walls of plant cells. This group of substances, generally known as *dietary fibre*, has been credited with many health-protecting properties over the years. Associations have been claimed between high fibre intakes and reduced incidence of CHD, hypertension, bowel cancer, appendicitis, constipation, diverticular disease and haemorrhoids (piles).

However, in 1991 the Department of Health Standing Committee on Medical Aspects of Food Policy cast doubt on these claims about fibre (they call it 'non-starch polysaccharides' or NSP). The committee reported that the methodological problems of most of the epidemiological studies were such 'that it is not currently possible to identify NSP as a major dietary factor in the aetiology of these diseases'. The committee also commented that '… NSP is not the major dietary determinant of blood lipid patterns' (that is, cholesterol levels), although they do also suggest there may be something other than fibre in oats and beans which may have a protective effect.

This is another nice example of an apparently simple idea that turns out to be complex. As with fat, the problem is one of multiple associations. High-fibre diets are by definition diets high in vegetables and fruit. Hence, they are nearly always *also* high in digestible starches and low in animal products. Like high intakes of fat, high intakes of fibre are better thought of as a *marker* of particular dietary (but therefore perhaps behavioural) patterns. The most convincing evidence of a causal role for fibre in protecting against illness is its value in reducing constipation. Both frequency and softness of stools increase with intake of fibre: but so does flatulence!

Antioxidants

Many of the chemical reactions that take place in the body as part of the normal processes of metabolism (the break-down of foods to release energy), also produce highly reactive chemical complexes known as *free-radicals*. If these substances are left un-combined or un-neutralised in some way, they will oxidise (usually this

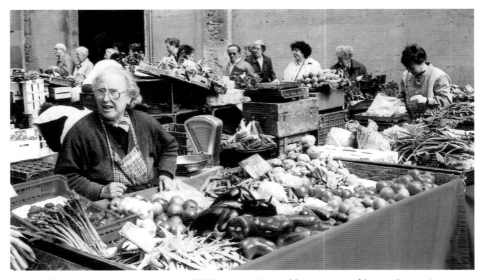

Vegetable market, Barcelona, Spain, 1999. Longevity and lower rates of heart disease in Southern Europe are attributed to the 'Mediterranean diet', low in meat, rich in fresh vegetables, fruit and olive oil washed down with a daily glass of red wine; but levels of physical activity may also be an important factor. (Photo: Mike Levers)

means 'rip hydrogen atoms away from') the structural proteins and fats of cells, rendering them gradually less able to fulfil their normal functions. (In rather the same way, hydrogen peroxide used unwisely can make hair brittle as well as blonde. Antioxidants are substances that can neutralise free radicals. There are many kinds which are effective in this way when ingested.

Some antioxidants are already recognised for their value as micro-nutrients. For example, vitamins C and E are both antioxidants as well as vitamins. Two other groups of antioxidants, which occur in common food items, are the *flavanoids* and the *carotenoids*. Flavanoids include compounds responsible for the red, blue and purple colours of many flowers, fruits and leaves — and tea, which contains large quantities of flavanoids. Black tea in particular, e.g. Lapsang and Darjeeling, contains significant amounts of several flavanoids, which have high potency as antioxidants. In a sample of 680 people, those who drank black tea were found to have a 44 per cent lower risk of heart disease than a comparable group of non-tea drinkers (Graziano *et al*, 1999, p. 162), although there may of course be some important feature of tea-drinkers *other than* their love of tea, which accounts for their lower CHD rates. Another member of the flavanoid group of antioxidants is responsible for the colour of the skins of black grapes. Several studies have suggested that red wine is more effective in reducing the risk of CHD than would be expected simply on the basis of its alcohol content (see below).

The carotenoids are another group of very potent antioxidants present in many foods, frequently the substances responsible for orange/red colours. Lycopene, the red pigment in tomatoes, is ten times as effective as vitamin E in neutralising free radicals.

The problem with these antioxidants is that they are not very soluble and, in addition, are often protected from digestion by the tough walls of the cells of the plants themselves. However, research at the Norwich Food Research Centre has shown that thorough cooking can free them from the cells, and this increases the amount that can be absorbed during digestion by four or five times. Thus, as a news report in *New Scientist* claimed (5 June 1999, p. 25), 'Soggy carrots and mushy broccoli could make you live longer'.

Alcohol

Considering their general enthusiasm for giving advice about personal behaviour, the health professions are remarkably coy about the fact that there is now very good evidence that alcohol *in moderate amounts* exerts a protective effect against CHD and other circulatory diseases. Studies in more than 20 countries show that moderate drinkers have CHD rates that are between 20 and 40 per cent lower than total abstainers, and that as a group, the death rate of moderate drinkers from all causes is lower than the average for their own country. Alcohol abusers are, not surprisingly at a higher risk of mortality from all causes — accidents and personal violence, in addition to liver disease, malnutrition, cancers of the alimentary tract, etc. Alcohol has what is called a 'J-shaped' risk relationship. Starting from zero intake of alcohol, the risks to health and life first decline as the amount consumed increases; the curve then passes through a minimum where drinking a bit more no longer has a beneficial effect, but it appears to do no harm (i.e. it has about the same health risk as being teetotal). But if you drink more than this minimum the risk to health rises steeply.

The problem for health communicators of course, is the fear that positively encouraging people to drink alcohol may result in an increase in alcohol addiction.

So what is a 'moderate amount' and does it matter what kind of alcohol you drink? The answer depends on the country you live in. The UK Department of Health recommends maximum daily intakes of pure alcohol of 30 ml (millilitres) per day for men (about the same amount of alcohol as in 1.5 pints of beer) and 20 ml (1 pint of beer equivalent) for women. The French equivalents are 60 ml of pure alcohol per day for men and 36 ml for women. There is still some dispute about whether some kinds of alcoholic drink are more protective than others: however, it is fairly clear that it is largely the alcohol *itself* that is responsible for most of the beneficial effect. However, since some of the substances responsible for red colours in the skins of fruits are also antioxidants, a preference for red wine might be a taste worth cultivating!

Functional foods

Finally, we should briefly mention the growing scientific and marketing interest in developing so-called **functional foods**, which have been modified in some way to function primarily as 'medicines' rather than as nutrients. These foods are designed to protect against, or reduce the negative effects of, specific disorders. Already on the market are a margarine that lowers blood cholesterol levels and yoghurt drinks that reduce the risk of gastro-intestinal infections. These products have not involved genetic modification (GM) of their ingredients, but GM technology will rapidly expand the range of functional foods on offer in developing as well as developed countries. By the year 2000, laboratory trials had already begun of around 40 GM food plants, including tomatoes and bananas, designed to act as *oral vaccines*. Genes from certain pathogens that cause disease in humans (e.g. the hepatitis B virus) have been inserted into the DNA of crop plants, which then synthesise proteins unique to the pathogen. When the plants, or processed foods made from them, are eaten, these unique proteins elicit an immune response in the consumer, who produces protective antibodies against the pathogen. It remains to be seen whether, over the next decade, it will become possible to immunise the populations of developing countries against some major infectious diseases by growing and eating GM bananas.

11.7   Food and health policy

So far in this chapter, we have alternated between the more narrowly focused issues of how diet affects the health of individuals, and the broader concerns about the social, economic, environmental and resource factors that ultimately determine a person's entitlement to food. These two aspects of the interconnecting web of issues concerning food point us inevitably towards the prospects for global sustainability in the future. In the next section, we shall try to integrate these aspects.

11.7.1   Food policy at the beginning of the twenty-first century

In reviewing opinions about the potential health benefits of following a 'prudent' diet, you have seen that initial hypotheses that a certain kind of illness might be associated with the intake of one of the normal constituents of diets, have often led — through further research — to a more complex picture. Many of the health problems of later life have been shown to be the outcome of multiple causes — many of which are only indirectly related to diet. In addition, some dietary problems seem to be serious only in individuals who have a particular constitutional tendency. 'Constitution' is used here to mean partly the genetic endowment, but also characteristics engendered by events in the early life-history of the person concerned.

● Can you think of some examples where variations in individual constitution determine the degree of sensitivity of response of an individual to dietary change?

■ We mentioned earlier that changes in salt intake only affect blood pressure in certain individuals who have a tendency to hypertension; similarly, blood cholesterol levels are only affected by the saturated fat content of the diet in people who already have very high cholesterol. In neither case does the evidence suggest that salt or dietary fat *causes* the elevated levels.

Interactions between diet and individual constitution mean that the effectiveness of dietary prescriptions depends to some degree on *who* is following the advice and on their willingness to consider not just one, but probably a whole range of adjustments of consumption and of general lifestyle. The implications of this complexity for government food policy in the UK are quite profound.

Changing what Britons eat

Until about the end of the 1980s, dietary change was considered to be a promising area in which *mass control measures* (i.e. measures applied across the board to whole populations), aimed at modifying behaviour, might lead to significant gains in the prevention of disease. The advocates of mass interventions argued that these measures could be justified even if they *also* affected people whose intakes (and hence levels of exposure to risk) were already low. The argument ran that low-risk individuals would benefit (even if only a little) from some further reduction because they followed the advice. Moreover, because of the large numbers of such low-risk subjects (they are in fact the vast majority of the total population), even a very small lowering of individual risk for each one of them would add up to a significant reduction in the total *social burden* of disease and mortality.

The practical and the ethical validity of this argument both depend of course on the correctness of the causal hypothesis — that, for example, reduced fat intake does indeed always result in some reduction of CHD or obesity. Furthermore, it assumes that most people, if informed of all the 'facts' in a convincing manner, would agree that the benefits to *society* (e.g. in terms of reduced health expenditure, or losses to industry from days off sick) would be worthwhile, despite the *individual* costs to themselves (economic, inconvenience, loss of pleasure, etc) of making a permanent change in eating habits.

In their report in 1983, the UK's National Advisory Committee on Nutrition Education (NACNE) claimed that the professional consensus about the causal role of dietary fat intake in respect of CHD was so strong that it was unnecessary to wait for further research before implementing policies designed to bring about reduced fat consumption by the population as a whole (Health Education Council, 1983). However, individual academics throughout the 1980s and early 1990s continued to challenge both the causal nature of the associations and the extent of the benefits likely to result from such a change. By the turn of the new millennium, there was no longer any consensus that a mass reduction in the fat content of the nation's diet would deliver the desired health benefits, *even if* people could be persuaded to do it.

Scepticism about dietary advice

This lack of certainty and the consequent frequent shifts in the content of dietary advice have combined to reinforce both public scepticism and government reluctance to take action on diet at the national level. According to a survey of attitudes towards diet conducted by the polling organisation MORI in 1992, although 95 per cent of the British public believed that eating healthy food was important for a healthy life, over 70 per cent thought that messages from health professionals on healthy eating were inconsistent. Over 40 per cent ignored food and diet advice and ate what they liked (National Dairy Council, 1992).

Since then, if there is an emerging consensus at all, it is about the sheer complexity of the role that diet plays in sustaining health. It is probable that most degenerative diseases are the outcome of multiple causes — some of which may be directly related to diet and some indirectly. Others may be connected to components of 'lifestyle', relatively few aspects of which may be within the individual's control, or to the constitution of the individual concerned which cannot be changed. Because of this complexity of interacting causes, advice on 'healthy eating' is increasingly given along with a whole set of advice about recreational exercise, avoidance of smoking and occupational stress, the proper use of drugs (both legal and otherwise), sexual fulfilment and much more. The list of what might contribute to 'healthy living' grows longer by the day.

Encouraging informed choice

Thus, the results of scientific research have presented us with a very subtle and complex picture of how the way we live affects our health. In order to understand how policy makers have responded to this, we also need to take account of the impact of two changes in social attitudes, which have taken place since the 1980s. The first is ideological. Anthony Giddens, in his book *The Third Way* (1998), describes this period as one in which Western governments of *all* political complexions saw the social problems of the post-war era as resulting (at least in part) from over-extensive involvement of the State in the social and economic life of individuals. The pendulum swung away from 'State planning' towards so-called 'neo-liberal' policies, which place maximum reliance on the operation of market forces that should, as far as possible, be left unsubjected to State regulation.

Against this background, it is not surprising that British governments in the 1980s and 1990s were reluctant to intervene directly to influence the consumers' choice of foods in the market-place. Instead, the trend has been towards regarding individuals as responsible for making their own choices of 'healthy' foods from the selection offered, while providing them with relevant information through appropriate labelling and marketing strategies. After some initial resistance, by the mid-1990s the food production and retailing sectors had adopted with enthusiasm the idea of promoting foods on the grounds of their positive contribution to health.

For those who can afford it, healthy eating can now be bought in convenient and clearly labelled packages. Competitive advantage is sought through labelling items as 'low fat' or 'very low fat' or 'virtually fat-free', together with suggestions that some brands are 'kinder' to one's health. British consumers in the 1990s used their purchasing power to assist lobbying organisations in campaigns against the widespread use of growth promoters and antibiotics in animals reared for meat. The availability of 'free-range' eggs, poultry and pork rapidly increased as consumers chose to buy them, even at higher prices, and demand for 'organically-grown' fruit and vegetables outstripped all market expectations.

These consumer trends were not simply due to a positive desire for more nutritious food; they were also a reaction against the perceived adulteration and contamination of food in the closed world behind the farm gate. This leads us to the second change in social attitudes towards government involvement in food and health.

11.7.2 But is it safe to eat?

The 1990s saw a marked increase in the level of public perception and anxiety about the problems of **food safety** in Britain. This anxiety fuelled the media outrage and political activity following well-publicised incidents in which safeguards appeared to have broken down, or to have been ignored. This in turn produced pressures that run strongly counter to the trend towards deregulation, which is a feature of the free-market ideology described above.

In Chapter 3, you saw that one of the more dramatic contrasts in the pattern of causes in morbidity and mortality between high-income and low-income countries, is the dominant role in the developing world of infectious diseases in general and of diarrhoeal diseases in particular. There is little doubt that a similar contrast would emerge if we compared these diseases in the UK population as it is now and as it was two hundred years ago. It is hard to disentangle the relative importance of 'hygiene' at the many different stages in food production, processing, storage and delivery, but Tobias Smollett's description of how household milk was delivered in London at the end of the eighteenth century, suggests how crucially important for public health the subsequent regulation and enforcement of food hygiene by the State has been.

> But the milk itself should not pass unanalysed, the produce of faded cabbage-leaves and sour draff, lowered with hot water, frothed with bruised snails; carried through the streets in open pails, exposed to foul rinsings discharged from doors and windows, spittle, snot, and tobacco quids, from foot-passengers; overflowings from mud carts, spatterings from coach-wheels, dirt and trash chucked into it by roguish boys for the joke's sake; the spewings of infants, who have slabbered in the tin-measure, which is thrown back in that condition among the milk, for the benefit of the next customer; and, finally, the vermin that drops from the rags of the nasty drab that vends this precious mixture, under the respectable denomination of milkmaid. (quoted in Drummond and Wilbraham, 1939, p. 194)

Over the two hundred years since then, government regulation, inspection and enforcement in the UK has not only brought more and more of the stages in the sequence from farm to plate under control, but has broadly kept pace with the steady growth in the overall size and complexity of what we now think of as the 'food system'. As a result, the incidence of all forms of infectious food-poisoning declined (along with other infectious diseases), to become a relatively low cause of mortality by the 1980s. To remind yourself about the *relative* significance of food poisoning, as compared to other causes of death, look back at Table 9.1.

⬤ How does food poisoning rank against other causes in terms of the chances of a fatal outcome?

◼ Averaged over the whole population of England and Wales, the risk of any kind of food poisoning to which an individual is exposed for a whole year is many times *less* likely to result in death than the non-infectious causes, such as heart disease, stroke, cancer or road accidents. Food poisoning ranks about the same as the results of inter-personal violence.

However, as you will see later, the incidence of food poisoning rose in the 1990s, to become a more significant risk to health, particularly among older people.

Assessing the risks

When people express their concerns about food safety and lobby the government to adopt policies to reduce the risks, they often over-estimate the risks associated with unsafe food. Psychologists have developed a number of hypotheses to account for this, which are applicable to other common 'misconceptions' in risk assessment. One idea is that people tend to think rationally of the risks they take in everyday life as being of two distinct kinds. Some risks are seen to be largely *unavoidable* 'acts of god' — like being struck by lightening. Others are felt to be either *acceptable* or *unacceptable*, depending on whether the person exposed feels the risk to be 'worthwhile' — like the greater risk taken when choosing to travel by car, as opposed to taking a train, because of the additional convenience or pleasure.

● How could this hypothesis explain the over-estimation of risks from unsafe food?

■ Lapses in food hygiene may assume exaggerated importance in our minds because we can see they are not 'unavoidable acts of god', nor are they 'worthwhile' since no benefit ensues.

There are two other very important factors. First, the *social context* matters: food is a vital part of individual and social life, playing a central symbolic role in the collective celebration of marriage, birth, death and worship. It is an unfailing source of pleasure, contentment and self-reward, and one of the most important symbols of social exchange and cultural communication. Guests receive food from their hosts and quite often bring it as presents; parents see it as central to their role of nurturing children.

Second, and perhaps most importantly of all from the point of view of social policy, is the suspicion that some apparently unavoidable risks are not really so at all, but are the result of the uncaring, incompetent or greedy actions of other individuals or commercial institutions. The possibility that some person might accidentally, negligently or deceitfully have caused items of food to be dangerous or unwholesome, gives rise not only to fear but to outrage. One American expert on risk communication argues that the strength of public reaction to a risk depends on two components: *hazard* — the measured chances of death or illness, and *outrage* — the extent to which someone or something can be blamed (Sandeman, 1997, pp. 21–2). The magnitudes of these two components can vary independently of each other, so that:

public perception of RISK = HAZARD + OUTRAGE

If this is so, then policy makers must learn to look beyond the rational scientific facts about food safety and ask more perceptively about what generates outrage.

Outrage against GM foods

The reaction of the British public in the late-1990s to the discovery that they were already eating **genetically modified foods (GM foods)**, without the option of choosing whether or not to do so, provides a good demonstration of the power of the 'outrage' factor to change public policy. Disclosure of GM components through food labelling became mandatory in the UK in September 1999. In the absence of watertight scientific evidence that there is *no* health risk from GM foods, many consumers in the UK and in several other European countries considered even the smallest possibility of such risks as unacceptable.

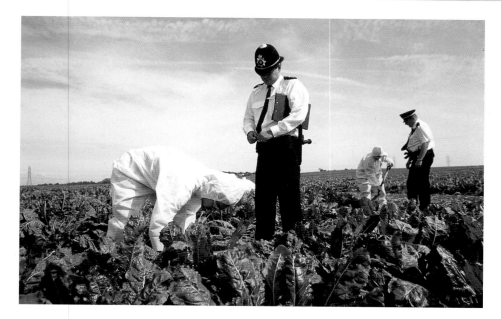

Police watch protesters uprooting genetically-modified crops on an Oxfordshire farm, England, 1999. (Photo: Nick Cobbing/ Still Pictures)

For example, in England in 2000, the arrival of a shipment of rape seed from Canada, which accidentally contained a minute proportion of GM seed, provoked outrage quite undiminished by assurances on the part of the *vendor* country that the seed met *its own* safety standards. The shipment was widely reported in the media to have been 'contaminated' by GM seeds which might (if grown) 'escape' into the environment — language that echoes public concerns of previous centuries about the pollution of food by contact with unclean sources. Farmers who had unwittingly sown the seed were instructed by the government to destroy the plants before they flowered. Protesters argued that GM pollen could drift onto nearby fields and fertilise non-GM plants, with possible consequences akin to the opening of Pandora's box. The conduct of field trials of GM crops and the assessment of their environmental impact has been subject to UK legislation since 1992.

Rational dialogue between the supporters and opponents of GM foods in terms of their relevance to high-income countries has been undermined by the 'outrage factor'. At the turn of the millennium, GM foods are widely believed to be 'unnatural' (the epithet 'Frankenstein foods' has been much used in the media). Among the issues that rarely find their way into public debate is the fact that in developed economies almost none of the food items in the diet could be described as 'natural' (unless you are a mushroom hunter in ancient woodlands). The species of plants and animals from which the Western diet is derived are the products of intensive interbreeding and selection for certain characteristics — in other words, they have been genetically modifed.

One difference between conventional plant breeding techniques and genetic engineering of new varieties has aroused more 'outrage' than any other. GM methods can transfer single genes, selected to add a particular characteristic, from one species to another, thereby combining genetic material from organisms that could not otherwise be induced to interbreed. The introduction of daffodil genes into a rice variety is one example. Such 'unnatural' combinations are held in deep suspicion by those who fear that our heritage of existing useful plant species will become genetically contaminated by GM pollen. The ability to select desirable traits so precisely is the key to the potential benefits from GM technologies, but it leads to another source of alarm.

Genetic engineering can also increase the resistance of crop species to being eaten by insects or infected by fungal or viral pathogens, and it can make them better able to withstand spraying with herbicides and pesticides. Opponents of GM technology argue that there is an unquantifiable risk of these resistance traits being transferred to other species (e.g. through cross-pollination), so GM crops should be banned in case — at some stage in the future — resistant weeds or insects or pathogens arise which could threaten the delicate balance of the ecosystem. Supporters of genetic modification point to the potential reduction in the use of agricultural chemicals, with benefits for wildlife and for the health of farm workers and consumers.

In addition to the 'outrage' factor, opposition to the introduction of GM foods into the markets of high-income countries is also fuelled by the fact that even a very small risk to the health of an individual consumer is not perceived to be 'worthwhile' because any compensating benefits are either trivial (e.g. GM strawberries might be a better colour or have a longer shelf-life), or if not trivial, accrue to someone else — farmers, seed companies, retailers, etc. But, as you have already seen, genetic modification of food crops could bring substantial direct benefits to individuals in poorer countries, many of whom suffer from debility and early death from micro-nutrient deficiencies. The question 'But is it safe to eat?' has a different meaning in these contexts. Given the opportunity to do so, these individuals might well decide that for them, the benefits of genetic modification of food crops could outweigh the risks. And as you will see later in this chapter, the threats to the delicate balance of the ecosystem from *conventional* food production methods are already immense and are unlikely to be indefinitely sustainable.

11.7.3   The collapse of public confidence in food safety

The furore over GM foods in the late 1990s may not have been as great had it not followed other food safety issues in Britain in the preceding decade, which greatly increased public concern, and illustrate a more general phenomenon in risk perception. The *suddenness* of events affecting (perhaps killing) people over a limited timescale, or the announcement that a previously unsuspected hazard exists, seem to generate and sustain far greater public anxiety than slower adverse trends, even though the latter may affect greater numbers in the long run. Two examples illustrate this: BSE and salmonella.

BSE

Bovine Spungiform Encephalopathy (BSE) was recognised in the late-1980s as a serious problem affecting cattle in Britain, which was transmissable between animals (although the agent, which consists of small protein molecules called *prions*, was not identified until much later). The possibility that the causal agent might be transferrable across species from cattle to humans was quite widely discussed in the media over several years, but was generally presented as a somewhat arcane dispute amongst scientists. The risk of BSE affecting humans was officially presented as vanishingly small, until the Minister of State for Health announced in the UK Parliament in 1996 that the link between BSE and its human version, variant Creutzfeldt-Jacob Disease (vCJD), could no longer be ignored. At the time, the total number of deaths attributed to vCJD was sixteen. The government statement triggered an incremental increase in public outrage, not only in the UK, but also among European countries such as Germany and France, which banned the import of British beef. By the middle of 2000 a total of 72, mainly young, Britons (but including a man of 74) had been diagnosed as suffering from vCJD, presumably from eating contaminated meat, and the majority of these had already died after experiencing particularly distressing symptoms. Although the annual death rate from vCJD is currently very small compared with other 'avoidable' causes (e.g. road accidents kill over 3 000 people a year in the UK), and is about the same as the death toll from lightning strikes, it has generated far greater anxiety. Uncertainty about the future emergence of more cases is part of the problem, with epidemiologists predicting anything from at most a few thousand to more than a hundred thousand cases (Ghani *et al.*, 2000).

Salmonella

Salmonella is the collective name for a number of related bacterial strains, which can cause severe diarrhoea and vomiting in humans. In the most susceptible individuals (usually the very young and the very old), whose immune system is not able to cope with the infection, the illness can lead to death. In 1988, a factually correct statement by a British Junior Health Minister (Edwina Currie), to the effect that salmonella is very common in commercial poultry flocks, caused an immediate substantial fall in egg and poultry consumption and the imposition of new safety regulations. More than a million hens were slaughtered and many small egg-producers went out of business. Ten years later, egg consumption in England and Wales (about 20 million eggs per day) was still 35 per cent lower than before that statement was made. Neither the actions taken to reduce the infection in poultry flocks, nor the reduction in egg consumption has had any discernible effect on the number of deaths — about 50 per year — from salmonella poisoning. The risk remains 1 death per million population, as Table 9.1 showed.

Food poisoning

Slow trends, by contrast, can lead to important changes in the level and pattern of risk exposure, but without much popular concern. From a more or less constant base-line over several decades, the period between 1987 and 1997 in the UK saw the level of *notified* cases of food poisoning from infectious causes of all kinds increase by about 5-fold, from 20 000 reported caes annually, to 100 000 cases (Department of Health, 1999). The incidence was still rising in 2000. Of the 397 people who died from food poisoning in 1998, 306 (86 per cent), were over the age of 65. Using the number of 70-year-olds in the population as the basis, we can calculate that the chances of a person dying of food poisoning in their seventieth year of life is about 1 in 6 800 — greater than their chance of dying in a road accident.

Despite the unpredictable nature of public responses, this sequence of incidents during the 1990s has produced an incremental change in public perception and level of anxiety about food safety (or more correctly the lack of it). Moreover, the political consequences of these incidents, together with the continuing upward trend in notified cases of food poisoning, have forced a sea-change upon the whole area of government food policy. Earlier pressure for intervention aimed at the possibility of improving health through changing national 'eating habits', has been eclipsed by the threatened collapse of public confidence in the safety of the whole food system.

Intense discussion in the UK about the need for a new government office to deal with all food-related health issues, led to the creation of the Food Standards Agency (FSA) in 2000. The Agency will be concerned primarily with the definition of standards of safety and the composition of foodstuffs, and with the research and development necessary for identifying and enforcing good practice. In order to restore public confidence, it is considered essential that the Agency is seen as independent, both from the food producers (farming and industry) and from either of the two powerful ministries, the Ministry of Agriculture, Fisheries and Foods (MAFF) and the Department of Health (DH), which have up to now rather uneasily shared responsibility for this area.

11.7.4 The ultimate rational choice?

We noted earlier that as knowledge has increased about the ways in which all elements of an individual's personal lifestyle interact in affecting their prospects for health, the more difficult it has become to articulate that knowledge in the form of simple rules and advice, which would be an effective recipe for all the members of a population. However, in the future, as a result of advances in the scientific understanding of human genetics, people in advanced industrial economies will probably have ready access to information about their own individual genetic propensities to particular health problems. This knowledge could, in principle, enable them to make rational choices about their diets, which could significantly benefit their health. In addition, if current trends continue, we can expect people to be faced with an even greater choice of foods and places to 'eat out' than they are at present. But the ability to make health-conscious decisions about what to eat rests on the assumption that people in the future will be able to *understand* a huge body of complex technical knowledge, far beyond anything we currently handle. How will the individual make sense of his or her personal genetic data, the nutrient composition and quantities of all items and dishes on offer, and the health implications of all possible choices?

- ● On the basis of the earlier discussion of British diets in the 1990s, explain why more detailed labelling of foods can have only a limited role to play in enabling each consumer to choose their own health-promoting diet in the future.

- ■ The average British family purchases more than a hundred different food items a week (as Figure 11.3 illustrated), and each family member chooses a sub-set of these to eat. There is a limit to how much time people will spend reading labels in an attempt to identify and add up the compositions and the amounts of all the food choices made in a single day (every day!), and match this to the 'best diet' indicated for their personal genetic profile. Moreover, the average family eats about 30 per cent of its food outside the home, where detailed labelling does not yet exist.

It is likely that computer technology in the future, coupled with the outcomes of the Human Genome Project, will lead to personal health-data profiles becoming available for those who can afford them, probably in the form of an electronic data base encoded on a 'smart' card. Supermarket check-out machines and restaurant menus could be made to provide detailed information on nutrient contents. Hand-held computers already exist which could 'read out' commentaries in response to all these inputs. Since all of this is technically feasible at a time when public anxiety about food has created a potential market, these products will probably become available. But will their use result in greater health for the individuals who take up the opportunity, or could it make people more anxious about the effects of the food they eat? Advanced computer programmes may be able to simplify the task, but how many of us will wish to punch in the details every time we eat or drink?

11.7.5 Global food markets and the amplification of risks

At the beginning of the nineteenth century, the British population was supplied with food by a large number of more or less independent producers, each one usually growing a whole range of foodstuffs, including cereals, vegetables, meat, dairy products and eggs, and operating on a scale ranging from large land-owners to individual 'cottage industries'. This diversified production has gradually given way to a food system in which the great majority of producers specialise in what they produce (e.g. beef, or cereals, but rarely both). Production has also intensified in relation to both land and above all labour, and is concentrated in far fewer — but much larger — farms. In addition, the distribution components of the food system now operate over distances ranging from local deliveries to international markets. To meet the large volume of demand for new products, the outputs of individual farms and units are combined and then further processed into a variety of forms, to regenerate diversity of choice closer to the final consumer. In other words, the food system has been transformed from a local industry to a global conglomerate, in which *horizontal integration* of the outputs from many different localities has taken place.

Horizontal integration has also occurred at the level of the *inputs* to primary food production. For example, dried and heat-treated slaughter house waste (including feathers) are used as protein supplements for animal feeding; farm land is fertilised with sterilised sewage sludge, which contains human excreta. Because of these activities, the food system now feeds back some of its outputs into its own primary production level. As you saw in Chapter 7, in the acceleration of food shortages in the 1974 Bangladesh famine due to panic buying, the existence of *positive feedback* in a system introduces the danger that the adverse effects of even quite small disturbances could be rapidly amplified by the system itself.

In addition, whilst concentration into smaller numbers of processing centres in some respects simplifies the tasks of monitoring, inspection and enforcement, it also greatly magnifies the size of the human population which could be placed at risk from any break-down. One of Smollett's 'milkmaids' could, and no doubt did, spread infections originating from a single sick human or cow throughout a street

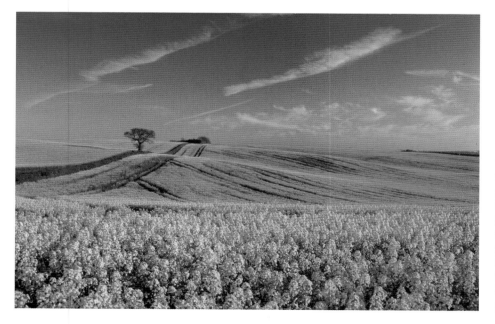

The trend in farming in Europe and North America since the 1950s has been towards ever-larger fields planted with a single specialised crop (monoculture); oil seed rape growing on a farm in Buckinghamshire, England in May 1996. (Photo: Mike Dodd)

or even a whole parish, causing outbreaks of cholera, typhoid or tuberculosis. Today, a single undetected or (worse still) unanticipated infection or accidental contamination can set at risk the population of a whole country. The most telling example was the triggering of the BSE epidemic, which may have originated in a single infected animal. The positive feedback of slaughterhouse waste tissues from a range of animal species in the form of processed cattle food, combined with the extensive transport of animals between producers, resulted in BSE spreading to almost the entire UK cattle population.

With this kind of horizontal integration now happening on a global scale, the population at risk from the effects of a breakdown in the food system can extend across national borders. Moreover, we can expect more problems of communicable disease transmission. In 1998, an outbreak of swine fever resulted in the deaths (mostly by slaughter) of 6 million of the 14 million pigs in the Netherlands. Swine fever is not known to affect humans, but influenza does and there is evidence that pigs, especially when housed at high densities, can breed new and possibly virulent strains of the influenza virus and pass them directly to humans (MacKenzie, 1999 p. 23). The future implications are not difficult to imagine.

Although from time to time there may be demands for some kind of 'food isolationism' (as in the banning of British beef exports in the 1990s), it seems unlikely that such policies will gain sufficient support to counteract the strong incentive for national governments to retain as big a share as possible in the growing profits from the global food trade. This means that the current trend among the industrialised countries to establish their own agencies for determining and enforcing food standards will quickly need to be complemented by an *international* food information network, which could encourage consistency of standards and methods and, most importantly, provide timely warning of trans-national emergencies.

11.8 The price of consumer sovereignty

Clearly, as in other areas of environmental health, prevention of food-related diseases will require *more* rather than *less* intervention on the part of national governments and international agencies, in order to protect the consumer. But along with the consumers' rights to safe food go obligations to safeguard the conditions of the world's poorest populations and to conserve the natural environment. It is to the difficult balance between these rights and obligations that we now turn.

11.8.1 The rich world's fancies

In the industrialised countries of Europe and North America, concerns about human health have ceased to be the only factors influencing what people choose to eat. Changes in attitudes have also arisen from the conviction that the food systems of industrial countries are (like industrial manufacturing processes) contributors to global warming and responsible for damaging the global environment. In addition to destruction of habitats, environmental pollution has been attributed to the waste products of animal production methods, particularly those that rely on the use of growth hormones (oestrogen-like products) and other growth-promoters, including antibiotics. These concerns, together with fears about the possible health consequences of eating food produced in this way, have reinforced the desire for more 'natural' methods of food production, a concern for 'animal rights', a sustained growth in demand for organic and 'free range' foods, and a powerful reaction against biotechnology in general and genetically-modified plant foods in particular (Teeman, 1999).

Concern for better animal welfare has not only brought a demand for less intensive and more humane methods of production. It has also increased the popularity of vegetarian foods and dishes among meat-eaters. Market research studies show that between 1985–2000 there was a small rise (about 10 per cent) in the number of people who claim to be eating less meat than they used to. However, the proportion claiming to be completely vegetarian over this period never rose above 5 per cent (Harrington, 2000). Perhaps a more significant change is that vegetarianism has become much more scientifically respectable. The same research that revealed the 'protein fiasco' of the 1960s also showed that there is no specific need for animal as opposed to vegetable protein in human diets. As you will see later, these trends are part of a general slowing down of the rate of growth of meat consumption in developed economies.

As we said earlier, per capita consumption of calories in the UK reached a peak some time ago and then began a gradual decline, in line with reduced physical activity. Since the number of consumers is also virtually constant, the food industry can only increase its profit by diversification of choice and by added value. For their part, consumers have the spending power to exercise choice over an increasing range of attributes — not only taste, texture and convenience, but also the circumstances of production. Consumers increasingly ask questions such as: 'Who grew it? Using what methods and inputs? At what cost to the environment? How humanely were the animals treated and what were they made to eat before we ate them?' Increased wealth also means more leisure and so extended direct contact with the natural environment, and this in turn increases first-hand experiences of the pressures exerted upon it by modern agricultural practices. People in higher-income groups are therefore increasingly able and willing to pay a premium for food produced by methods that are presented as more environmentally-friendly. An indication of the flexibility of choice open to such consumers is that on average in the UK at the beginning of the twenty-first century, only about 9 per cent of disposable income is spent on food.

Finally, for the producers of food, the most problematic feature of agriculture in Europe now, is *over-production*. Intensification of production methods, increasing openness to imports, combined with a population with a fixed and normally sated appetite, means that demand for primary commodities has also reached a peak. Small and medium-sized traditional family farms are faced with stark choices, such as lobbying politicians for even greater levels of subsidy from the public purse; diversifying production towards the niche markets for high-value specialist foods; or abandoning food production altogether and converting their land to recreational uses — tourism, golf courses, leisure parks, etc.

11.8.2 The poor world's ambitions

In low-income countries, the food and economic situations are different and in some ways opposite. Consumers there have also experienced rapidly rising incomes, tripling on average during the past 30 years (*World Resources*, 1998, p. 38). However, even where household incomes are relatively low, the effect of any increase in income on total demand for food is different from that seen in the high-income countries.

● Can you suggest why?

■ First, because average income starts from a very much lower baseline, a major proportion of any additional income is spent on essential items, especially on food. Second, the number of people living in the low-income countries is very large (four times as many as in the high-income group), with numbers still growing at an average rate of 1.8 per cent per year.

Of course, the gains in income have been very unevenly distributed within these populations, so that typically about one-fifth of people are close to *absolute* poverty (i.e. lacking the means to sustain life). More than 80 per cent of whatever small additional income these less fortunate people achieve is likely to be spent on extra food. With a large part of the growth in incomes arising from employment in activities still dependent on human physical labour, dietary energy needs are high and jaded appetites are definitely not a problem. The overall picture in the low-income countries therefore, is one of strong and steadily rising demand for the *basic* products of agriculture — cereals, meat, eggs and dairy items, with competition primarily focussed on *price*.

The contrasting food situations of the high as compared to low income countries, are well illustrated by the figures for past and projected future consumption of meat shown in Table 11.9.

Table 11.9   Consumption of meat by countries at different income levels, over the period 1983 to 2020. ('Meat' includes pig, beef, sheep and poultry.)

National income level	Meat consumption per head (kg per year)			Total meat consumption (million tons per year)		
	1983	1993	2020	1983	1993	2020
high	74	78	81	88	99	113
middle and low	15	21	31	51	89	193
total world	**30**	**34**	**40**	**139**	**188**	**306**

Data derived from Delgado, C. L., Courbois, C. B. and Rosegrant, M. W., Global food demand and the contribution of livestock as we enter the new millennium, in British Society of Animal Science (1998) *Food, Lands and Livelihoods*, Occasional Publication No. 21, p. 31.

In the high-income countries, meat consumption per head changed little during the period 1983–1993, and despite increasing prosperity, is expected to rise at an even slower rate in the first 20 years of the twenty-first century. The figures for *total* consumption show larger rates of increase, but these reflect the combined effects of income change and population growth.

● How does this compare with the pattern of consumption in the rest of the world?

■ Consumption of meat in the middle and low income countries has always been comparatively low, but this underlies a very strong desire to increase it, a desire which will continue for a long time and make first call on any extra income. In addition to the strong income effect, these populations are growing rapidly in numbers, with the result that total annual meat consumption rose by 75 per cent (from 51 to 89 million tons annually) during the ten years from 1983 to 1993, approaching the levels of the rich countries. Providing the current trends in human fertility and in income continue, it will more than double again by 2020.

These huge increases are expected, despite the inclusion in the calculations of countries such as India, whose future demands for meat will continue to be restrained by the traditions of their large vegetarian populations. However, this will be more than counterbalanced by the meat eating cultures of the Far East. Overall, some 30 per cent of the total world increase by 2020 will be accounted for by China alone.

11.8.3 A global free-trade market and equal rights to food?

The predictions of meat consumption rest on the assumption that world population will continue to grow, but will reach a peak of around 9 billion in 2050. In October 1999, the United Nations announced the birth of the 6 billionth consumer. What practical problems does the world face in attempting to feed an additional 3 billion by the middle of the twenty-first century? A serious prospect indeed, but considerably better than some of the prophesies of doom which were common in the early 1990s. If these additional numbers of people could be persuaded to meet their nutritional needs from a largely vegetarian diet, this would require the current production of cereals and other vegetable crops to increase by 50 per cent. However, if income growth in the developing world continues to follow its current course, it would be more sensible to assume that the demand for *meat* will also continue to grow along the trajectory indicated by the figures in Table 11.9. If the demand for meat continues to rise to this extent, a major part of the increase is likely to continue to be met in the form of pigs and poultry, rather than grazing animals which need large pastures.

● How will this pattern of demand and supply for meat affect the world needs for cereal production? (think about the efficiency of conversion of plant fodder into meat.)

■ You saw earlier that plant fodder is converted into meat at a rather low efficiency (around 20 per cent only), so every additional unit of 'meat energy output' will require 5 additional units of 'plant fodder input'. Greater livestock production at the levels projected for 2050 will in fact require a *doubling* of the current world cereal crop output.

It is of course tempting, especially for vegetarians, to urge that the vegetarian choice would be 'better' for the global environment, particularly in view of what we said earlier about the nutritional adequacy of such diets. The irony is that, leaving aside those populations whose cultures are already vegetarian by tradition, the most enthusiastic advocates for a vegetarian solution to the problem of global food security are largely to be found in the industrialised countries (Tansey and D'Silva, 1999). In contrast, the model on which the predictions in Table 11.9 are based, assumes that people in the poorer countries who are at the moment enjoying unprecedented growth in their real incomes, have a lot of 'catching up' to do and will go on wanting to eat more of the commodities that represent the most desirable diet in their own cultural traditions. For the majority of the world's poor, this means eating more meat. As you will see shortly, although a doubling of world cereal production by 2050 is probably achievable, it may not be easy to do this in a sustainable way without incurring serious damage to the natural environment.

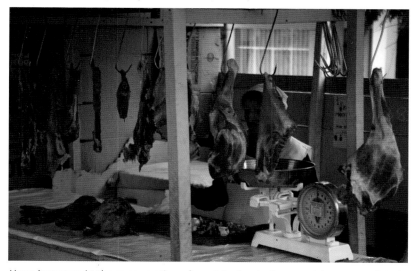

Huge increases in the consumption of meat in developing countries are predicted in the early twenty-first century, placing growing pressure on the environment as pristine habitats are cleared for fodder. Meat market, Villa el Salvador, Peru, 1999. (Photo: Andy Crump/WHO/HPR/TDR)

Throughout this book, we have stressed the importance of seeing the problems of hunger and malnutrition as aspects of *poverty*: symptomatic of social exclusion and economic disparity. It has become generally accepted that we should expect the emergence of such disparities *within countries* as a probable — even perhaps inevitable — part of economic development. Such inequalities require national governments and international assistance agencies to pursue policies that are deliberately aimed at securing entitlement to food for the poorest of the poor (Department for International Development, 2000).

During the present phase of globalisation, international trade is becoming increasingly important as the engine of economic growth, already accounting for 25 per cent of global GDP. You saw one of the adverse features of this in Chapter 7, namely the emergence of growing disparities *between* poorer countries, in respect of their ability either to produce sufficient food to meet the needs of their own populations, or to obtain it through international trade. In other words, whole countries as distinct from individual households, are now in danger of experiencing a failure of 'entitlement'. For such countries, the majority of which are in the Sub-Saharan region of Africa (e.g. Zimbabwe), avoiding famine is likely to be increasingly dependent on their ability to pay the going world market price for food.

Meanwhile, countries like China are now in a position to choose between investing more in local cereal production or alternatively, more in manufacturing goods with which to trade for food. If they choose to do the latter, they will be in a position to dominate the world food market, to the detriment of those countries of the Sub-Saharan African region whose food security is already fragile. If the next 50 years are to see a significant reduction in the extent of world hunger, this will only come about through new international initiatives in trade regulation, designed to protect the poorest countries and regions from the worst effects of markets, which are either unregulated, or regulated in ways that give further comparative advantages to countries which are already better off. The point of course is that we have to have the economic growth in the first place and moreover, that this must be achieved in a sustainable way.

11.9 Feeding humans and preserving the environment

We conclude this chapter by asking two final questions. First, will it be possible to double world cereal production by 2050? And second, if so, will it be possible to do so without destroying what remains of the biodiversity of the natural environment?

It would take another volume of this size to review the arguments about these two questions. There are quite a few followers of Malthus, who believe that the Earth's sustainable carrying capacity has already been exceeded, or inevitably soon will be. There are many others however who will answer yes to both, but strictly subject to some conditions. It all depends on *how* the increased production is achieved. The 'Green Revolution' which has so far been successful in raising food production in line with population growth, has operated by increasing crop *yields per hectare*, by introduction of new varieties, extending irrigation and increasing levels of fertilisers. As a result, cereal yields per hectare have risen steadily since the middle of the twentieth century.

However, there is now disturbing evidence of a '**yield plateau**', or 'yield stagnation' in global cereal production (*World Resources,* 1998–99, p. 152). Inevitably, overall production increases will, in future, depend more on extending the *area* under cultivation. Past extensions of agriculture have already occupied most of the high quality land, (for example as you saw in Chapter 4, in Bangladesh), so that increased yields in future will be progressively more and more dependent on conversion of the remaining forest, grass and wetland regions for agricultural uses.

This means that we all, as inhabitants of the global ecosystem, may be faced with a profound choice. If we rely on existing conventionally-bred crop varieties, fertiliser inputs and pest control techniques, 'feeding the world' will make much greater inroads into the habitats currently sheltering most of the world's remaining biodiversity. Alternatively, a new phase of the 'Green Revolution' could apply the new methods of biotechnology to modify and extend the genetic potential of food plants, increasing yields per hectare on land already under cultivation (Food and Agriculture Organisation, 2000b). GM technology also has the potential to reduce the need for fertilisers, herbicides and pesticides, the manufacture of which is a major consumer of energy. It could also make possible significant increases in crop production on land which is currently in use, but which has low or moderate fertility. For example, one-third of the world's arable land has levels of aluminium that restrict the yields of current varieties of cereal crops to as little as 20 per cent of their potential maximum. In Mexico, varieties of maize have been developed by genetic modification, whose roots secrete citric acid into the soil, converting the aluminium to insoluble aluminium citrate, thus reducing the uptake of aluminium by the plant and increasing its growth.

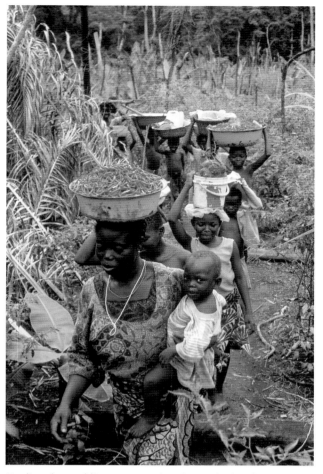

Feeding the world's poorest nations increasingly relies on destruction of virgin habitats, as here in Nigeria, where local families grow vegetables in clearings they have hacked from the forest. (Photo: Mark Edwards/Still Pictures)

Obviously, the choice of conventional or GM crops is not mutually exclusive, but the human species may be facing a 'trade off' in the very near future between — on the one hand — rejecting the genetic modification of food plants on account of as yet unquantified risks, and on the other hand preserving as much as possible of the world's biodiversity (Goklany, 1999, p. 256). In facing the challenge of fulfilling our obligations to 'feed the world and still save the planet', it will be of crucial importance to be aware of what is known and what is not yet certain about the limits within which humans can adapt to different patterns of diet, without incurring unacceptable risks to health. Exploring the current state of that knowledge has been a primary objective of this chapter.

We conclude our exploration with two thoughts. First, that the important question for nutritional science to answer is not so much 'what is the composition of a diet which is optimal for health?' but rather, 'what will be the health implications of a diet which is sustainable around the globe in the long run, assuming also an acceptable degree of equity?' And this in turn, prompts a concluding question for all of us: what will be the health implications of some way of *living* which is sustainable around the globe in the long run, assuming an acceptable degree of equity? For the prevailing patterns of world health and disease as set out in this book would be regarded by few people as acceptably equitable. Moreover, increasingly urgent questions of equity and sustainability are raised by the present trajectory of world population growth and economic development.

OBJECTIVES FOR CHAPTER 11

When you have studied this chapter you should be able to:

11.1 Define and use, or recognise definitions and applications of, each of the terms used in **bold** in the text.

11.2 Make a critical assessment of the evidence for the role of food availability and food consumption in accounting for current differences in health between the developed and the developing countries.

11.3 Discuss the ways in which environmental factors give rise to adaptive changes in adult body size through influencing the developmental process in children.

11.4 Describe the main changes that have taken place since the 1880s in the patterns of food entitlement and consumption in the United Kingdom.

11.5 Discuss the changes that have taken place in the relationship between human work inputs and the energy outputs of food production systems, from prehistoric times to the present day, and identify the significance of these for global climate change.

11.6 Describe the problems involved in using (a) epidemiological techniques, and (b) laboratory measurements, to find the relative importance of nutrition, genetic constitution and other environmental factors in determining human health.

11.7 Identify the consequences for food safety of the industrialisation and globalisation of food supplies, and comment on the conflicting forces that promote either more regulation or fewer controls.

11.8 Discuss the problems to be faced and the choices to be made in the future, in securing the food entitlement of the populations of the developing countries, while at the same time sustaining the biological diversity of the planet.

QUESTIONS FOR CHAPTER 11

1   (*Objective 11.2*)

What kind of evidence would be needed to show that the health of a population was limited by its supply of food?

2   (*Objective 11.3*)

Contrast the significance for food and health policies in a developing country, of (a) small average stature of adults, (b) interrupted growth of children of less than two years.

3   (*Objective 11.4*)

If a family of today were transported back two hundred years in time to become a typical agricultural household in Britain, in what ways would their energy consumption and energy output be different?

4   (*Objective 11.5*)

How has the increased productivity of farm workers been achieved during the twentieth century? What kinds of changes in the food systems of the industrial countries might limit their adverse effects on the global environment in the future? What are the likely consequences of these changes for consumers in high-income countries?

5   (*Objective 11.6*)

Why is it so difficult to interpret 'standardised' laboratory tests on human subjects so as to understand more about how the food we eat influences our health?

6   (*Objective 11.7*)

How have people's attitudes towards the health risks caused by the contamination of foods changed in England since the eighteenth century? In what ways do you think they could change further during the twenty-first century?

7   (*Objective 11.8*)

Why do you think there could be a conflict of interests between the need to meet rising levels of food demand in the more rapidly developing countries and the desire of people in the already developed countries to see less intensive methods used for food production?

References and further sources

References

Abdullah, M. and Wheeler, E. (1985) Seasonal variations and the intrahousehold distribution of food in a Bangladeshi village, *American Journal of Clinical Nutrition*, **41**, pp. 1 305–13.

Adnan, S. (1998) Fertility Decline Under Absolute Poverty: Paradoxical Aspects of Demographic Change in Bangladesh, *Economic and Political Weekly*, **XXXIII** (No. 22) 30 May, pp. 10 337–49.

Aldous, P., Coughlan, A. and Copley, J. (1999) Report of a MORI survey of public attitudes towards the use of animals for drug tests, *New Scientist,* 22 May, pp. 26–31.

Asian Development Bank (1997) *The Dancing Horizon: Human Development Prospects for Bangladesh.* A Joint Publication by 11 Agencies for International Assistance, ADB, Dhaka, Bangladesh.

Bairoch, P. (1982) International industrialization levels from 1750 to 1980, *Journal of European Economic History*, **11** (2), pp. 269–333.

Bangladesh Bureau of Statistics (1995) *Bangladesh Health and Demographic Survey*, Ministry of Planning, Dhaka, Bangladesh.

Bangladesh Institute of Nutrition (1981) *Bangladesh National Nutrition Survey, 1981*, Bangladesh Institute of Nutrition, Dhaka.

Bayliss-Smith, T. P. (1982) *The Ecology of Agricultural Systems,* Cambridge University Press, Cambridge.

Beaton, G. H. (1989) Small but healthy? Are we asking the right question? *Human Organization*, **48** (1), pp. 31–7.

Benjamin, B. (1989) Review article: Demographic aspects of ageing, *Annals of Human Biology*, **16** (3), pp. 185–235.

Berthoud, R. (1986) *Selective Social Security*, Policy Studies Institute, London.

Bobadilla, J. L., Cowley, P., Musgrove, P. and Saxienian H. (1994) Design, content and financing of an essential national package of health services, in Murray, C. J. L. and Lopez, A. D. (eds) *Global comparative assessments in the health sector: Disease burden, expenditures and intervention packages*, WHO, Geneva.

Bone, M., Bebbington, A. C., Jagger, C., Morgan, K. and Nicolaas, G. (1995) *Health expectancy and its uses*, HMSO, London.

Braudel, F. (1981) The Structures of Everyday Life: the Limits of the Possible, Collins, London.

British Geological Survey and Mott Macdonald UK (2000) *BGS Report on Groundwater Studies of Arsenic Contamination in Bangladesh*, BGS, UK.

Brownell, K. D. (1982) Obesity: understanding and treating a serious, prevalent and refractory disorder, *Journal of Consultant Clinical Psychology,* **50**, pp. 820–40.

Burnett, J. (1966) *Plenty and Want,* Nelson, London.

Caldwell, J. C. (1986) Routes to low mortality in poor countries, *Population and Development Review*, **12** (2), pp. 171–220.

Charlton, J. and Murphy, M (eds) (1997) *The Health of Adult Britain 1841–1994*, ONS, Series DS No. 12, The Stationery Office, London, 1997.

Cipolla, C. (1974) *The Economic History of World Population,* 6th revised edn, Pelican, London.

Coale, A. J. (1991) Excess female mortality and the balance of the sexes in the population: an estimate of the number of 'missing females', *Population and Development Review*, **17** (3), pp. 514–24.

Cobbett, W. (1823) *Cottage Economy*, reprinted in 1974 by Landsman's Bookshop, Bromyard, Herefordshire.

Cobbett, W. (1830) *Rural Rides*, reprinted in 1967 by Penguin English Library, Penguin, London.

Davey, B., Gray, A. and Seale, C. (eds) *Health and Disease: A Reader*, 2nd edn 1995; 3rd edn 2001, Open University Press, Buckingham.

Dawkins, R. (1976) *The Selfish Gene*, Oxford University Press, New York.

Delgado, C. L, Courbois, C. B. and Rosegrant, M. W. (1998) Global food demand and the contribution of livestock as we enter the new millennium, in Gill, M., Smith, T., Pollot, G. E., Owen, E. and Lawrence, T. L. J. (eds), *Food, Lands and Livelihoods — Setting Research Agendas for Animal Science*, British Society of Animal Science, Occasional Publication No. 21, BSAS, Edinburgh.

Department for International Development (2000) *Eliminating World Poverty: Making Globalisation Work for the Poor*, White Paper on International Development, CM 5006, The Stationery Office, London. (Also accessible at http://www.globalisation.gov.uk)

Department of the Environment (1999) *English House Condition Survey 1996*, The Stationery Office, London.

Department of Health (1991a) *Manual on Dietary Reference Values*, HMSO, London.

Department of Health (1991b) *Standing Committee on Medical Aspects of Food Policy*, HMSO, London.

Department of Health (1996) *Hospital Episode Statistics, Volume 1*, Department of Health, London.

Department of Health (1997) *Health Survey for England*, The Stationery Office, London.

Department of Health (1998a) *Health and Personal Social Services Statistics for England, 1998*, The Stationery Office, London.

Department of Health (1998b) *Independent Inquiry into Inequalities in Health* (The Acheson Report), The Stationery Office, London.

Department of Health (1999) *Saving Lives: Our Healthier Nation*, The Stationery Office, London.

Department of Health (2000) *Health Survey for England 1999, Preliminary Report, Ethnic Health*, The Stationery Office, London.

Department of Health and Social Security (1980), *Inequalities in Health*, Report of a Working Group (the 'Black Report'), DHSS, London.

Diamond, J. (1991) *The Rise and Fall of the Third Chimpanzee*, Vintage, London. An edited extract 'Agriculture's two-edged sword' is reproduced in Davey, B., Gray, A. and Seale, C. (eds) *Health and Disease: A Reader*, 3rd edn 2001, Open University Press, Buckingham.

Drever, F. and Bunting, J. (1997) *Patterns and trends in male mortality*, pp. 95–107 in F. Drever and M. Whitehead (eds) *Health inequalities: Decennial supplement*, Government Statistical Service, Series DS No. 15, The Stationery Office, London.

Drever, F. and Whitehead, M. (eds) (1997) *Health Inequalities: Decennial Supplement*, Government Statistical Service, Series DS No. 15, The Stationery Office, London.

Drèze, J. and Sen, A. (1989) *Hunger and Public Action*, Clarendon Press, Oxford. An edited extract 'Entitlement and deprivation' is reproduced in Davey, B., Gray, A. and Seale, C. (eds) *Health and Disease: A Reader*, 2nd edn 1995; 3rd edn 2001, Open University Press, Buckingham.

Drummond, J. C. and Wilbraham, A. (1939) *The Englishman's Food: A History of Five Centuries of English Diet*, Jonathan Cape, London.

Dubos, R. (1979) *Mirage of Health*, Harper and Row, New York.

Dye, C., Scheele, S., Dolin, P., Pathania, V. and Raviglione, M. C. (1999) Global burden of tuberculosis: estimated incidence, prevalence and mortality by country, *Journal of the American Medical Association* (JAMA), **282** (7), pp. 677–86.

Engels, F. (1845, first published in German; 1892 first English edition; 1969 first paperback edition, Panther Books, London) *The Condition of the Working Class in England.* An extract 'Health: 1844' is reproduced in Davey, B., Gray, A. and Seale, C. (eds) *Health and Disease: A Reader,* 2nd edn 1995; 3rd edn 2001, Open University Press, Buckingham.

Ehrlich, P., Ehrlich, A. and Holdren, J. (1970) *Ecoscience: Population, Resources and Environment,* Freeman, New York.

Epstein, P. R. (1999) Climate and health, *Science,* **285** (5 426), pp. 347–8. This article is also reproduced in Davey, B., Gray, A. and Seale, C. (eds) *Health and Disease: A Reader,* 3rd edn 2001, Open University Press, Buckingham.

Flinn, M. W. (1965) *An Economic and Social History of Britain 1066–1939,* Macmillan, London.

Fogel, R. (1994) Economic growth, population theory and physiology: the bearing of long-term processes on the making of economic policy, *American Economic Review,* **84,** pp. 369–95.

Food and Agriculture Organisation of the United Nations (1996) *The Sixth World Food Survey,* FAO, Rome.

Food and Agriculture Organisation of the United Nations (2000a), *FAOSTAT database,* FAO, Rome.

Food and Agriculture Organisation of the United Nations (2000b), *Agriculture: Towards 2015/ 30 — Interim technical report of the Global Perspectives Studies Unit,* FAO, Rome. (Also accessible at http://www.fao.org/WAICENT/FAOINFO/ECONOMIC/ESD/gstudies.htm)

Forbes, T. R. (1979) By what disease or casualty: the changing face of death in London, in Webster, C. (ed.) *Health, Medicine and Mortality in the Sixteenth Century,* Cambridge University Press, Cambridge.

Fox, J. and Goldblatt, P. (1982) OPCS Longitudinal Study, 1971–5, *Socio-Demographic Mortality Differentials,* Series LS, No. 1, HMSO, London.

Fox, J., Goldblatt, P. and Jones, D. (1990) Social class mortality differentials: artifact, selection or life circumstances? in OPCS (1990) *Longitudinal Study: Mortality and Social Organisation,* HMSO, London, pp. 99–108.

Frenk, J., Bobadilla, J. L. and Stern, C. (1991) Elements for a theory of the health transition, *Health Transition Review,* **1** (1), pp. 21–38.

Fries, J. F. (1989) Compression of morbidity: near or far?, *Milbank Quarterly,* **67,** pp. 208–32.

Fry, J. (1983) *Common Diseases,* 3rd edn, M.T.P. Press, Lancaster.

Ghani, A. C., Ferguson, N. M., Donnelly, C. A. and Anderson, R. M. (2000) Predicted vCJD mortality in Great Britain, *Nature,* **406,** pp. 583–4.

Giddens, A. (1998) *The Third Way: The Renewal of Social Democracy,* Polity Press Cambridge.

Goklany, I. M. (1999) Meeting global food needs: the environmental trade-offs between increasing land conversion and land productivity, pp. 256–89 in Morris, J. and Bate, R. (eds) *Fearing Food: Risk, Health and Environment,* Butterworth Heinemann, Oxford.

Goodman, A., Johnson, P. and Webb, S. (1997) *Inequality in the UK,* Oxford University Press, Oxford.

Government Statistical Service (1998) *Mortality Statistics: Cause 1998,* Series DH2 No. 25, The Stationery Office, London.

Griffiths, M., Payne, P. R., Stunkard, A. K., Rivers, I. R. W. and Cox, M. (1990) Metabolic rate and physical development in children at risk of obesity, *Lancet,* **ii,** pp. 76–8.

Halstead, S. B., Walsh, J. A. and Warren, K. S. (1985) *Good Health at Low Cost: Proceedings of a Conference held at the Bellagio Center, Bellagio, Italy,* 29 April–2 May 1985, Rockefeller Foundation, New York.

Harding, S., Bethune, A., Maxwell, R. and Brown, J. (1997) Mortality trends using the Longitudinal Study, Chapter 11 in Drever, F. and Whitehead, M. (eds) *Health Inequalities: Decennial Supplement*, Government Statistical Service, Series DS No. 15, The Stationery Office, London.

Harrington, G. (2000) *The Future of the Pig Industry: Local and Global*, Harper Adams, University College, Newport.

Harrison, P. (1979) *Inside the Third World*, Penguin, London.

Hartmann, B. and Boyce, J. K. (1983) *A Quiet Violence*, Zed Press, London.

Hawkes, S. and Azim, T. (2000) Bangladesh's response to HIV–AIDS (Health care systems in transition III; Bangladesh, Part II), *Journal of Public Health Medicine*, **22** (1), pp. 10–13.

Health Education Council (1983) *Report of the National Advisory Committee on Nutrition Education* (NACNE), HEC, London.

Hill, M. J. (1998) Meat or wheat for the next millennium? Meat and colo-rectal cancer, *Proceedings of the Nutrition Society*, **58**, pp. 261–4.

HMSO (1997) *Health Survey for England, 1997*, Her Majesty's Stationery Office, London.

Hobsbawm, E. (1969) *Industry and Empire*, Weidenfeld and Nicolson, London.

Hughes, R., Adnan, S. and Dalal-Clayton, B. (1994) *Floodplains or Flood Plans? A Review of Approaches to Water Management in Bangladesh*, International Institute for Environment and Development, London, and Research and Advisory Services, Dhaka.

Institute of Nutrition, Dhaka (1971 and 1981) *Bangladesh National Nutrition Surveys*, Institute of Nutrition, Dhaka.

Jette, A. M. (1980) Health status indicators: their utility in chronic disease evaluation research, *Journal of Chronic Diseases* **33**, pp. 567–79.

Jones, J. R., Hodgson, J. T. and Osman, J. (1997) *Self-reported working conditions in 1995: results from a household survey*, HSE Books, London.

Kelly, A. C. (1988) Economic consequences of population change in the Third World, *Journal of Economic Literature*, **XXVI**, pp. 1 685–728.

Kempson, E., Bryson, A. and Rowlingson, K. (1994) *Hard Times? How poor families make ends meet*, Policy Studies Institute, London.

Keys, A. (1980) *Seven Countries: a Multivariate Analysis of Death and Coronary Heart Disease*, Harvard University Press, London.

Kinnersley, P. (1974) *The Hazards of Work: How to Fight Them*, Pluto Press, London.

Kuhn, T. S. (1970) *The Structure of Scientific Revolutions,* University of Chicago Press, Chicago.

Kunst A. E., Groenhof, F. and Makenbach, J. P. (1998) Mortality by occupational class among men 30–64 years in 11 European countries, *Social Science and Medicine*, **46** (11), pp. 1 459–476.

Laslett, P. (1971) *The World We Have Lost*, 2nd edn, Methuen, London.

Latham, R. E. (1968) Introduction, in *The Travels of Marco Polo*, Pelican edition, London.

MacKenzie, D. (1999) This little piggy fell ill, *New Scientist*, 12 September, pp. 18–19.

Malcolm, L. A. (1974) Ecological factors relating to child growth and nutritional status, in Roche, A. F. and Falkner, F. (eds) *Nutrition and Malnutrition*, Plenum, New York.

Malthus, T. R. (1798) *An Essay on the Principles of Population*, reprinted in 1970 by Penguin, London.

Marmot, M. G. (1986) Social inequalities in mortality: the social environment, in Wilkinson, R. G. (ed.) *Class and Health: Research and Longitudinal Data*, Tavistock, London, pp. 21–33.

Marmot, M. G., Adelstein, A. M. and Bulusu, L. (1984) *Immigrant Mortality in England and Wales 1970–78*, OPCS Studies on Medical and Population Subjects No. 47, HMSO, London.

McEvedy, C. and Jones, R. (1978) *Atlas of World Population History*, Penguin, London.

McKeown, T. (1976) *The Modern Rise of Population*, Edward Arnold, London. An edited extract, 'The role of medicine', is reproduced in Davey, B., Gray, A. and Seale, C. (eds) *Health and Disease: A Reader*, 2nd edn 1995; 3rd edn 2001, Open University Press, Buckingham.

McNeill, W. (1976) *Plagues and People*, Basil Blackwell, Oxford.

Medical Services Study Group (1978) Deaths under 50, *British Medical Journal*, **2**, pp. 1 061–62. This article is also reproduced in Davey, B., Gray, A. and Seale, C. (eds) *Health and Disease: A Reader*, 2nd edn 1995; 3rd edn 2001, Open University Press, Buckingham.

Ministry of Agriculture Fisheries and Food (1999) *National Food Survey 1998: Annual Report on Food Expenditure, Consumption and Nutrient Intakes*, The Stationery Office, London.

Morgan, M. (1980) Marital status, health, illness and service use, *Social Science and Medicine*, **14A**, pp. 633–43.

Moser, K., Goldblatt, P. and Jones, D. (1990) Unemployment and mortality, in *OPCS Longitudinal Study 1971–81: Mortality and Social Organisation*, HMSO, London, Chapter 5.

Moss, R., Watson, A. and Ollason, J. (1982) *Animal Population Dynamics*, Chapman & Hall, London and New York.

Mudur, G. (2000) Half of Bangladesh population at risk of arsenic poisoning, *British Medical Journal*, **320** (7 238), p. 826.

Murray C. J. L. and Lopez A. D. (eds) (1994) *Global comparative assessments in the health sector: Disease burden, expenditures and intervention packages*, WHO, Geneva.

National Centre for Health Statistics (1999) *National Vital Statistics Reports*, **47**, No. 19, 1999, Hyattsville, Maryland.

National Dairy Council (1992) *Food and Health: What Does Britain Think?* National Dairy Council and MORI, London.

National Food Survey Committee (1983) *Household Food Consumption and Expenditure, 1981: Annual Report of the National Food Survey Committee*, HMSO, London.

Nickson, R. T., McArthur, J. M., Ravenscroft, P., Burgess, W. and Ahmed, K. M. (2000) Mechanism of arsenic release to groundwater, Bangladesh and West Bengal, *Applied Geochemistry*, **15**, pp. 403–13.

Notzon, F. C., Komarov, Y. M., Ermakov, S. P., Sempos, C. T., Marks, J. S. and Sempos, E. V. (1998) Causes of declining life expectancy in Russia, *Journal of the American Medical Association*, **279**, pp. 793–800.

O'Brien, P. M., Wheeler, T. and Barker, D. J. (1999) *Fetal programming: influences on development and disease in later life*, Proceedings of the 36th Royal College of Obstetricians and Gynaecologists' Study Group, RCOG, London.

ONS (various years) *Annual Abstract of Statistics*, The Stationery Office, London.

ONS (1998a) *Living in Britain: Results from the 1996 General Household Survey*, The Stationery Office, London.

ONS (1998b) *Mortality Statistics: Cause 1997*, ONS Series DH2, No. 24, The Stationery Office, London.

ONS (1999a) *Mortality Statistics: Cause 1998*, ONS Series DH2, No. 25, The Stationery Office, London.

ONS (1999b) *Regional Trends No. 34*, The Stationery Office, London.

ONS (2000a) *Living in Britain: Results from the 1998 General Household Survey*, The Stationery Office, London.

ONS (2000b) *Social Trends No. 30*, The Stationery Office, London.

OPCS (various years) *Adult Dental Health: Great Britain*, HMSO, London.

OPCS (1991) *General Household Survey 1989*, OPCS Series GHS, No. 20, HMSO, London.

OPCS (1995) *Occupational Health: Decennial Supplement*, The Registrar General's decennial supplement for England and Wales, edited by F. Drever, HMSO, London.

OPCS (1996) *General Household Survey 1994*, OPCS Series GHS No. 25, HMSO, London.

OPCS (1997) *General Household Survey 1995*, OPCS Series GHS, No. 26, HMSO, London.

OPCS (1998) *General Household Survey 1996*, The Stationery Office, London.

Open University (1982) D301 Historical Data and the Social Sciences, Units 5–8 *Historical Demography: Problems and Projects*, The Open University, Milton Keynes.

Parker, C. J., Morgan, K., Dewey, M. E. *et al.* (1997) Physical illness and disability among elderly people in England and Wales: the Medical Research Council cognitive function and ageing study, *Journal of Epidemiology and Community Health*; **51** (5), pp. 494–501.

Parkes, C. M., Benjamin, B. and Fitzgerald, R. G. (1969) Broken heart: a statistical study of increased mortality among widowers, *British Medical Journal*, **1**, pp. 740–43.

Phelps Brown, E. H. and Hopkins, S. V. (1956) Seven centuries of the prices of consumables compared with builders' wage-rates, *Economica*, **23**, pp. 296–314.

Phillimore, P. and Morris, D. (1991) Discrepant legacies: premature mortality in two industrial towns, *Social Science and Medicine*, **33** (2), pp. 139–52.

Pierce, J. T (1990) *The Food Resource: Themes in Resource Management*, Longman Scientific & Technical, Harlow, England.

Polo, Marco (1968 edn) *The Travels of Marco Polo*, translated by Latham, R. E., Penguin, London.

Powles, J. (1973) On the limitations of modern medicine, *Science, Medicine and Man*, **1** (1), pp. 1–30.

Pryer, J. (1990) *Socioeconomic and environmental aspects of undernutrition and ill health in an urban slum in Bangladesh*, PhD thesis, London University.

Rappoport, R. A. (1968) *Pigs for the Ancestors: Ritual in the Ecology of a New Guinea People*, Yale University Press, New Haven.

Registrar-General (various years) *Annual Abstract of Statistics*, The Stationery Office, London.

Rockney, B. P. (1991) *Soviet Statistics since 1950*, Dartmouth, Aldershot, UK.

Rosenbaum, S., Skinner, R. K., Knight, H. and Garrow, J. S. (1985) A survey of heights and weights of adults in Great Britain, *Annals of Human Biology*, **12**, pp. 115–27.

Royal College of General Practitioners/OPCS/DHSS (1995) *Morbidity Statistics from General Practice: Fourth National Study*, OPCS Series MB5, No. 3, HMSO, London.

Sahlins, M. (1974) *Stone Age Economics,* Tavistock, London.

Sandeman, P. M. (1997) Risk Communication: facing public outrage, *EPA Journal* (American Environmental Protection Agency Journal), November, pp. 21–2.

Sen, B. (1997) *Health and poverty in the context of country development strategy: a case study of Bangladesh*, WHO, Geneva.

Sesso, H. D., Gaziano, J. M., Buring, J. E. and Hennekens, C. H. (1999) Coffee and Tea intake and the risk of myocardial infarction, *American Journal of Epidemiology*, **149,** pp. 162–7.

Shellard, P. (1970) *Factory Life in 1774–1885,* Evans Bros, London.

Simon, J. (1981) *The Ultimate Resource*, Princeton University Press, Princeton.

Singer, B. H. and Manton, K. G. (1998) The effects of health changes on projections of health service needs for the elderly population of the United States, *Proceedings of the National Academy of Sciences of the USA*, **95** (26), pp. 15 618–22.

Smith, J. and Harding, S. (1997) Mortality of women and men using alternative social classifications, pp. 168–83 in Drever, F. and Whitehead, M. (eds) *Health inequalities: Decennial Supplement*, Government Statistical Service, Series DS No. 15, The Stationery Office, London.

Smith, L. C., Pashon, H. and del Ninno, C. (2000) Intra-household food distribution in the aftermath of the 1998 floods in Bangladesh (Conference presentation abstract 356.10), *FASEB Journal,* **14** (4), p. A503.

South African Institute of Race Relations (2000), *South African Survey, 1999/2000,* South African Institute of Race Relations, Johannesburg.

Southon, S. (1999) Soggy carrots and mushy broccoli could make you live longer, *New Scientist*, 5 June, p. 25.

Strassburg, M. (1982) The global eradication of smallpox, *American Journal of Infection Control,* **19,** pp. 220–5. An edited version of this article is reproduced in Davey, B., Gray, A. and Seale, C. (eds) *Health and Disease: A Reader,* 2nd edn 1995; 3rd edn 2001, Open University Press, Buckingham.

Szreter, S. (1988) The importance of social intervention in Britain's mortality decline c. 1850–1914: a re-interpretation of the role of public health, *Social History of Medicine*, **1,** pp. 1–37. An edited version of this article is reproduced in Davey, B., Gray, A. and Seale, C. (eds) *Health and Disease: A Reader,* 2nd edn 1995; 3rd edn 2001, Open University Press, Buckingham.

Tansey, G. and D'Silva, J. (eds) (1999) *The Meat Business: Devouring a Hungry Planet*, Earthscan Publications Ltd., London.

Teeman, T. (1999) The most important issue of our time, *The Times Weekend*, Saturday 6 November, p. 3.

Thompson, E. P. (1967) Time, work-discipline and industrial capitalism, *Past and Present*, **38,** pp. 56–97.

Townsend, P. (1979) *Poverty in the United Kingdom*, Penguin, London.

Townsend, P., Davidson, N. and Whitehead, M. (1990) *Inequalities in Health*, Penguin, London.

United Nations (1999a) *United Nations Demographic Yearbook 1997*, UN, New York,

United Nations (1999b) *The Demographic Impact of HIV/AIDS*, ESA/P/WP.152, UN, New York.

United Nations (1999c) *Levels and Trends of Contraceptive Use as Assessed in 1998*, UN, New York.

United Nations (1999d) *World Population Prospects 1998*, Volume 1 (ST/ESA/SER.A/177), UN, New York.

United Nations Children's Fund (1998) *The State of the World's Children*, Oxford University Press, Oxford.

United Nations Development Programme (1991) *Human Development Report 1991*, Oxford University Press, Oxford and New York.

United Nations Development Programme (1992) *Human Development Report 1992*, Oxford University Press, Oxford and New York.

United Nations Development Programme (1999) *Human Development Report 1999*, Oxford University Press, Oxford and New York.

Van Rossum, C. T., Shipley, M. J., van de Mheen, H., Grobbee, D. E., Marmot, M. G. (2000) Employment grade differences in cause specific mortality. A 25-year follow up of civil servants from the first Whitehall study, *Journal of Epidemiology and Community Health*, **54**, pp. 178–84.

Velazquez, A. and Bourges, H. (eds) (1984) *Genetic Factors in Nutrition,* Academic Press, London and New York.

Webster, C. (ed.) *Health, Medicine and Mortality in the Sixteenth Century*, Cambridge University Press, Cambridge.

Westoff, C. F. (1974) The populations of the developed countries, *Scientific American*, **231** (3), September, pp. 108–22.

Wilkinson, R. G. (1986a) Occupational class, selection and inequalities in health: a reply to Raymond Illsley, *Quarterly Journal of Social Affairs*, **2**, pp. 415–22.

Wilkinson, R. G. (1986b) Socio-economic differences in mortality: interpreting the data on their size and trends, in Wilkinson, R. G. (ed.) *Class and Health: Research and Longitudinal Data*, Tavistock, London.

Wilkinson, R. G. (1986c) Income and mortality, in Wilkinson, R. G. (ed.) *Class and Health: Research and Longitudinal Data*, Tavistock, London.

Winter, J. M. (1982) The decline of mortality in Britain, 1870–1950, in Barker, T. and Drake, M. (eds) *Population and Society in Britain, 1850–1950*, Batsford Academic and Educational, London.

World Bank (1982) *World Development Report 1982*, Oxford University Press, Oxford and New York.

World Bank (1991) *World Development Report 1991*, Oxford University Press, Oxford and New York.

World Bank (1993) *World Development Report 1993: Investing in Health*, Oxford University Press, New York

World Bank (1999) *Global Economic Indicators Database*, Washington DC.

World Bank (2000) *Entering the 21st Century: World Development Report 1999/2000,* Oxford University Press, Oxford and New York.

World Cancer Research Fund (1997) *Food Nutrition and the Prevention of Cancer: a Global Perspective*, AICR, Washington DC.

World Health Organisation (1958) *Constitution of the World Health Organisation*, WHO, Geneva.

World Health Organisation (1978) *The Declaration of Alma Ata,* WHO, Geneva.

World Health Organisation (1990) *Diet, Nutrition and the Prevention of Chronic Disease*, Report of a WHO Study Group, WHO Technical Report Series, No. 797, Geneva.

World Health Organisation (1997) *Obesity: Preventing and Managing the Global Epidemic,* WHO, Geneva.

World Health Organisation (1999) *World Health Report 1999: Making a Difference*, WHO, Geneva.

World Resources, 1998–99 (1999) A joint publication by The World Resources Institute; The United Nations Environment Programme; The United Nations Development Programme; The World Bank. Oxford University Press, Oxford and New York.

Wrigley, E. A. and Schofield, R. S. (1989) *The Population History of England 1541–1871: a Reconstruction*, paperback edn, Cambridge University Press, Cambridge.

Yusuf, H. R., Akhter, H. H., Rahman, M. H., Chowdhury, M. E. E. K and Rochat, R. W. (2000) Injury-related deaths among women aged 10–50 years in Bangladesh, 1996–97, *Lancet*, **355** (9 211), pp. 1 220–24.

Further sources

For those interested in world health, population, development and environment, the following *annual* publications are always worth referring to, for information, commentary, analysis and references to other research:

Human Development Report (United Nations Development Programme, Oxford University Press, Oxford and New York, also available along with other data and publications at http://www.undp.org/indexalt.html) gives an overview of social and economic development around the world during the past few decades and of the prospects for the future;

World Development Report (World Bank, Oxford University Press, Oxford and New York, and at http://www.worldbank.org/) concentrates more on economic development. It is an essential source of economic, demographic and health-related data, with annual features on topics such as environment, debt or population;

World Resources: A Guide to the Global Environment (World Resources Institute, Oxford University Press, Oxford and New York, and http://www.wri.org/wri/index.html) provides a wealth of information on conditions and trends in the global environment.

Other invaluable web sites, with news, downloadable reports and databases include the World Health Organisation (http://www.who.int/), the Food and Agriculture Organization (http://www.fao.org/), the United Nations Population Fund (http://www.unfpa.org/index.htm), the United Nations Population Information Network (http://www.undp.org/popin/), and the International Food Policy Research Institute (http://www.ifpri.org).

A selection of books and articles with particular relevance to specific topics covered in this book follows:

Global comparative assessments in the health sector: Disease burden, expenditures and intervention packages (1994, WHO, Geneva), edited by C. J. L. Murray and A. D. Lopez, gives a full account of the DALY approach to estimating the global burden of disease.

Using Bangladesh as a case study, *Out of the Shadow of Famine: Evolving Food Markets and Food Policy*, edited by R. Ahmed, S. Haggblade and T. Chowd (2000, Johns Hopkins University Press, USA), describes how new approaches by governments of the South Asian subcontinent to food policy and food market reforms, are helping to free the region from the constant threat of famine.

A very entertaining and accessible speculation on palaeopathology, the hunter–gatherers and the influence of our evolutionary past is *The Rise and Fall of the Third Chimpanzee*, by Jared Diamond (1992, Vintage, London).

Also by Jared Diamond, *Guns, Germs and Steel: a short history of everybody for the last 13 000 years* (1998, Vintage, London), suggests how the original natural distribution of plants and animals that humans were able to adapt for food, together with the lethal pressures of the contagious diseases that co-evolved with them, might have contributed to the very uneven distribution of power and wealth amongst nations and cultures that we see in the world today.

In *Changing the Face of the Earth: Culture, Environment, History* (2nd edition, 1996, Blackwell, Oxford and Cambridge, Mass.) I. G. Simmons gives a most enjoyable and wide ranging account of how the human species, throughout its evolution, has continuously modified its own environment.

A clear overview of the development process and its relation to health, deprivation and hunger is set out in *Development as Freedom* by Amartya Sen (1999, Oxford University Press, Oxford).

Robert Fogel's lecture on receiving the Alfred Nobel Memorial Prize in Economic Sciences, entitled 'Economic growth, population theory, and physiology: the bearing of long-term processes on the making of economic policy' (1994, *American Economic Review*, **84**, pp. 369–95) gives an accessible overview of research linking economic development to changes in health and human physiology since 1700.

An authoritative study of England's historical experience of mortality, fertility, population, famine, marriage and related topics is *The Population History of England 1541–1871: a Reconstruction* by E. A. Wrigley and R. S. Schofield (1989, Cambridge University Press, Cambridge), and its companion volume *English Population History from Family Reconstitution 1580–1837* by E. A. Wrigley, J. E. Oeppen, R. S. Davies and R. S. Schofield (1997, Cambridge University Press, Cambridge).

The two volume collection of material entitled *The Health of Adult Britain 1841–1994*, edited by J. Charlton and M. Murphy (1997, ONS, Series DS no. 12, The Stationery Office, London) offers an excellent commentary and overview of morbidity and mortality in Britain over the last 150 years, as seen through official statistics.

Understanding Health Inequalities (Graham, H., ed., 2000, Open University Press, Buckingham) is a collection of articles by leading researchers whose work is directed towards explaining and reducing inequalities in health in the UK. The book is edited by Hilary Graham and is divided into four sections: ethnicity, gender and socio-economic status; how health is shaped by experiences and exposures over the lifecourse; how home and neighbourhood may have an additional influence on health; and assessing the impact of public policy on inequalities in health.

Agriculture: Towards 2015/30, FAO Technical Interim Report (April 2000) is a massive report by the Food and Agriculture Organisation (over 300 pages, but all downloadable from *www.fao.org/WAICENT/FAOINFO/ECONOMIC/ESD/gstudies.htm*). It reviews the technical problems and resource demands facing the world's farmers, in continuing to produce as much food as the increasing and — gradually wealthier — global population can afford to buy, projecting up to 2030. It builds up the picture from country level and sketches out in considerable detail the prospects for increased production of vegetable, meat, fish and dairy foods. Finally, it reviews the impacts and costs on the natural environment and the finite resource bases (land, water, fertilisers etc.) of using conventional intensive farming methods, and comments on the potential that GM crops may have to reduce the pressure on these resources and hence lessen the destruction of habitats.

Internet database (ROUTES)

A large amount of valuable information is available via the Internet. To help OU students and other readers of books in the *Health and Disease* series to access good quality sites without having to search for hours, the OU has developed a collection of Internet resources on a searchable database called ROUTES. All websites included in the database are selected by academic staff or subject-specialist librarians. The content of each website is evaluated to ensure that it is accurate, well presented and regularly updated. A description is included for each of the resources.

The URL for ROUTES is: http://routes.open.ac.uk/

Entering the OU course code U205 in the search box will retrieve all the resources that have been recommended for *Health and Disease*. Alternatively if you want to search for any resources on a particular subject, type in the words which best describe the subject you are interested in.

For example, the Office of Health Economics (OHE) commissions research and publishes reviews of UK health data, with an emphasis on economic aspects (http://www.ohe.org/). Data collected, analysed and published by the Office for National Statistics (ONS) can be accessed via the UK government's National Statistics website (http://www.statistics.gov.uk/).

Other useful websites include the Department of Health (http://www.doh.gov.uk/) and the electronic British Medical Journal (http://www.bmj.com/).

Answers to questions

Chapter 2

1 (a) This is a straightforward calculation. All that is required is to add the percentages of the female population in the age bands from 65 upwards. Obviously this can only be done roughly from Figure 2.1, but the percentages in the age groups above 65 in the Russian Federation add up to almost 16 per cent. This is a smaller figure than for, say, Sweden, where the comparable figure is over 20 per cent, but is much larger than the proportion in South Africa or China. Such profound differences have serious implications for patterns of disease, as you will see in Chapter 3, and for the organisation of health care.

(b) From Figure 2.9:

(i) The pyramid in Figure 2.9a indicates a population in which birth and death rates have been low for many years, and in which the proportion in older age-groups — particularly females — is high. These features suggest a country that has been industrialised for a long time. The country is the United Kingdom in 1997. The pyramid in Figure 2.9b indicates a population in transition from the pattern typical of a developing country to an industrialised one. The narrowness at the top of the pyramid suggests there has been high mortality and fertility in the past. However, the shape at the bottom suggests that child and infant mortality rates have been falling, and the indentation right at the bottom suggests a decline in fertility, perhaps as a result of a family planning programme. Taken together, these features suggest a developing country that is industrialising fairly rapidly. The country is the Republic of Korea in 1997.

(ii) Because of the relatively large number of older people in the UK, we might reasonably expect the crude death rate there to be fairly high, but the age-standardised death rates to be low. This is typical for industrialised countries. In contrast, the reverse would be expected in the Republic of Korea in 1997. With its young population it would be expected to have a low crude death rate but higher age-standardised rates. In fact, the crude death rates for the UK and the Republic of Korea were respectively 11 and 5 per 1 000. However, if the Republic of Korea had the *same* age–sex structure as the UK, but the present age- and sex-specific death rates, its crude death rate would have risen to 18 per 1 000.

(c) This would only be possible if the conditions in the country were to remain constant over the lifetime of the child. For many countries this is not so. A population pyramid is a snapshot of the population at a given time — it is based on cross-sectional data. The predictions it makes about the evolution of a system over time must be treated with great scepticism.

2 At first sight, you might expect the crude death rate to be the more useful measure in that it covers deaths occurring in the entire population, whereas the infant mortality rate only measures deaths in a very narrow age-band. However, because the crude death rate covers the entire population, it is influenced by the age- and sex-structure of the population; consequently it may be misleading to compare the crude death rates in two different countries if their populations do not have a similar age–sex structure. Because the infant mortality rate only covers those aged up to 1-year-old, it does not suffer from this problem. A country's infant mortality rate may not be an accurate guide to more general levels of mortality in that country, but normally it provides a rough indication.

3   The absolute difference between the IMR in Brazil and the average for the more developed world has narrowed, from around 179 to 33 per 1 000 live births. However, the *relative* difference has widened substantially, from 2.4 times higher in 1950–55 to 4.7 times higher in 1995–2000. In other words, the IMR in the more developed world has been falling at a faster rate than it has in Brazil.

Chapter 3

1   In general, the chapter showed that the so-called 'tropical' diseases are not in fact the major cause of death in developing countries, and that the major causes of death in these countries also occur in industrialised countries — good examples are the respiratory diseases such as pneumonia, influenza, measles, bronchitis and whooping cough. The mortality differences between developing and industrialised countries arise in part from the very different impact these diseases have. In addition, the different age structure of the populations in industrialised countries, with a much higher proportion of older people, means that the degenerative diseases contribute a higher proportion of deaths there than in the developing countries.

2   'Years of potential life lost' weight deaths according to the age at which they occur. 'Disability adjusted life years' (DALYs) also give weight to the age of death, combined with a measure of healthy life lost from disability. As infant and childhood deaths are very much more common in developing countries than in industrialised countries, both these measures are very good at emphasising this difference.

3   Diseases create substantial costs. For example, malaria is expensive to control and results in many lost days of work. In addition, there is evidence that high morbidity lowers productivity and compounds poverty, thus slowing economic development. So investment in health care can be an investment in economic development.

4   Zoonotic diseases are shared by humans and other species and are transmissable to humans from the disease reservoir in these species, either directly or by a disease vector (an intermediary animal, most often an insect). Examples of zoonotic diseases include brucellosis, rabies, plague, tuberculosis, gastroenteritis and typhus. Rabies is an example of a directly transmitted disease, and yellow fever is a vector-borne disease, transmitted from monkeys and rodents to humans by certain kinds of mosquito. Zoonotic diseases may be difficult to control because reservoirs of infection exist in other species and these may be hard to detect and eliminate.

5   You may have used data from Table 2.3 from the previous chapter alongside Table 3.6 in this chapter.

   (a) Expectation of life at birth in Bangladesh is similar for males and females, at 59 years. In the UK females have a significantly longer life expectancy at birth — 79 years compared with 74 years for males.

(b) In Bangladesh males have a slight advantage from birth to around 30 years, but by the age of 50 the difference has disappeared. In the UK the female advantage in life expectancy at birth persists at all ages.

(c) One consequence of these gender differences in expectation of life (and of other factors such as male and female birth rates) is that Bangladesh has a population structure in which the actual ratio of males to females is higher than might be predicted from the demography of African, Latin American or European countries, and in 1981 this was estimated to be equivalent to 1.6 million 'missing' women (Table 3.5).

6   To decide what to include it would be best to consider the cost in relation to the health improvement obtained by each intervention: that is, to calculate cost-effectiveness. For example, Table 3.8 showed that the cost of AIDS prevention was $112 per person receiving care but the cost per disability adjusted life year gained was only $3–5. By contrast, acute services only cost $6 per person who would benefit but the cost per DALY was $200–300. Consequently, if the objective is to get as much health gain as possible with the budget, it would be best to concentrate on AIDS prevention. Just knowing the cost per person receiving care is insufficient to make rational decisions.

Chapter 4

1   The narrative profile gave important insights into the processes that undermine the health and security of poor rural families, and may even threaten their lives. For example, the unresolved dispute with Sophi's brothers over the ownership of the half-acre of land inherited from her father adds to the family's insecurity. The underlying reasons for the stunting and wasting of the children are revealed by the inability of this small plot to provide enough food for the family, particularly in the 'hungry' season before the main harvest, by the strenuous physical labour contributed by the children, and by stories of their repeated bouts of infection at an early age. Through the eyes of Sophi's sister, we gain a glimpse of life in the city for migrants from the rural population who have been forced to seek work there in the textile mills. These qualitative accounts 'bring alive' the statistical information and suggest areas for potential intervention; all good case studies should have practical applications. The limitation and potential danger of a narrative profile such as this one is that it must be representative of the lives of the rural poor in general; if it is not, it risks distorting the readers' understanding of health and disease in Bangladesh.

2   At the top of the list must come the extent of the population in absolute poverty, lacking the basic essentials of clean water and sanitation, adequate food, shelter from the extremes of climate, and even the bare minimum of education and health care. These features of rural life are also found in urban squatter camps, where the proximity of people living in destitution increases the transmission of measles, the diarrhoeal diseases and parasite infestations to which so many children succumb. Undernutrition increases susceptibility to infectious diseases, and though smallpox and plague are distant memories, cholera and TB are growing threats. The discovery that water from bore-holes is contaminated with arsenic may increase the use of polluted surface water and trigger further epidemics. Malaria has begun to return as mosquitos and parasites become resistant to chemical controls and traffic from heavily-infested neighbouring states increases. Although HIV rates are currently very low, syphilis is already prevalent in the substantial 'high-risk' population of sex workers, migrant

labourers and injecting drug-users; condom use is rare (contraception is primarily via the female contraceptive pill), so all the pre-conditions for wildfire spread of HIV are present.

3   For a small farming family in Bangladesh:

(a) Improved access to basic health services would have an impact on child survival (e.g. through better immunisation programmes) and this could be expected to increase the survival of girls to levels comparable with that of boys. It would also reduce the risk of maternal mortality through the provision of contraceptive services and ante- and post-natal care. Easier availability of essential drugs, especially antibiotics, would benefit all age groups and might especially reduce the risk of loss of production or employment through illness at critical times of the year.

(b) Improved food security would mean not only the ability to avoid seasonal hunger and reduce the impact of infectious diseases by improving resistance, but it would also reduce indebtedness and perhaps even allow families to build some reserves of cash or credit against the risk of natural disasters. It might make investment possible — in education for a child perhaps.

These two kinds of improvements are not mutually exclusive, but to have any meaning, both have to be treated as investments in a future. The 'twist' to the question of course is that the food security of such households could only be improved in a sustained way by structural changes in the security of land tenure and the availability of secure employment and reasonable credit — in other words by laying the foundations for the future.

4   Achieving a 'replacement' rate of fertility (i.e. close to 2.2 children per female in the population), at the earliest possible date, must rank as one of the highest development aims of the country. The longer it takes for this to happen, the larger will be the final equilibrium population size and this in turn will imply greater demands on agricultural production of food and hence greater pressure upon the natural environment — to the detriment of both human and wild-life populations. However, the cost of achieving population stabilisation through family planning services will be massive and is estimated at three times the current health budget annually until at least 2045. If Bangladesh is to afford such an ambitious population control programme, it implies such a substantial increase in industrial and agricultural development will be needed to fund it that the sustainability of the natural environment is sure to be threatened.

Chapter 5

1   Infectious diseases such as measles cannot remain endemic in very small and scattered populations. The Agricultural Revolution increased food production and so populations increased and agricultural areas became more densely populated. This provided the conditions under which many new types of infectious diseases could have a fairly constant presence (for example, food stores attract vermin).

2   This is a broadly accurate statement in relation to the human population in total, which was probably remarkably stable over long periods with a very low growth rate. However, the 'punctuation marks' of sudden changes in death rates were very frequent: data from France indicates up to 13 general famines occurred in the course of the eighteenth century. And at the local level there may well have been substantial sharp fluctuations in population numbers.

3 Changes in real wages can affect mortality rates (as wages rise, mortality falls and vice versa), thus changing the population size as represented in the upper loop in the Malthusian model (Figure 5.5). Real-wage changes also alter nuptiality, which in turn affects the fertility rate (as wages rise, so too do nuptiality and fertility, and vice versa), thus changing the population size as represented in the lower loop in Figure 5.5.

4 The Industrial Revolution was driving changes in the social structure of people's lives that greatly increased the importance of coordinated routines and time-keeping. Technological change was also cheapening certain goods such as watches, making them available to a mass market. Finally, many industrial towns were accumulating sufficient wealth to erect public buildings as symbols of civic pride and opulence.

5 Many people were being forced to leave rural areas as a result of landlessness due to enclosures or unemployment, and had nowhere to go but to the cities. Also, although conditions were appalling in the cities, they may have been no better in many rural areas because of the changes the Industrial Revolution was making to the country as a whole. The riots in the countryside by people on the verge of starvation testify to this.

Chapter 6

1 The most likely cause is autonomous infectious disease (exogenous epidemics) — the evidence in the chapter indicates that 'crises of subsistence' only increased the mortality rate by three or four times, whereas the mortality crises in the years listed in the question are six to ten times greater than the underlying mortality rate.

2 We managed four reasons:
   (i) Changes have occurred since 1550 in the definition of what constitutes hysteria (a subject discussed in detail in Chapter 6 of the first book in this series, *Medical Knowledge: Doubt and Certainty* (2nd edition 1994; colour-enhanced 2nd edition 2001; Open University Press, Buckingham); in particular, there has been the gradual disappearance of 'hysteria' as a medically-recognised disease category in Western countries;
   (ii) Changes have also occurred in the social construction of the condition, largely driven by doctors through the ages; for example, a medieval interpretation of hysteria would have been in terms of the 'wandering womb', but this was supplanted in the nineteenth century by the failure to find any physical lesions in the body that could cause hysteria; the incorporation of Freudian theory into medical practice in the twentieth century led to the acceptance of psychological causes;
   (iii) In comparison with today, in 1550 there were few qualified practitioners to make the diagnosis and few people had access to them, so prevalence would have been under-recorded;
   (iv) Another huge problem is the lack of adequate and reliable records surviving from the sixteenth century, to show what people suffered from.

3 A rise in fertility and a decline in mortality both contributed to the expansion in the population of England between 1680 and 1850. However, the evidence in Chapter 6 suggests that the rise in the birth rate *contributed two and a half times as much* to the increase in population as did the decline in the death rate.

4   According to Szreter, McKeown's thesis runs as follows: declines in air-borne diseases were the main factor in reducing mortality during the nineteenth century; there is no evidence of effective public health measures to contain or combat them during this period; therefore the population must have become more resistant to them, and the most likely way this happened was by improved *nutrition*. However, Szreter argues that McKeown has *over*-emphasised the decline in air-borne diseases and *under*-estimated the decline in water-borne diseases during the nineteenth century. Szreter suggests that *public health measures* against water-borne disease in the nineteenth century and against air-borne diseases in the twentieth century were of great importance, and that the role of nutrition as an isolated factor is less clear than McKeown concluded.

5   As Figure 6.2 shows, the period from 1541 to the start of the eighteenth century was one in which birth rates and death rates both oscillated, but broadly birth rates were falling while the death rate was static or rising. This pattern does not fit any of the stages of the model of demographic transition precisely: stage 1 of the model is characterised by a high death rate and a high birth rate. However, almost by definition, models are simplifications of reality and often put erratic and irregular events to one side. And this particular model does fit the broad pattern of events in England from the eighteenth century onwards.

Chapter 7

1   In 1800, manufacturing production in the UK was only a small fraction of manufacturing production in the developing countries. Even in 1850 UK production was only *half* that in the developing countries, so in this sense it was not 'the workshop of the world'. However, the phrase is more accurate in conveying the notion of a great concentration of manufacturing production in one not very populous country. Furthermore, as Table 7.1 shows, by 1880 the UK was producing more manufactured goods than all the developing countries combined, and continued to do so until the late 1950s.

2   It is true that a country's level of GNP per person is not always a reliable guide to standards of health, education or other aspects of human development. This is partly due to the fact that a nation's wealth may be unequally distributed across the population or may be directed to other policy objectives and areas of spending, such as military expenditure or industrial expansion. The Human Development Index (HDI) does go some way to take account of health, education and income distribution, and so does move away from 'means' towards 'ends'. However, it does not take account of important issues such as civil liberties. There is in fact a broad association between the GNP and HDI measures. To view the question from a different perspective, some people may consider that education and health are not 'ultimate ends', but are themselves means to attaining an end, such as prosperity or security.

3   The developing countries do have a much larger population than the industrialised countries: in fact 85 per cent of the world's population are in low-income or middle-income countries. But these countries are so much poorer that their *share* of world GNP is very small indeed: as the text noted and Table 7.2 showed, the 60 per cent of the world's population in the poorest (low-income) countries accounts for just 6 per cent of world GNP. Even when their share is adjusted for 'purchasing power parity', it still only amounts to 20 per cent of the world's wealth.

4   The two most important shared difficulties are that:

(a) Production may go unrecorded because it is in the subsistence sector, or within the family, or is bartered or exchanged unofficially;

(b) The *average* food production per person and the *average* GNP per person are both likely to disguise inequalities in distribution, so that many people may not in fact get the average or anything like it.

5   No. Sen and Drèze stress that food availability *must* be one of the factors that determine entitlement. They list four ways in which the two may be linked:

• subsistence farming can be thought of as 'direct entitlement';

• entitlement is influenced by the price of food, which is influenced by food availability;

• food production can be a major source of employment;

• a stock of available food in a public distribution system can be an important instrument to combat starvation and improve entitlement.

However, their central point is that a range of *other* factors also influence the command over food that different sections of the population can exercise.

Chapter 8

1   It is true that population change is subject to many factors and uncertainties, some of which are poorly understood. And projections frequently have turned out to be inaccurate and have had to be revised substantially. However, most population projections include a range of different assumptions (for example, high, middle or low projections, given different rates of fertility decline). Moreover, populations have a fair degree of momentum built into them, so that short-term projections are unlikely to be very wide of the mark. Finally, projections are not always intended as predictions, but rather as illustrations of what might happen if present trends continue. Their merit is in illustrating a possible outcome against which informed public debate can take place.

2   The developing countries have followed the broad path of demographic transition characterised by high birth rates and death rates, followed by falling death rates and continued high birth rates, and then a fall in birth rates. However, the rate of population growth in developing countries has been much higher than anything experienced in the past in England or other industrialised countries. In addition, the fall in death rates in England and other industrialised countries occurred over a long period of time, whereas in the developing countries it has been compressed into a few decades. Finally, the industrialising countries of the nineteenth century exported a large portion of their population growth in the form of international migration to former European colonies and the USA; this has not happened (so far) to anything like the same extent in the current developing countries.

3   The main factors are: the overall level of development; education levels, especially female literacy; rates of child survival; the cultural setting, including the influence of particular religions; government population policies, including family planning programmes and the availability of acceptable and affordable contraception.

Education levels (particularly female literacy) and child survival are among the most important factors, but innovative family planning programmes can be successful (as in Bangladesh).

4   It is true that the objective of most developing countries is low mortality in absolute terms. But as Table 8.2 showed, the 'superior health achievers' — countries that have achieved a lower *relative* mortality rate than might have been predicted on the basis of their income level — have also achieved lower mortality and longer life expectancy in *absolute* terms than the 'inferior health achievers' — the group of countries doing particularly badly in relation to their income level. The relevance of the superior health achievers is in demonstrating that low mortality is not an automatic spin-off from rising levels of income.

Chapter 9

1   Although skin diseases are not mentioned in the chapter among the important causes of death, and are not a common reason for admission to hospital (Figure 9.5), they do cause considerable morbidity. They are one of the commonest reasons for consultations in general practice (Table 9.2 and Figure 9.5). Skin diseases do not appear to cause much physical impairment (Figure 9.7), though people who suffer severe skin conditions may well experience considerable social handicap.

2   Almost certainly not. The younger cohort are unlikely to experience the same rate of dental decay suffered by the older cohort. For instance, the younger groups may have benefited from using fluoride toothpaste, eating less refined sugar and receiving better dental care, so a higher proportion may retain their teeth than was true for the older cohort who were born around 1910 and have not enjoyed these benefits. Figure 9.6 contains some evidence of such cohort effects: for example, 64 per cent of the group who were aged 55–64 in 1968 had already lost all their teeth, but ten years later, when they were aged 65–74, this had increased a further 10 percentage points to 74 per cent. In comparison, 48 per cent of the group aged 55–64 in 1978 had lost all their teeth, but ten years later, when they were aged 65–75, this percentage had barely increased at all. So at the same stage of the life cycle, the groups born more recently were more likely to have some of their own teeth and were losing teeth at a much slower rate.

3   Table 9.3 only gives information grouped into manual and non-manual classes. However, it does broadly support the argument that mortality rates are lower amongst married than unmarried men and women, whether in manual or non-manual social classes. It appears from the table that being unmarried has a greater adverse effect on women in manual social classes than in non-manual classes. However, information on statistical significance would be required to support this statement.

4   First, it should be noted that minority ethnic groups are not a homogeneous group, and that there are difficulties of definition and measurement. In general, migrants to England and Wales experience excess mortality in comparison with the population as a whole (Table 9.4). Many minority ethnic groups also give lower self-assessments of their general health than does the population as a whole (Table 9.5). Overall, GP consultation ratios amongst minority ethnic groups are higher than those for the population as a whole (Figure 9.13). The limited information available on reasons for consulting a GP suggests that minority ethnic groups differ from the general population mainly in the degree to which they consult, rather than in the kind of conditions they bring.

5   (a) For a biological explanation, you may have suggested the influence on the human body of climatic or geological factors, such as hours of sunshine or water hardness.

   (b) A social explanation could be variations in housing standards or in income or occupation.

   (c) A life-history explanation might be alcohol or tobacco consumption (although this is also a social explanation as levels of consumption may be affected by income).

6   The only exception to the 'health gradient' in social class mortality mentioned in the chapter was that of breast cancer mortality (Figure 9.17), which is higher in social classes I&II than in social classes IIIN and IIIM; however, the rate is still highest in social classes IV&V. Although other exceptions do exist, the vast majority of diseases either show no social class gradient or are commoner in lower social classes. This is true whether mortality, morbidity, or disability is being measured.

7   Low-back pain is likely to increase with age due to biological 'wear and tear' on the backbone and its musculature, but the increase will be greatest in those regularly engaged in occupational or domestic heavy lifting, i.e. those in the manual social classes. Thus the *combined* influence of age and social class needs to be taken into account, and an analysis of either factor alone would distort the apparent distribution of back pain in the population.

8   The large size of the total sample and the high proportion of people from ethnic minorities who were included (almost half the total sample) tend to give confidence that the data on health and health-care use within each group is statistically robust. Note that the sample is not representative, in the sense that the proportions of people in the sample from ethnic minority groups are deliberately much higher than in the general population. However, the point of the survey was not to establish how many people there are in ethnic minority groups, but to see how similar or different they are from the whole population in their health and health-care use.

   Confidence in the *reliability* of the survey would be further increased by knowing that the numbers of respondents in each of the different ethnic groups surveyed was sufficiently large to allow statistical significance tests to be carried out on the results (it was). Therefore, we can be fairly confident about generalising the results from this sample to the various ethnic minority populations as a whole.

   The combination of two different methodologies — questionnaire-based interviews which reveal the self-perceptions and reports of the respondents, and objective measurements of e.g. height, weight and blood samples — further increase confidence in the *validity* of the survey (i.e. that the conclusions are *valid* reflections of the actual health status of the respondents). Confidence in the validity of the results would also require that interviews were conducted by native-speakers in the appropriate language, or at least that interpreters were present (they were).

Chapter 10

1   Figure 10.1 shows that health inequalities widened across social classes for men aged 20–64 over the period 1970–72 to 1991–93. It has been suggested that these *cross-sectional* data, which are based on Decennial Supplements,

might be prone to various measurement errors (as described in Section 10.2), for example that the classification of social classes may have altered between one census and the next. The OPCS Longitudinal Study (Table 10.1) avoids most of the potential measurement errors because it tracks the same individuals over time, and it too shows that health inequalities across the social classes have widened among men and women from 1976–81 to 1986–92. The fact that two different ways of tracking the size of the 'health gradient' produces the same results increases confidence in the conclusion that health inequalities really did get worse from the 1970s to the 1990s.

2   Table 10.2 does show that the proportion of the population in the lowest social classes (classes IIIM, IV and V) fell from 54 per cent in 1981 to 49 per cent by 1991. These are the social classes with the poorest health experience. However, there are at least two reasons why this does not necessarily imply that health inequalities must have declined also. First, there are inequalities *within* social classes as well as between them. Second, many measures of inequality do not simply count the proportions at the lowest end of the distribution, but attempt to assess the degree of inequality *above* as well as *below* the average. The highest social classes with the best health experience have grown substantially in size, and so, on most measures, inequality in health has not diminished. In fact, the answer to Q.1 above showed that it has increased.

3   Patterns of smoking vary substantially by social class, with higher rates found in lower social classes (Table 10.5). As smoking is a major cause of death (Chapter 9), this is likely to be reflected in mortality differences between social classes, although it may take many years for *current* patterns of smoking to appear in mortality rates, particularly among women who generally took up smoking later than men (the audiotape on the global health impacts of smoking refers to this). The influence of drinking is less certain: as Figure 10.4 shows, the proportion of men who can be classified as heavy drinkers is higher in the lower social classes, but so is the proportion who do not drink at all. Among women, drinking appears to be more prevalent in the higher social classes.

4   Occupation is a useful classification because it contributes to morbidity and mortality both in *direct* ways (e.g. injury and death rates are much more common in manual occupations such as construction work than they are in professional or managerial occupations), and also in *indirect* ways through the health consequences of income, housing standards, quality of nutrition, stress levels, etc. associated with different occupations. Occupation itself may account for up to 20 per cent of the health gap between top and bottom social classes. We can estimate this by standardising death rates between occupations.

5   The first quote, from RoSPA, emphasises individual responsibility for accidents and largely blames defects in personal behaviour such as carelessness or irritability (although it does mention working conditions, in passing). This view echoes that of the Medical Services Study Group in attributing deaths under 50 to 'self-destructive' habits such as smoking and drinking. The second quote stresses the influence of physical conditions at work and the way in which the work is organised (a viewpoint we discuss in depth in another book in this series — see Chapter 8 of *Birth to Old Age: Health in Transition*, 2nd edn 1995; colour-enhanced 2nd edn 2001; Open University Press, Buckingham). This 'structural' view of the causes of accidents at work is similar to one you will meet in Chapter 5 of that book, in a study of accidents to children on the Corkerhill Estate in Glasgow; the authors concluded that parents were

knowledgeable about accident prevention but were defeated by the extent of the environmental hazards facing their children.)

Chapter 11

1   A sustained deficit of energy, affecting a significant proportion of the population, would imply the existence of famine — continuing loss of body weight and a rising death rate from starvation. If the situation then stabilised, with a fixed, but reduced supply, there would be many very thin people and deaths from starvation would reduce population growth to zero. If there were none of these signs of energy deficit, then some other nutrient in the food supply might be limiting health, and the information needed would be the prevalence of some deficiency disease.

2   (a)   Small average stature of the adult population *per se* has few implications for health policy, since nothing can be done to correct it. It may simply be a reflection of adverse factors or circumstances when those adults were very young.

    (b)   Frequent faltering of growth of children under two-years-old is evidence of impoverished home environments, leading to a high risk of infections and/or low levels of care, including inadequate feeding. The policy implications are for better access to basic preventive health services, better housing and sanitation, and better employment conditions and education, especially for women. More food in the house would help, but it would probably be more effective to raise household income and hence make available more time and resources for child care, rather than to provide more food. The real problem would be deciding which of all these to concentrate on first.

3   They would all have to engage in work that was *physically* much harder — probably the man at labouring and the woman and children at growing, preserving and preparing whatever food the man's wages would not cover so their energy consumption would go up. However, they would probably lose some body weight and because of that, would reduce their 'maintenance' needs for energy, hence raising their work efficiency. If Cobbett's figures are correct, after these adjustments, they would be eating about 30 per cent more food than before their time trip.

4   The increased productivity has been achieved partly by improved farming practice — improved varieties of crops and the use of fertilizers (dung, and later chemicals); partly by more efficient management of human labour, leading to economies of scale; but mainly by a large increase of energy inputs (lately in the form of fuel oil). One consequence has been a large net production of carbon dioxide, with adverse effects on the global climate. Changing this contribution to global warming will entail improving the energy efficiency of agricultural practices, by using lower energy techniques — e.g. less working of soils, more sparing use of high-energy chemical inputs, and (as part of a general response to the need to reduce carbon emissions) using more renewable energy sources. Another change would be to farm subsidies which promote 'food mountains'; yet another would be to limit consumers' choices to more locally-produced foods, thus reducing the energy costs of transporting produce around the world. One outcome would be a lot less meat and dairy production, and in

turn much higher prices for these foods! Another consequence would be a reduction in the availability of strawberries in England in December.

5   Most of the things nutritional scientists would like to know more about involve tests and measurements over long periods — ideally, over an appreciable fraction of the human lifespan. Since everything interacts with everything else, we need to try to keep as many factors of the environment and of behaviour as constant as possible. People in nutritional studies either end up living in a way which bears almost no resemblance to real-life, or start cheating. Poor James Lind's subjects, after months on a diet without fruit or vegetables, probably got their relatives to pass them a few things through the window!

6   People in the 18th century knew nothing of the germ theory of disease (as already discussed in the first book in this series, *Medical Knowledge: Doubt and Certainty* (2nd edn 1994; colour-enhanced 2nd edn 2001; Open University Press, Buckingham; see particularly Chapter 4). But, as Tobias Smollett's description of the quality of milk delivered in the streets of London illustrates, they were deeply concerned with the contamination of food. (And, as a later book in this series describes — *Caring for Health: History and Diversity*, 2nd edn 1993; 3nd edn 2001; Open University Press, Buckingham — they were also outraged by the fraudulent dilution of foods, or the substitution of cheaper and less wholesome ingredients.) However, in sharp contrast to the present-day population, people in the eighteenth century would have laid the blame for such practices on the immediate purveyors — shopkeepers, street traders, etc. In the absence of any health-related inspection system, it would not have occurred to them to hold the primary producers (e.g. farmers), the Government or other institutions responsible for any ill-effects they may have believed they suffered from eating the normal foods of the time.

By the end of the 20th century, with mandatory labelling of contents and inspection of quality, Western populations had become more inclined to regard dilution of their food or the inclusion of additives as simply requiring the buyer to 'beware'. They had, however, become very much more sensitive towards the possibility of contamination of food with biological disease agents, chemical toxins or genetic material introduced from other species (GM foods). The public increasingly laid responsibility for food-related diseases at the door of food producers (e.g. British farmers who used recycled animal protein as cattle fodder, thus spreading BSE), or of local or national governments for failing to enforce food-safety legislation. In the twenty-first century, these attitudes are likely to develop into demands for an increasingly effective global system of monitoring of food supplies, enabling the tracing of items right back to the point of primary production and providing early warning of contamination with an ever-expanding range of known or suspected hazardous substances. The establishment of the Food Standards Agency in the UK in 2000 is one step in this direction.

7   The population sizes of the developed countries (which account for 20 per cent of the world's population) are, for the most part, stable or declining in numbers. On average, these populations are spending only about 10 per cent of their disposable incomes on food, so over the next few decades they will be able to afford to be increasingly selective in regard to its origin and mode of production. If present trends in food choices in the developed economies continue, there will be a greater demand for foods with lower intensity of production, less

dependence on chemical inputs, better standards of welfare for meat-producing animals, and more land area set aside for nature conservation.

By contrast, the other 80 per cent of the world's population in the developing countries is facing a further doubling of their numbers by the middle of the twenty-first century, and a huge expansion of economic demand for the 'quality' components of their diets — meat in particular. The developing countries' dilemma is that they cannot avoid the choice between either increased intensity of production per unit of land area, or of greater extension of agriculture into the remaining areas of wild-life habitats. Thus, a conflict of aims and values seems likely to intensify, with the developing countries adopting intensive farming methods and new technologies (including GM crops and animals), while the developed world's consumers exert purchasing pressure *against* these practices.

Acknowledgements

Grateful acknowledgement is made to the following sources for permission to reproduce material in this book:

Figures

Figure 1.1 Mark Edwards/Still Pictures; *Figure 3.3* Eye of Science/Science Photo Library; *Figure 3.4* Werner, D. (1979) *When There Is No Doctor*, Hesperian Foundation, © David Warner; *Figures 4.1 and 4.8* Jorgen Schytte/Still Pictures; *Figure 4.3* Shoeb Faruquie/DRIK; *Figure 4.4* Fred Hoogervorst/Panos Pictures; *Figure 4.5* Gil Moti/Still Pictures; *Figures 4.6 and 4.10* Shehzad Noorani/Still Pictures; *Figure 4.7* Vanya Kewley/Camera Press; *Figure 4.9* Abir Abdullah/DRIK; *Figure 5.2* adapted from McEvedy, C. and Jones, R. (1978) *Atlas of World Population History*, Penguin Books, reproduced by permission of Curtis Brown Ltd, London on behalf of Colin McEvedy and Richard Jones. Copyright Colin McEvedy and Richard Jones 1978; *Figure 5.3* Mark Edwards/Still Pictures; *Figure 5.4* Courtesy of Haileybury and Imperial College, Hertfordshire; *Figure 5.6* Bridgeman Art Library; *Figure 5.8* © Museum of English Rural Life, University of Reading; *Figure 5.9* The Mansell Collection; *Figures 6.3 and 6.4* Forbes, T. R. (1979) By what disease or casualty: the changing face of death in London, in Webster, C. (ed) *Health, Medicine and Mortality in the Sixteenth Century*, Cambridge University Press; Figure 6.5 © Bodleian Library, MS Ashmole 216, Folio 116r; *Figure 6.7 Annual Abstract of Statistics 1999*, Office for National Statistics. © Crown Copyright 2000; *Figure 11.2* Andrew Davidson/Camera Press; *Figure 11.3* The Mansell Collection; *Figure 11.4* © Museum of English Rural Life, University of Reading;

Tables

Table 3.3 Data from World Health Organisation (1999) *World Health Report 1999: Making a Difference*, Annex, Table 3; *Table 3.5* Coale, A. J. (1991) 'Excess female mortality and the balance of the sexes in the population: an estimate of the number of 'missing females'', *Population and Development Review*, **17**, (3), pp. 514–24, The Population Council; *Table 3.7* Data from World Health Organisation (1999) *World Health Report 1999: Making a Difference*, Annex, Table 7; *Table 3.8* Bobadilla, J. L., Cowley, P., Musgrove, P. and Saxienian, H. (1994) Design, content and financing of an essential national package of health services, Table 2, p. 175, in Murray, C. J. L. and Lopez, A. D. (eds) *Global comparative assessments in the health sector: Disease burden, expenditures and intervention packages,* WHO, Geneva; *Table 6.1* Forbes, T. R. (1979) By what disease or casualty: the changing face of death in London, in Webster, C. (ed) *Health, Medicine and Mortality in the Sixteenth Century*, Cambridge University Press; *Table 6.2* adapted from Szreter, S. (1988) The importance of social intervention in Britain's mortality decline, c.1850–1914: a re-interpretation of the role of public health, *Journal of the Social History of Medicine*, Oxford University Press; *Table 7.5* Data from Notzon, F. C., Komarov, Y. M., Ermakov, S. P., Sempos, C. T., Marks, J. S. and Sempos, E. V. (1998) Causes of declining life expectancy in Russia, *Journal of the American Medical Association, 279*, pp. 793–800; *Table 7.8* Drèze, J. and Sen, A. (1989) *Hunger and Public Action*, Oxford University Press; *Table 8.1* United Nations (1999) *The Demographic Impact of HIV/AIDS*, ESA/P/WP.152; *Table 9.2* Derived from Fry, I. (1983) *Common Diseases*, M.T.P. Press, with kind permission from Kluwer Academic Publishers; *Table 9.3* Data from Harding, S., Bethune, A., Maxwell, R. and Brown, J. (1997) Mortality trends using the Longitudinal Study, pp. 143–55 in Drever, F. and Whitehead, M. (eds) *Health Inequalities: Decennial Supplement*, Government Statistical Service, Series DS No. 15, Office for National Statistics; *Table 9.5* Data from *Health Survey for England 1999 (Preliminary Report)*. Crown copyright is reproduced with the permission of the Controller of Her Majesty's Stationery Office; *Table 10.1* Data from Harding, S., Bethune, A., Maxwell, R. and Brown, J. (1997) Mortality trends using the Longitudinal Study, pp. 143–55 in Drever, F. and Whitehead, M. (eds) *Health Inequalities: Decennial Supplement*, Government Statistical Service, Series DS No. 15, Office for National Statistics; *Table 10.2* Drever, F. and Whitehead, M. (eds) *Health*

Index

Entries and page numbers in orange type refer to key words which are printed in **bold** in the text. Indexed information on pages indicated by *italics* is carried mainly or wholly in a figure or a table.